"It's All In Your Head"

Patient Stories from the Front Lines

Intimate Aspects of Chronic and Neuropsychiatric Lyme Disease

Book I
Large Print Edition

by PJ Langhoff

Foreword by Dr. Joseph Jemsek

About the cover artist:

A contest was held for artwork for the front cover of the Lyme patient story books, with the stipulation that the work was to be created by a Lyme disease patient. Many artists submitted works from the U.S. and Canada. One of the cover art pieces chosen from these entries was created by Lyme patient Valerie White, a resident of Toronto, Canada and graduate of The Ontario College of Art and Design, and Lyme patient. I chose her artwork because of its vibrance, and terrific representation of the many facets of Lyme disease.

Valerie has this to say about Lyme disease and her art: "This artwork represents my experience of the slow but gradual slide from the happiness of enjoying life and nature, into the confusing mire of Lyme disease. At one point, life is very simple and then suddenly you are confronted with an array of diverse symptoms, leading to ambulances and emergency rooms, referrals to numerous doctors, multiple diagnoses, and a multitude of prescriptions and therapies."

"I have always enjoyed painting wildlife and landscapes, but have been restricted in this activity in the past few years due to Lyme Disease. I am unsure as to where I contracted Lyme, but it was possibly while on painting/camping excursions in Arizona, California, Pennsylvania or the lake lands of Ontario, including Long Point on Lake Erie."

"I never had a rash, and for many years I was troubled with a wide variety of seemingly unrelated and disturbing symptoms. After several years and perhaps 17 doctors, I was fortunate to find an LLMD here in Toronto. Sadly, there are only a few in this country. Now after 2 years of a variety of antibiotics, I find myself 90% better on a good day, with a few recurring symptoms, and I have resumed drawing and painting."

"When you finally find someone who can diagnose you correctly, (by sending your blood to the USA), for a moment you realize, 'I'm not crazy, I have Lyme disease!' But you find yourself in a mysterious and discouraging world, where most of the medical profession doesn't believe in Lyme Disease, and the government downplays its existence, by establishing unresearched guidelines for treatment."

"You hear stories of government-approved bio-warfare testing. So you research spirochetes and learn how insidious they are and 'unkillable.' You discover that the few, brave doctors who genuinely want to treat you are unsure what that treatment is. The whole thing is more than confusing when you're not thinking straight to begin with due to Lyme disease."

You are so right Valerie, Congratulations to you and thank you for your delightful artwork and a job well done!

To view more of Valerie's work, visit: www.bigchickenart.com

"It's All In Your Head" – Patient Stories from the Front Lines:
Intimate Aspects of Chronic and Neuropsychiatric Lyme Disease – Book I

Front cover art by Valerie White, Ontario, Canada

Published by Allegory Press, Hustisford WI, USA
ISBN: 978-0-9654580-2-3
First Edition, Large Print

Printed in the United States of America.

For more information, and/or to contact the individuals contributing their stories to this book: indicate which story author you wish to contact, and provide your contact information so that it may be forwarded to the appropriate parties.

Write the author at:

PJ Langhoff
c/o Allegory Press
PO Box 444
Hustisford, WI 53034, USA

Stories and other items are reprinted with gracious permission from the authors.

To the brave physicians treating Lyme sufferers despite controversy,
Thank you for saving lives in a system trading illness for private agenda.

With a special dedication to the families of:
Roger D. Stikeleather and Ryan Guerin*

Two Lyme patients who recently took their own lives...
...one due to the intractible nature of this insidious illness,
and the other specifically lost hope when
his beloved physician was forced to close his practice
due to a decision by a state medical board
which doesn't understand the complexity of Lyme disease
And because the doctor treated outside the "standard of care,"
daring to cure severely ill Lyme patients when no one else would.

May they rest in peace and their families find comfort.
And let these tragedies mark the turning point for patients who
have thus far received little credence from the medical community at large.

For my precious children, who in time will mature, and with that
comes many gifts, none the least of which are understanding, patience, and
the knowledge that you are always loved completely and without question

**Ryan's story is told herein by his family*

Contents

Disclaimer

The author is not a medical physician and has no credentials which would constitute being an expert in any medical field. Those submitting stories for publication are not to be considered medical experts, though some may have physician credentials. Nothing in this book is offered as any form of medical advice, recommendation, treatment therapy, suggestion, nor for the diagnosis or treatment of any disease or disorder, but is included solely for informational purposes and independent patient study. Always seek the advice of a qualified medical professional before attempting any treatment, taking any test, or starting or stopping any medications, diets, herbs or "alternative" therapies. Persons attempting to self-medicate should not do so. Information herein is presented solely as personal opinion and has not been verified as, nor should be deemed as, accurate.

DO NOT FOLLOW ANYTHING WRITTEN WITHIN THIS BOOK without consulting with a qualified medical provider first. Following any procedures, treatments, medications or other therapies without consulting with a medical professional is done solely at your own risk. Certain content of this book is not necessarily the opinion of those contributing personal stories, and statements made by contributors are not necessarily the opinion of the author or publisher. References cited in this book are not necessarily the personal opinion of the author and are reported solely for education and independent evaluation. Any errors or inaccuracies in this publication are accidental and apologies are extended in advance from the author, who has done the best job possible while being disabled by tick-borne infections. Any laboratories, tests, physicians or healthcare practices (public or private), mentioned in this book are solely referenced by the author and/or patients submitting stories, and the test results, interpretations thereof, processes, opinions of the patients or their families, and the contents of this book are not necessarily the opinion of the laboratories, physicians or clinics mentioned.

This book should be considered "opinion." It should be noted that the author is a patient with Lyme and co-infections, and should not be held responsible for the content of this book as the thoughts, expressions and opinions herein may have come about while under the influence of these illnesses. *Any errors or omissions should be considered fundamental proof that the author and those submitting their stories, are suffering from Lyme and other tick-borne illnesses, which make logic, focus, and communication, difficult.*

In fact, since *Borrelia burgdorferi* are regarded as somewhat "intelligent" organisms, there is no substantiated proof that the organisms themselves did not influence the authors' writing style and/or content, nor attempt to communicate to a larger audience through the authors in some manner. If the reader finds any portion of this disclaimer *inappropriate or ridiculous in nature,* keep in mind that the Lyme patient is forced to accept a "diagnosis" equally ridiculous each time they must deal with a physician who is not Lyme-literate, and any others who attempt to ignore or dismiss our collective illness, telling us "It's All In Your Head."

Note: All medications listed herein are considered registered or trademarked products of their respective manufacturers whether marked as such, or not.

❖ ❖ ❖

Acknowledgements

To everyone who participated in the making of this book, for sending me your very personal and private patient stories, and for your bravery and honesty – you give me additional reasons to fight for all, each day. To everyone who helped me find important information, for connecting me with others, or for simple encouragement, I humbly and gratefully thank you, you know who you are. Thank you to Open Eye Pictures for courageously creating a documentary film which reveals the truth about Lyme disease. (www.openeyepictures.org/underourskin/index.html).

Special thanks to the Dr. "J's" and Dr. "B's" of the world for your efforts on behalf of suffering Lyme patients despite tremendous controversy and personal loss; and three in particular for your general advice, friendship and ongoing support – you are the salt of the earth. To everyone else I have failed to mention, I humbly thank you as well. To my LLMDs, thank you for putting your necks on the line and treating Lyme patients despite the sociopolitical risks. It took me over a dozen years to find you, and I will treasure you always for saving my life.

To "T" for your endless emails making me chuckle; may peace travel with you from this point forward, I admire your strength and sense of humor. To Scott, thanks for being there as well as you were able. For all the other unwitting impetuses to this project, thanks for reading and liking what you see; and encouraging me to continue despite disability. To JR, my heart goes out to you always.

Thank you to *Borrelia burgdorferi*, my unwelcome, but constant "companion" and double-edged sword. You were the needle in the haystack that took doctors a dozen and a half years to "find," though I recognized you from the start. You managed to destroy everything in my life that *was* my life prior to being innocently infected. All my goals, ability to function, family life, work, understanding of medicine and politics, and my love of the outdoors have been permanently altered. You have brought years of pain, suffering, starvation, anaphylaxis, fear, anxiety, disability, immobility, dysfunction, anguish and loss. You turned my life completely upside down and forced me to reinvent myself to accommodate you – the destroyer who thinks of nothing but its own survival. Thanks to you, my life has taken a much harder road than I ever would have imagined, or chosen for myself. And yet by your presence, I have learned the kindness of many, and the graces of humility, patience, courage, strength, and a renewal of spirituality. You give me the motivation to get up in the morning and fight you each day, to help raise consciousness of the devastation you bring to your victims, in the hopes that one day you will no longer threaten human life – and for that, you deserve acknowledgement.

And of course, thank you God for giving me the challenges I must overcome daily to grow in strength and service to others, in Your name. And thank you to my nasty-piece-of-work ex-husband, who through his meanness and abuse of a family court system which is currently clueless about chronic illness, has taught me to stand firmly on the principle of truth, and believe in myself despite anything he (and they) could ever possibly do to harm my children or myself. Just because you collectively said and did what you did, does not make it the truth. May God forgive you all for what you have done to this family, and to the many families who will find themselves in a similar situation, in the name of ignorance, and in the name of chronic Lyme disease.

❖ ❖ ❖

Foreword

By Dr. Joseph Jemsek

The truth in life is always troubling to those who bother to question what happens around them. For those who seek truth, those who have curiosity about a more profound meaning, and for those who have the time and resources to question the truths in their lives, the conclusions are troubling, or should be.

Truth is often the only thing which gives comfort and relief to the human species when we find ourselves experiencing pain in our incontrovertible dilemmas. Truth is "the strongest argument" (Sophocles). It is the "aim of the superior man," (Confucius) and the "highest compact we can make with our fellow man" (Ralph Waldo Emerson).

In spite of all that occurs in our fleeting lifetimes, the truth must be let out. It must be revealed in our lifetimes or in the lifetimes of the generations which follow, lest the gases resulting from the fermentation of lies perpetrated by purveyors of non-truth burst forth, splatter about, and necrotize us all.

If one does not embrace the truth, the forces at hand will disfigure truth in a manner which changes lives so they become existence without meaning. Ignoring truth forces lives to lose purpose; lives which last 3-4 decades and then end; lives which fade into insignificance regardless of to whom they belonged. "Is that all there is?" (Peggy Lee).

In our modern world, our assault on the "truth," as spoken by Wall Street of CNN, is translated to the temporary advantage of wealth and influence. The advantage goes to those who strictly adhere to human law and follow a human-endorsed, ordained ability to legislate, mandate, and judge – all those who have a vote make the rules…fair or unfair.

PJ Langhoff writes in a consummately researched and articulately expressed work, about the sins against truth in Lyme Borreliosis Complex and related disorders. She argues that these sins should be rejected. She argues that this deceit should not be accepted by adults, nor accepted for our future generations – our children. Our children have no choice about dealing with congenitally acquired, and/or environmentally acquired life-altering illness; chronic illness which may doom a child to an unfulfilled life. A parent's heart aches for the child who is afflicted and who suffers from an illness in which the truth is bandied about as those who buffet a political football.

The sorrow is this, and this sorrow will resonate throughout all of Congress one day: "many families will be afflicted by the time that this message fully impacts American consciousness. There is an epidemic. Please look into my son's eyes, my daughter's eyes...your son's eyes, your daughter's eyes."

When did we lose our soul in this country?

What will it take for this country to again live up to the precepts which made it great? There is no greater sorrow on earth than a parent who watches helplessly as their child suffers, without hope.

Truth is "the foe of tyrants and the friend of man" (Thomas Campbell). Truth is the straight line we necessarily follow when we, as finite beings, wish to be most sure and most safe against the nuances and vagaries of nature; which are often most harsh and final, and to which we all will eventually succumb.

I applaud PJ Langhoff...and please join me in this. What a gifted and inspirational lady she is. We have to celebrate our special people and she is one. So please sing out loudly about the effort that this gifted advocate/author has brought to your consciousness about the complex and controversial issues at hand. But, please be aware that PJ cares less about any credit than she does knowing she's on the right track for the rest of us. If you love PJ like I do, then please let her know.

Be blessed,

– JGJ

"In all we do, we must remember that the best health care decisions are made not by government and insurance companies, but by patients and their doctors."

— President George W. Bush State of the Union Address January 23, 2007

In August of 2007, it was announced in several news articles, that the President of the United States was infected with Lyme disease, in **2006.** As Americans witness his actions and notice progressive symptoms subsequent to "appropriate" treatment, fellow Lyme sufferers are asking the hard questions:

- Did he receive the same type of treatments Lyme patients receive which have left many with continued, disseminated illness?
- Was the President told his Lyme disease was "*all in his head*?"
- Is the President *still sick* but is he being told he is now "cured" of Lyme, but that he rather has *something else?*

One recent private communication via email assured me that the President had consulted with an ILADS-treating physician. This offered him a secondary look at Lyme disease from a different treatment perspective than what current Infectious Disease guidelines might recommend. That information was somewhat reassuring to me, but I wonder what kind of treatment he received.

Of course the public is wondering whether or not President Bush is being told what patients collectively have learned to be the truth about Lyme disease – that it is a complex, systemic, debilitating illness often leaving patients with a lifetime of health issues and complications when inappropriately treated, because current diagnostics and treatment therapies are falling short and failing patients.

We hope our unfortunate President will not become the "poster child" for an illness whose acknowledgement is long overdue. We wish the best to President Bush, and we hope his Lyme disease process will not progress in a manner similar to the hundreds of thousands who have been left untreated, under treated, misdiagnosed, or ignored, and told, *"It's All In Your Head."*

❖ ❖ ❖

Gems from "Friends"

"In the country of the blind, the one-eyed man is king"

– From an IDSA 2004 annual meeting slide show presentation on Performance of clinical trials in private practice.[1]
(The title of this particular slide was "Budget Considerations.")

❖ ❖ ❖

"Among B. burgdorferi-infected patients,
a prior history of depression or anxiety seems to be
a risk factor for the development of Chronic Lyme disease...
a counterculture has emerged regarding Chronic Lyme disease."

– IDSA 2006 Guidelines co-author Dr. Allen C. Steere et al.[2]

A "counter-culture?" Lyme disease is not "all in our heads."
You mean we dare to disagree – "we" being the *patient majority*!

Lyme patients, their treating physicians, a growing body of scientific evidence, and epidemic numbers of victims suffering from infectious disease will *not* be denied or dismissed forever.

Indeed, there is much work to be done
to reeducate those whose thinking is entrenched in
the mindset such as in the examples above.

– PJ Langhoff

"Objectivity does not need a diploma to express itself.
We have it or we don't."

– Chris LeHérou, Belgium,
a Lyme patient whose story
is told in book 2 of this series.

Before We Begin

Lyme disease and tick-borne illnesses have had their share of controversy in the past 50 years. There have been allegations that Lyme disease has been a product of U.S. government biological warfare research, and that Lyme-infected ticks were released either deliberately or "accidentally" into the United States, off Plum Island (NY).[3] There have been rumors of covert military air drops of ticks on unsuspecting populations to study vector transmission and epidemiology[4]. We do know that as early as 1970, the military was testing the MI1HX helicopter for the application of 10% DDT dust in areas of tick-borne encephalitis foci. They found the method and delivery system highly effective, though the general public, for the most part, were not made aware of tick-borne illness risks during this time period.[5]

[Author note: I recall from my own childhood the practice of routine "spraying" by truck, of the suburbs of Chicago for "mosquitoes" in the late 1960's-early 1970's. I wonder now if ticks weren't also a problem that were perhaps being covertly addressed during those "mosquito" control measures.]

In some books we may read about how tick-infested birds, deer, small mammals, and even rats hopped aboard shipments for the fur trades in earlier decades, and flocks of migratory birds are postulated as to how tick-borne illnesses have spread throughout the United States.[6]

Since the 1940's, biological agents such as *Borrelia burgdorferi*, (the spirochete causing Lyme disease), have been studied for their potential to infect populations and disable, rather than eliminate them. When civilians are ill and disabled and forced to rely on government agencies for medications, livelihood, disability, and healthcare, then whole populations may be easily controlled. Ticks and other bio-agent carriers were studied by governments abroad as well as in the United States and bio-agent research is still taking place today, in U.S. laboratories and abroad. Meanwhile, innocent civilians fall victim to disease-carrying organisms making their way into the population by whatever means they do, while patients are denied diagnoses and treatment opportunities, for various reasons, which are too large in scope to fully address herein.

In current Lyme treatment, antibiotics that are used to treat early infection differ in efficacy than those required for later forms of the same disease, and those medications and treatments currently have no standardized approach. In fact, due to the extremely variable nature of the illness itself, Lyme disease is a complex organism and every patient's disease course and infection load different, so no standardized approach may be possible. The methods used to treat patients command flexibility for every patient, even for the same illnesses, no matter where in the world these patients live. There are many factors which affect treatment. Individual body types, biochemical makeup, infection "menu," immunology issues and even patient compliance are all issues needing consideration in each case.

In Lyme disease testing, results have been shown to be at times, unreliable in accuracy, and patients and physicians alike are often left with many unanswered questions. Whether or not a patient has Lyme disease often becomes a bone of contention between physicians and their patients, because the patients know that they are ill, but the physicians often rely upon testing as the last word in differential diagnoses. As a result, many Lyme patients are often dismissed, ignored, or even called "crazy" by researchers, insurance companies, some of their own physicians, family members, and friends. As a consequence, those infected are left to deal with the destruction and devastation of an illness which slowly or perhaps rapidly descends upon their lives, leaving a wake of uncertainty and despair in its path.

This book is not an attempt to seriously debate the opposing sides of what I will deem the "Lyme Wars;" which includes those who have the disease (or are treating same), and those who agree with a handful of Infectious disease researchers attempting to set prevailing diagnostic and treatment policies to physicians, patients, medical boards, government bodies, and disability and insurance companies. As a Lyme patient who couldn't get a proper diagnosis for more than a dozen years for myself and my two children who "allegedly" have Lyme, it would be obvious to assume which side of that debate I might stand firmly behind.

Still patients inherently know what is happening inside of their own bodies, even if they lack the ability to define what that illness actually is. Most of us have to resort to internet research only **after exhausting every effort** to extract meaningful information or a valid diagnosis from our doctors – doctors who perhaps perform limited testing, but who, more often than not, leave patients with little more than shrugged shoulders and an offer of anti-depressants. It is sad that in this day and age to know that when a physician cannot define the cause of an illness, that the patient is often dismissed and/or ridiculed – the doctor doesn't know what is wrong so therefore the patient is perceived as "delusional" or "hypochondriacal." Dismissing patients because a physician doesn't have time or a diagnosis for them is unacceptable; and ridiculing them for any reason, is unforgivable. Ignoring research which more than remotely supports the position of large numbers of patients having the chronic form of an illness, is **unconscionable.** Any doctor who routinely accuses his or her patient of fabricating their illness when the evidence of that illness is staring them in the face; or who refers them to psychiatry rather than investigate that patient's concerns, is truly clueless as a physician.

It is for the explicit purpose of educating those who are dismissing Lyme patients and their symptoms that we collectively offer our patient stories in this series, as told by the patients themselves – people from all walks of life. They are not members of some delusional internet or activist groups, but patients who have stepped forward to courageously offer their personal viewpoints about dealing with tick-borne illnesses which are routinely ignored by those in the medical field. Although each story is unique, their continuity of a lack of credence provided to them, is astounding and leaves us to question why they have been so cruelly ignored.

For researchers and clinicians telling us "It's All In Your Head," we collectively state that **hundreds of thousands of patients are not delusional. Chronic Lyme disease is not mass hysteria brought about by internet research,** or depressed or prior personally traumatized patients who are in need of sympathy. We are not anecdotes, but rather **people who are suffering from real illness that a handful of influential "experts" in the medical world simply refuse to acknowledge.**

Our symptoms were present long before we knew with what we were dealing; followed by our efforts to research our illness and give it a name – not the other way around. And contrary to what some people have claimed, **Lyme patients don't care what you call this disease, they are merely sick and just want to be made well.**

We must all remember that the evolution of Lyme medicine is constantly changing. As in cancer and AIDS research, until quality long-term data and clinical experience is properly collected and evaluated, the practice of treating chronic Lyme patients remains an art, and not a definitive science. More research is needed and medicine must remain open-minded with objective studies which report all findings, not just carefully spun propaganda created by self-interested parties.

The fact of the matter is that **Lyme, an endemic infectious disease, is rapidly outpacing medical science.** The responsible clinician needs objective direction so they may offer patients intelligent solutions. In fact, **direct patient experience is rapidly overruling clinical research,** and one reason why infectious disease doctors and treating physicians need to listen to their patients – the voices of those doing the practical "field work." As a Lyme patient myself, in my experience, patients and doctors alike are best served when medical science selects an open-minded, middle-of-the-road approach; and when doctor and patient work together to explore and correct health issues.

To Lyme patients, limiting the process of diagnosing and treating us by relying on narrowly defined, and/or restrictive guidelines or "recommendations" that limit a physician's ability to do their job effectively, and which are counterproductive to the ability of patients to be made well, is akin to tying the hands and feet of an ill and weakened patient and throwing them into the deep end of a pool. Neither one can do anything about their situation; and the end result is exactly the same – a dead patient. **Killing patients for profit is certainly not objective medicine.**

Lyme patients have been still and silent long enough, and want their voices to be heard now more than ever before. We cannot continue to relax and watch the political debate in the arena of Lyme disease. We are demanding answers for our illness, and we certainly deserve them. We are demanding that our insurance companies pay for our serious illness in exchange for the premiums we pay, and ask that our caretakers and insurance companies alike refrain from trading profit for human lives.

To illustrate the effects of our very real and devastating diseases, we offer our personal stories for further analysis. If recommended tests and treatments did not serve us in the past, then those same treatments are going to continue to fail us in the future, especially as diagnostic and treatment guidelines grow more restrictively defined. Patients want everyone to understand Lyme disease from the patients' perspective – those who have to suffer daily with this illness.

We are not statistics, nor have we invented our illnesses. Lyme disease is real, and chronic Lyme exists. **We are real patients dealing with real disease, and we deserve a voice, and a choice.**

❖ ❖ ❖

The Reality of Lyme

Whatever initiated the current Lyme disease political firestorm, fortunately for the patient, there are many physicians with compassion enough to recognize our serious illness, and they sincerely want to help the very ill, for whom practically no one else lends any credence. In my experience, it is these compassionate physicians, (often themselves personally touched by Lyme), whom become highly motivated to treat others in this specialized area of medicine.

Unfortunately, many of these Lyme-friendly physicians are finding themselves face-to-face with medical boards who want to know why they are treating patients outside the current "standards of care." And while being a governing body for medical care providers is beneficial, board members must be extremely careful when evaluating individual circumstances and "standards." They must ignore prejudice and allow flexibility in treatments which may be considered "experimental" or outside the mainstream in emerging infectious diseases. If they do not, medicine will simply neither advance nor improve and people will die.

Doctors should never be prosecuted for being *willing to treat*, or for thinking "outside the box" in medicine; indeed, that is how medicine has moved forward throughout history. No treatment which is "standard" should remain static, but rather should be open-ended and as variable as the patients these doctors treat. Let us not forget that the practices of using leeches, and bloodletting were once "standards of care," as well.

It is sad too, that so many physicians still know nothing about Lyme disease, especially since in this "information age," so much information is readily available. If the patients have access to it, physicians do so, as well. Whatever the reason for the "average" physician's inability to reliably recognize and diagnose Lyme disease, (whether lack of education, threatened with sanctions by insurers, poor testing, or provided with strategic misinformation or other reasons), it is nevertheless important for the patient to be their own advocate if they are ill. This holds true for any disease, but especially with Lyme, the fastest growing vector-borne infectious disease in the United States. We must do our homework and help our doctors find the source of our ills before what might be a shortened illness turns into years of debilitating disease simply because an uneducated or apathetic doctor did not take us seriously or have the wherewithal to deal with us. We must educate our physicians if they will not educate themselves.

It has sadly become a common theme among Lyme patients that they must wait on average, *at least 2 years* and make 10-20 visits to various doctors before finding one who can *correctly diagnose* them. Sadly, even when properly diagnosed by one or more doctors, subsequent physicians will attempt to argue that Lyme disease "doesn't exist" in these patients. We ask, "why all the denial?" In actuality, many Lyme patients have seen upward of 50 or more physicians before finding an accurate diagnosis which fits their symptom and tick exposure history. By that time, not only have many of them **never been treated** for Lyme, but their illnesses have progressed to such an extent that patients are forced to deal with perhaps years of constant, or debilitating illness that relapses and remits, but which never seems to completely disappear.

Worse, many physicians have no idea of the importance of testing for so-called tick-borne "co-infections." These are additional infections which can be life-threatening in their own right, and which make up the complex of Lyme borreliosis – and which complicate the treatment and recovery therefrom.

Since Lyme is the "great imitator," it presents a myriad of symptoms which mimic many other illnesses, leading physicians to misdiagnose patients with MS, Lupus, CFS, RA, Alzheimer's, ALS, hypochondria, Munchausen's, Anorexia and even psychiatric disorders like ADHD, bi-polar disorder and severe depression. Symptoms of Lyme disease routinely get lumped into syndrome categories for which doctors prescribe "band-aid" pharmaceuticals such as in "restless leg syndrome," depression, ADHD, or for sleep disorders, or reproductive problems, all of which may be caused by Lyme and/or co-infections.

As a matter of fact, by the time most patients are diagnosed, most of them no longer fit within the purposes of the current Infectious Disease Society of America (IDSA) diagnostic and treatment guidelines for Lyme, which then casts these patients into a future of chronic illness and disability. Since there are no definitive tests to reliably detect if a patient unequivocally *has* Lyme or *if they have been cured*, (and research bears that Bb persists after treatment), the patients' futures therefore hold a most uncertain outcome. And because of these guidelines, the majority of patients who are not diagnosed or who are misdiagnosed but who still have symptoms following treatment but are told they are "cured," (and despite progressive disability), are left without any treatment options whatsoever.

Indeed, the myriad of symptoms which overlap between Lyme disease and its many "co-infections" can and do leave even sincere, educated physicians scrambling for answers. To make matters worse, the complex and variable nature of the Lyme spirochete alone leaves many current lab tests lacking in both sensitivity and accuracy. Physicians are being fed misinformation about emerging infectious diseases that they don't necessarily have the time to research and for which they were taught minimally or not at all, during academic medical training.

From the patient's perspective, the existing published "mainstream" information seems designed to purposely prevent the diagnosis and treatment of Lyme. As currently established, it saves money for insurance companies and helps generate revenue for diagnostic manufacturers, laboratories, and research scientists studying these diseases. Undiagnosed illness would seem to ensure the availability of a steady consumer market for the pharmaceutical industry as well. Instead of curing the underlying diseases, symptoms are masked through prescriptive use of "band-aid" treatments, and patients are told their illness is "all in their head" – a huge cost-savings for all, except for the patient who is left dealing with chronic illness. In the end, the only person failing to profit from this scenario, is the patient.

The controversy over diagnosis and treatment of Lyme disease and tick-borne illnesses is a hotly debated issue. One Lyme "camp" which consists of researchers and a handful of Infectious Disease (IDSA) physicians (some of whom were present and helped identify the illness in the 1970's and testing and CDC surveillance criteria in the 1990's), seem to infer to some degree that the illness is perhaps "hard to catch" and "easy to treat." They have set forth what many call overly restrictive guidelines to diagnose and treat Lyme and other tick-borne illnesses, and may be working diligently on some levels to discredit competitive laboratories, Lyme-treating physicians and patients alike. Of course this is only my opinion, but it is echoed by many.

One has to ask the question of what would motivate them to do so if this were indeed the case? Also, while the President of the IDSA reports a membership of about 8,000 members, in truth, only a small minority of these individuals actually stand behind the new IDSA Lyme treatment guidelines. Some of these individuals are noticeably behind the "machine" of defending same, and from a patient perspective, beyond apparent logic and existing research. Many patients feel these guidelines seem to address only certain cases of tick-borne illness, and subjectively deny the existence of the majority of others, despite research clearly proving that these patients exist, and why – including research written by some of these minority IDSA members themselves.

Another "camp" is quick to cite research articles which support the fact that Lyme disease is a complex illness which may be chronic, and that open-ended treatment therapies are beneficial to patients. This camp is made up of Lyme patients, their treating physicians, researchers, advocates, support groups and even IDSA members. They contend that patients are not treated "successfully" with a 21-30 day antibiotic regimen and that the "wait and see" approach is not only dangerous for the patient, but helps to entrench the very illnesses these patients are attempting to have eradicated. They know from experience that an open-ended treatment process is more effective for the elimination of the symptoms of Lyme disease and other tick-borne illnesses.

Many Lyme patients feel discriminated against merely because they have a disease that some factions in the medical community do not wish to openly acknowledge. These patients are tired of hearing "it's all in your head," and that they are a mass of delusional, attention-seeking hypochondriacs. They often hear this from insensitive, under educated or extremely biased physicians who are perhaps motivated by other self-interested parties. They are also frustrated that court systems and social services prefer to think the worst of having a chronic illness instead of becoming more educated therewith so they can exercise diligence when making decisions which adversely affect families. They are disgusted with Psychologists, Counselors and Psychiatrists who are unaware of Lyme disease and the manifestations which tick-borne illness can take, causing psychiatric disorders and depression. They are tired of merely being handed anti-depressants, being told they are under too much "stress" and that they have no business researching their illness on the internet when medical science offers them no practical solutions for a cure.

Although there is division and extreme controversy with the treatment of tick-borne illnesses, one thing is abundantly clear. **Patients having legitimate tick-borne illness are failing to receive timely diagnoses and are having difficulty finding treatment options, insurance cov-**

erage, disability awards, and credence in the medical system as a whole – and this trend must change.

In fact, Lyme patients will be the first to tell you how many times they have tried antibiotic treatments recommended by doctors (or as in the IDSA guidelines), only to learn very quickly that those treatments do little, if anything, to eradicate a very complex series of infections. This becomes especially true if they have multiple infections, and have never been correctly diagnosed, or "appropriately treated" as the guidelines repeatedly speculate about these patients. In actuality, the number of patients who know they have been bitten by ticks, and who then develop symptoms, and go to their doctors and get accurately diagnosed and treated immediately, at onset of their illness **are the scant, minority few.** The majority of patients are unaware of tick exposure, many do not exhibit the characteristic *erythema migrans* (EM) rash; most doctors can't recognize an EM rash when they see one, and most patients go on to have disseminated disease which becomes Lyme in its most destructive, chronic form.

It is interesting that the highest-profile American public servant, the President of the United States George W. Bush, was recently reported to have suffered from Lyme disease in August of 2006, but that it was "cured." Yet the President is still indicated to be suffering a year later from other health issues such as "imbalance," "unsteadiness," "otitis media," and "vestibular neuronitis," all of which may also be attributed to Lyme disease, the President's previously reported medical condition,[7-12] (symptoms which occur when Lyme is disseminated and under treated). Lyme patients immediately wonder if the President was treated using the same, standard IDSA 2006 treatment guidelines many of our doctors have used, and which have, (according to many Lyme patients), failed miserably. If so, this may leave Mr. Bush with disseminated disease likely to be dismissed as some "other" illness like "MS, Alzheimer's, Parkinson's or "ALS" in the decades to come. Remember former U.S. President Ronald Reagan's Alzheimer diagnosis? I now wonder at the possible cause of his illness, as Bb has been found in biopsies of the brain tissues of some deceased Alzheimer patients.

We may never know for sure if our current President's Lyme disease was "cured," but from the point of view of Lyme patients, it is highly interesting that he "still" has reported health issues which happen to mirror those of chronic Lyme sufferers. To be sure, Lyme patients and their treating physicians will be watching very closely, the health of the leader of the United States of America, following this recent revelation. And yet, the patients can't help but wonder if, or how hard those who dismiss chronic Lyme disease might attempt to bury the President's illness, dismissing any ongoing symptoms as "other" health concerns. We wonder will he be told he suffers from some "post-Lyme syndrome," a "diagnosis" many Lyme patients have been handed by their own physicians, echoed by a handful of IDSA guidelines authors and their associates, some of whom are not treating physicians.

Naturally, our best wishes are extended to the President with the hope that his recovery from Lyme disease is swift and complete – unlike those whose stories are highlighted within the pages of this book series and the hundreds of thousands around the world whose diagnoses have gone ignored, ridiculed, dismissed, or accidentally overlooked; whose stories are never heard.

To those who wholly state that Lyme is "easily treatable" or "curable" when no real tests exist to determine that actual process, we would like to suggest that this thinking be immediately re-evaluated. Medical science is an art, and one which is ever-evolving, not stagnant. Assuming that all Lyme patients are treated, even inadequately, is inappropriate, especially since Lyme disease is so misunderstood, and often not recognized or diagnosed by physicians. For those who say Lyme is a "knee," "arthritis," or "rash" illness occurring in a subset of patients, you are missing the majority of Lyme cases. Some identify post-treatment illness as "post-Lyme syndrome." This is exceptionally narrowminded thinking when you consider that there is currently no test to determine if treatment has been effective, or if spirochetes have been eliminated. To those who dismiss patients legitimately suffering from an illness which is not their fault, and without considering valid research and patient/doctor input proving persistence, I say you are woefully shortsighted and perhaps even medically or scientifically irresponsible.

In addition, setting forth treatment guidelines authoritatively contraindicating treatments which have proven effective in the past for more than just a few individuals, is wholly irresponsible in my opinion. Existing research proves contrary to some of the current IDSA guidelines claims; and shows that patients with a chronic form of Lyme disease can, and do, exist. The number of patients and existing research bears that Lyme is a complex syndrome affecting the entire body. Unfortunately certain individuals seem to choose to ignore the facts – even those which lay within their own past research.

Medical societies routinely publish guidelines for the diagnosis and treatment of diseases. But sometimes their colleagues rush to publish similar articles and guidelines which serve to mislead the public into thinking *an entire additional medical society has jumped on a supportive bandwagon*. This seems to be the case with the Infectious Disease guidelines as well as the new guidelines issued just months later by the American Academy of Neurology (AAN) for the treatment of "nervous system Lyme disease." Physician John J. Halperin was the first author on the latter, but he also co-authored the IDSA guidelines. Unfortunately the above practice hopelessly underestimates the intelligence of the public – especially with IDSA guidelines already mired in controversy. Patients know there is something wrong within their bodies and will not be easily dismissed by "friends" trumpeting support for one another through subjective media manipulation. Appropriately, the public doesn't perceive this "support" as *independent* support.

In the end, the unfortunate reality is such that the collective medical opinion *doesn't completely understand Lyme disease*,[13] and to minimize current available choices, or recommend the denial of treatments that *do work* without sufficient research to support those contraindications, is a serious disservice to all patients, whether chronic or newly infected. Patients need advocates for their care, and have the right to be made well. And yet in the arena of Lyme disease, those rights are being taken away and the patients want to know why. Why would medical science ignore an illness it knows exists – one which is the fastest growing vector-borne illness in the world?

The answer may well be that private industry and academicians may be trading profit for human life, which is deplorable and inexcusable in my opinion. If current trends continue, than I predict that anyone perpetrating the removal of patient and doctors' rights, will be sadly disappointed when they find themselves infected with these very same diseases, (because in time they will). Then following "standard" treatment, they will wonder why they have become disabled. Then they will be saddened beyond belief when they discover that there is quite literally no one left on earth who can, or will, be allowed to treat them. And then they will die – not only from Lyme disease, but a death with the realization that it was perhaps of their own making.

Patient Responsibility

Patients must be realistic and choose an advocate for their wellness if they are not clear-thinking due to their disease. With Lyme that process can become quite challenging, as patients lose insight into their own behavior and intellectual capabilities during various stages of their disease processes – even deteriorating on a daily basis, in many cognitive areas. Admittedly, we must acknowledge that sometimes it is the patient who is at fault for being unrealistic about the treatment and/or recovery process, and sometimes that is due in part, to the disease process itself. Anxiety, frustration, phobias, irrationality and other problems arise in infections which attack the brain, rendering patients with hostility and clarity of thinking (even on "good" days), that falls short of "normal" behavior. Patients look at life through a most difficult window, what I call the Lyme "filter" – and patients are judged harshly by those around them who misunderstand the reason for their "behaviors," especially those which may appear objectively hostile or inappropriate. And yes, patients often expect doctors to have all the answers, and tend to think that if they take medication, that the medication will be safe, and that they should automatically be made well as a result. Treatment fatigue in chronic illness is a fact of life for patients and their families.

When one is desperate for a cure, especially in an illness at times as debilitating and expensive as Lyme, some people will try anything for an immediate "cure," and may even risk their lives in the process of becoming well. I have personally listened to extremely ill patients tell me of "new" treatments they discovered through one source or another. In one case, this included a woman who spent $2,000 of her savings on a man she had never met who resided in a different state, who offered no credentials, business license, nor web site. In fact he told me personally that he will "never" have a web site. This man managed to sell a patient little more than a vial of some sort of "water," a suggestion of coffee enemas, and a deliberately blocked cell phone "support" number.

Upon hearing the patient's story, I recognized a scam, but sadly I did not learn about the situation until well *after* this charlatan had bilked the woman out of her dough. The poor patient gave me the cell number of the salesman, so I called him and I proceeded to pursue a line of questioning designed to determine the man's true motivations. One comment he made to me was startling, and certainly underscores the importance of checking out your sources before paying good money for, quite frankly, who knows what. "Look," he began. "I am under the assumption that if I give my patients water that contains nothing more than *carpet fibers*, and if it makes the patient feel better, then there is nothing wrong with that." *Carpet fibers?* The man was reported to authorities, but that's not the point.

In life we have heard the phrase "buyer beware," and in the realm of treatments, (even those proven), we must do our homework. Patients and their doctors must be permitted to make individual decisions about the risks and benefits of pursuing any treatment therapy; not only in Lyme but in other illnesses as well. While general guidelines are good as a suggestive device, attempts to ridicule other therapies or research offering realistic options, is a deliberate disservice to all and certainly not objective medicine. Once doctors lose their objectivity, then the patients' interests are not being served. Isn't that why one would become a doctor in the first place – to heal the sick and not to harm them?

Problems occasionally do occur in treatment, such as ineffective doses, human error, drug interactions, side-effects, varied responses to treatments, and opportunistic infections which can, and do manifest with some therapies (oral as well as intravenous). Often these cannot be avoided due to the patients' depressed immune system leaving them wide open to infections. Also an overgrowth of organisms already present in the body will awaken during times of stress, illness and depressed immunity. Inflammatory processes will combine with mold and other biotoxin loads to wreak havoc on the body during treatments. This will also heighten "herxheimer" reactions and further blur the line between allergies, drug reactions, and the natural healing process. Patient compliance is always an issue, and it falls upon the patient to take medications as directed, report problems to physicians or even keep access ports for IV medications sterilized (though a reasonable request, not always possible nor the patient's fault).

There are no quick solutions to some of these problems which can be universally applied to *all patients in all disease categories.* Sometimes patients try antibiotics or other therapies and blame their doctors for their inability to get well, (treatment failure), drug reactions, or other, more serious consequences. Sometimes, as soon as a patient's expectations are not being met, they become the ones pointing the finger at the treating physician, much to the delight of those on the other side of the Lyme debate who are quick to exploit these failures, regardless of circumstances, and help medical boards "discipline" these often faultless doctors.

Where has it ever been written that medicine is an exact science? With any treatment, there are inherent risks and side-effects, and this is not necessarily the doctor's fault. Nor is it a reasonable expectation that the physician can adequately inform his/her patient before treatment *of all possible risks or side-effects,* even through copious amounts of paperwork and disclaimers. Physicians are not super-human, though we many expect them to be.

Patients must read the package inserts for medications where are listed some of the possibilities for risks or complications that exist before treatment is undertaken. That information is there for a reason, and it *does* apply to you, the patient. If you don't have the package insert for a medication, ask your Pharmacist or Chemist for it the next time you pick up your medications. If you don't know much about a treatment therapy, do the research. There is the internet, the library, book stores, and you can ask your doctor for more information. Get a second opinion, or a third, until you understand what you are facing. Have an advocate to help you make intelligent decisions before treatment. Patients must accept responsibility for the choices that they make, even when relying on their physician for input. And the physician should be responsible for informing the patient about potential risks as well as benefits to these therapies before undertaking them, *to the best of his or her ability.*

The other side of the patient coin is one of having to face physician ignorance about their illness and the humiliation that patients feel when confronted by physicians who argue with them and refuse to acknowledge their illnesses or complaints, even when they have legitimate positive test results. Logic and suffering dictates to these patients that their symptoms are real, and yet some doctors openly ridicule them for trying to discover what is going wrong within their own bodies. In addition, some physicians and medical society members ridicule cutting-edge laboratories for simply producing positive test results. They will argue every angle possible against these test results, and choose to dismiss what is staring them in the face.

This is a world-wide problem, especially for women, the elderly, and disabled persons, who are routinely dismissed in private practice, or made to feel stupid, childish, or hysterical for thinking "something" might be seriously wrong with them. And yet these patients are keenly aware when they are not feeling well, but merely lack the ability or "acceptable" laboratory tests to prove it. As one physician actually said to this author, **"I'm not going to hold your hand every time you think there is something wrong with you." Why not? I ask, because the physician is so much better at the craft when he or she listens to the patient.**

In some cases, physician attitudes are undeservedly harsh toward their patients because *by nature of the illness itself, the ability to express anxiety, fear, and even basic communication can at times be quite challenging for the Lyme patient.* Doctors quickly perceive a Lyme patient's confusion, frustration, or determination about their illness as overt hostility or even lunacy and immediately lose their patience, often growing sarcastic or hostile themselves. At times patients are ridiculed as if they are fabricating extensive "stories" of illness which on the surface, sound far-fetched (to those unfamiliar with Lyme), but are sadly, harsh reality. If physicians would step back and realize that Lyme patients are sometimes unable to "check" their tone of voice, or understand that they have lost insight into their own behavior or communication skills by virtue of the neuropsychiatric aspects of their illness, or that they tend to ramble on with scattered thoughts during conversation, then the patient will be far better served.

Instead, some doctors lacking patience and empathy quickly dismiss these patients from the very care they so desperately need, and actually become obstacles to their wellness. If the physician can just ride over the initial humps of illness with these patients, they may be pleasantly surprised to find incredibly grateful, clearer-thinking and quite pleasant people on the other side following treatment. Rather, some doctors tend to "fire" any patients they find not immediately "easy," leaving very ill patients without treatment options through no reasonable fault of their own – except that they have a brain infection. I say that this is *inhumane treatment of patients.*

Then there is the whole can of worms whereby many patients do not have any private or government health insurance coverage. Unfortunately, (and largely due to insurance, medical board micro management, government monitoring of patient medical records, and red tape issues), many Lyme-treating physicians do not accept insurance of any kind. As a result, large fees often are required up front, or the patient cannot initiate or continue treatments at that clinic. This is not faulting the doctors for those practices, as they have valid concerns and expenses, but it does point out the problems which many Lyme patients face. And when patients are disabled and unable to work, it becomes more than a little difficult to afford even routine healthcare or specialty testing in any amount.

If the patient has insurance and access to decent healthcare, additional roadblocks may arise. Problems obtaining prescription drug coverage, treatment therapies and problems with insurance coverage often complicate an already difficult situation. Then there can be problems tolerating antibiotics used to treat their illnesses, and this only adds to the frustration patients feel. I have personally been in many of these situations and when one is already fighting for their life (which is hard enough). Patients don't have energy to also fight insurance companies, doctors, pharmacists or even family members.

Lyme patients simply do not receive the credence they deserve, in any arena, period – **and this practice is completely unnecessary and must stop.** Why are chronic acne patients, for example, allowed long-term treatment with potent drugs their insurance companies are happy to cover, and these patients are never questioned about their need for treatment, while individuals with life-threatening tick-borne illness are dismissed and discredited for believing that they are ill? Why must we first "look sick" before we get any credence?

Ultimately patients must be responsible for their own healthcare. If they have no advocate, they must find one. We also must resist the urge to deify physicians. They are highly educated, though fallible human beings; and they are often doing the best they can in a world of medicine that is ever-evolving, has numerous constraints, and is more than difficult. Unfortunately it is a fact that not every doctor is qualified to treat and I shudder to think there are many who should not be allowed to practice medicine of any sort, but the majority of physicians are both qualified and sincerely trying to work within the confines of a broken healthcare system.

And just because physicians attempt to treat patients outside what is being presented as the *routine standard of care* in medicine does not make those physicians "quacks!" It simply means that they are courageous enough to pursue treatment therapies for their legitimately ill patients and they are doing the job they are hired to do.

Perhaps the problem is that the standard of care needs to be modified to address the needs of the patients – not the needs of a few researchers, insurance and pharmaceutical giants, and/or others who are entrenched in their ideologies for their own self-serving purposes.

Medical boards which attempt to, and succeed at, closing the doors of treating physicians under pretenses that those who treat Lyme patients long-term are doing something "wrong" or "dangerous," need to come to grips with the fact that **Lyme disease exists and its patients will not go away.** These people will continue to require treatments for their illnesses, no matter what those illnesses are labeled. **Call it "Lyme" or illness by any other name, someone is going to have to pay for these patients to become well.** Ignoring the problem makes it ever so much more costly for everyone involved. The effects of current practices will become more obvious over time. It will become abundantly clear that the current medical "standards" for treating Lyme disease are failing miserably. Perhaps under pressure from subscribers and/or lawsuits, insurance companies will have to respond and begin covering these illnesses or be doomed to loss of subscribers and hence, profits. Perhaps through the publication of stories such as those in this book series, the voices of the Lyme patients will finally be heard.

In a practical world, physicians humble themselves a bit so they can better relate to their patients, and give them the respect and attention they are entitled to. Despite time constraints, it does not cost anything to be compassionate towards patients, (even on a tight schedule), and extend to them the kindness and respect which they rightly deserve. **Physician and patient need to work together as a team to make the patient well.** Humiliating patients through the use of insensitivity is simply inappropriate, unfair, and shameful. Perhaps the real problem is that the doctors who utilize these tacts needs more education – both in scope of disease processes, as well as bedside manner.

Issuing restrictive guidelines based upon carefully selected research and/or relying solely on interpretations of double-blind, randomized clinical trials to determine healthcare options for millions is counterproductive to treating ill patients with real disease. It doesn't matter what you label an illness, illness is illness, and patients should not be forced by medical societies, boards, insurance, governments, or pharmaceutical companies, to remain ill.

Last, when medical boards begin to pursue doctors for *failing to treat and failure to diagnose,* instead of against doctors who are *willing to treat* patients, then doctors and patients alike will be properly served.

❖ ❖ ❖

The Lyme Rubicon:
A Bit About the "Bug"

Rubicon – A limit, that when passed or exceeded, permits no return, and typically results in irrevocable commitment.

Lyme Disease – An illness which, when contracted, permits no easy return to wellness and typically results in irrevocable commitment to find a Lyme-literate physician and open-ended, long-term treatment therapies.

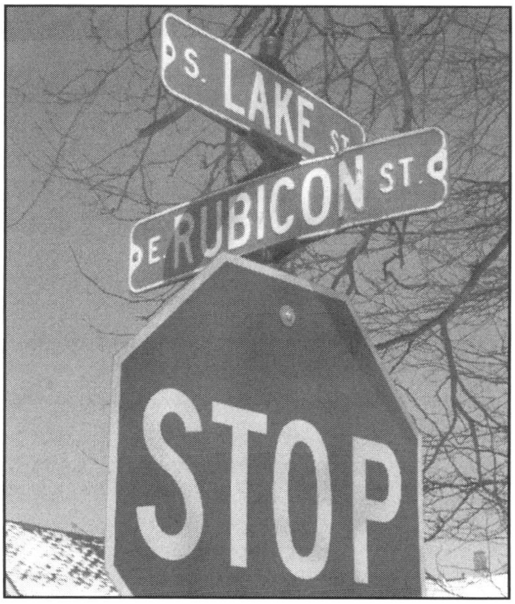

This photograph is from a lake in Wisconsin, near the author's home, in an area known to harbor ticks which carry Lyme disease.

To the author, the combined three signs evoke an eerie warning to take heed that a visit to the lake doesn't perhaps yield more than is anticipated.

Most people have never heard of a tick named Ixodes (Ĭcks-zō-dēēz). I know I never heard about ticks as I grew up, let alone ever saw one personally, nor read about them in any literature. I had no clue what ticks even looked like, let alone where they lived. It was only when I became an adult and moved to Wisconsin that I first grew respectfully aware of these tiny creatures, and the impact that their life-altering bites have on otherwise healthy human beings.

Ticks are tiny, eight-legged, blood-meal feeding external arthropod parasites. This animal, a member of the order *Acarina* which includes mites, is sometimes as small as the period at the end of this sentence, but when engorged, is roughly the size of a small raisin, and can have tough outer bodies, or soft, smoothly wrinkled, leather-like bodies. Ticks carry Lyme disease in their saliva and can transmit the organisms that cause Lyme within moments of feeding.[14] Lyme disease is transmitted by the bite of ticks, like the hard-bodied, slow-feeding *Ixodidae*, of which there are over 200 member species.[15]

Ticks have very few predators, and are more likely to succumb to heat and low humidity. Unfortunately, due to their small size, ticks and their bites more often than not go undetected by their victims, making the discovery of Lyme disease and accompanying illnesses (what are often called co-infections), more than a little challenging. The symptoms which accompany tick-borne infection are as unique and varied as the individuals affected by those bites and the infectious diseases transmitted to them. Ticks typically attach to human hosts, birds, and animals such as deer, rodents, and domestic pets – any warm-blooded creature that can offer a blood meal.

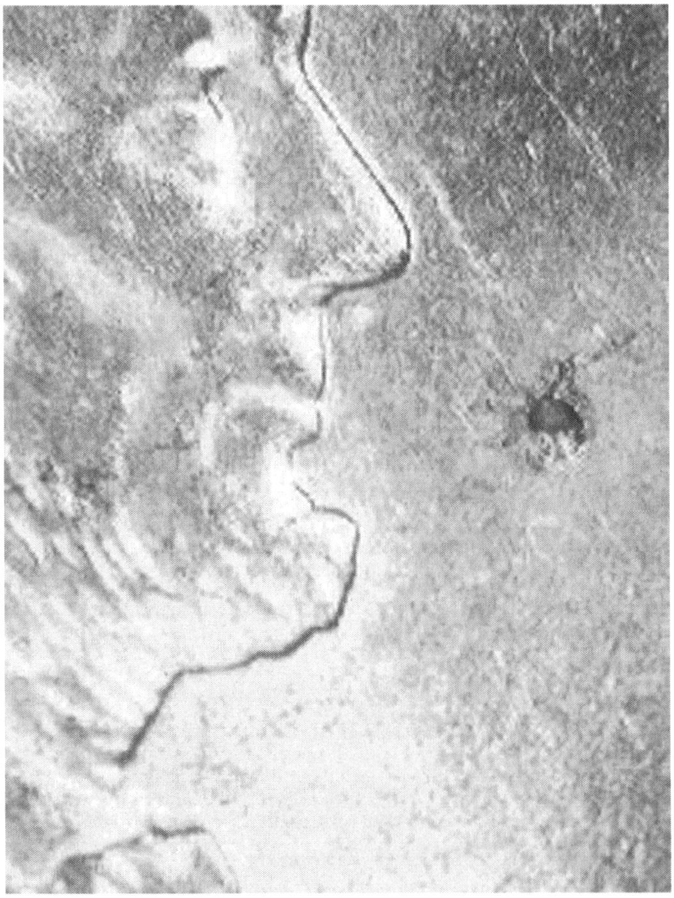

Deer tick larvae on U.S. coin (penny) to illustrate the extremely small size. Reprinted with permission from Marc G. Golightly, Ph.D., Stony Brook University School of Medicine, New York.

Any way you look at them, ticks are ugly little critters, both inside and out. They carry within their bodies any of a number of infectious diseases, many of which can be, and sometimes prove to be, fatal. Lyme disease, Ehrlichiosis (Anaplasmosis), Babesiosis, Bartonella, Q-Fever, Relapsing fevers, Encephalitis, Mycoplasma, Tularemia, Rocky Mountain Spotted Fever, Helicobacter pylori, Epstein-barr, Herpes, other viruses, and yeasts are some of the many illnesses transmissible by ticks.[16] Some persons also believe that a newly emergent disease named Morgellons is possibly a vector-borne, tick-transmissible illness.

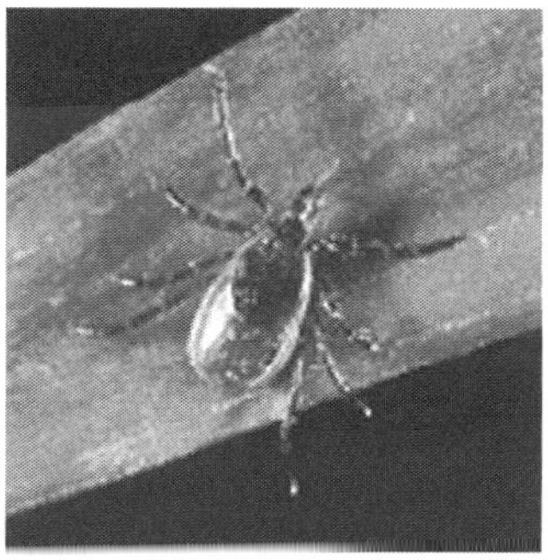

Left: Adult female *Ixodes scapularis* (black legged tick). Courtesy CDC.

Right: Adult female *Ixodes pacificus* (western black legged tick). Courtesy CDC.

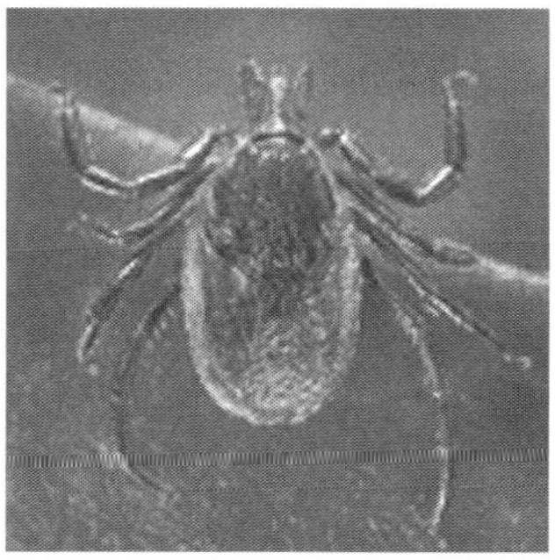

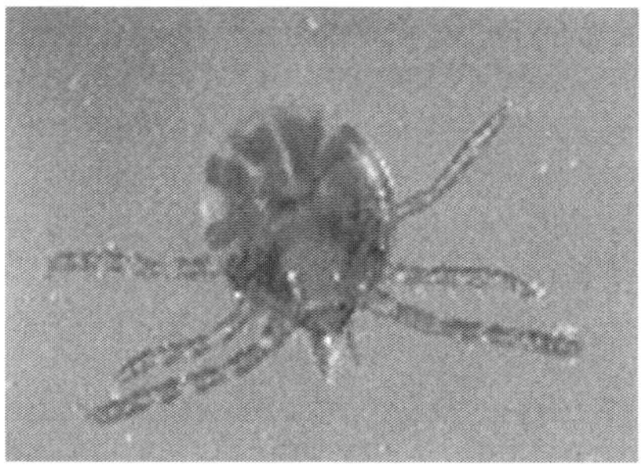

Left: Deer tick larvae at high power. Note only 6 legs on nymph as opposed to 8 for adults. Image used with permission of Marc G. Golightly, Ph.D., Stony Brook University School of Medicine, NY.

Right and below right: Dog Ticks (*Dermacentor variabilis*). Adult Female top. Adult Male, bottom. Reprinted with permission of Marc G. Golightly, Ph.D., Stony Brook University School of Medicine, NY.

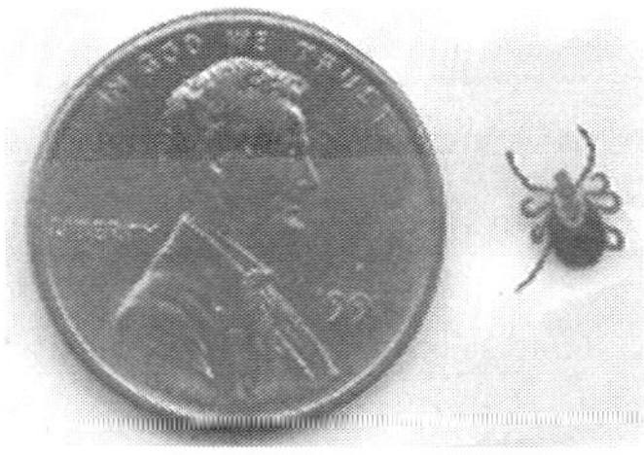

Below left: Two members of *Amblyomma* genus. Note elongated mouth parts, distinctive to North American hard-body ticks. CDC photo.

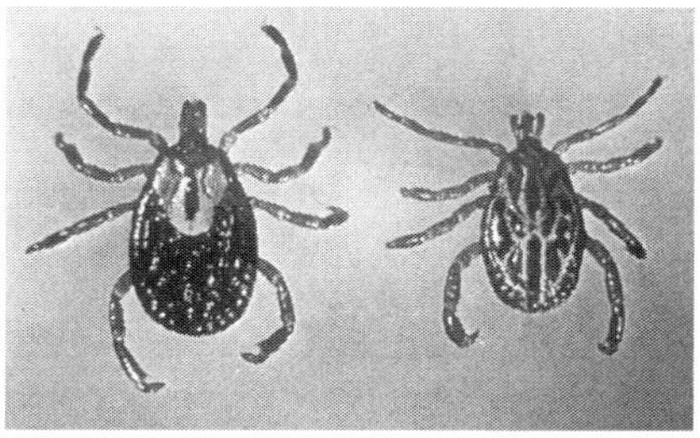

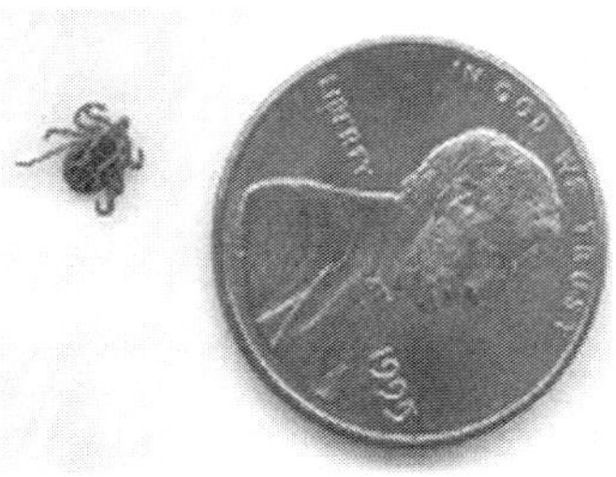

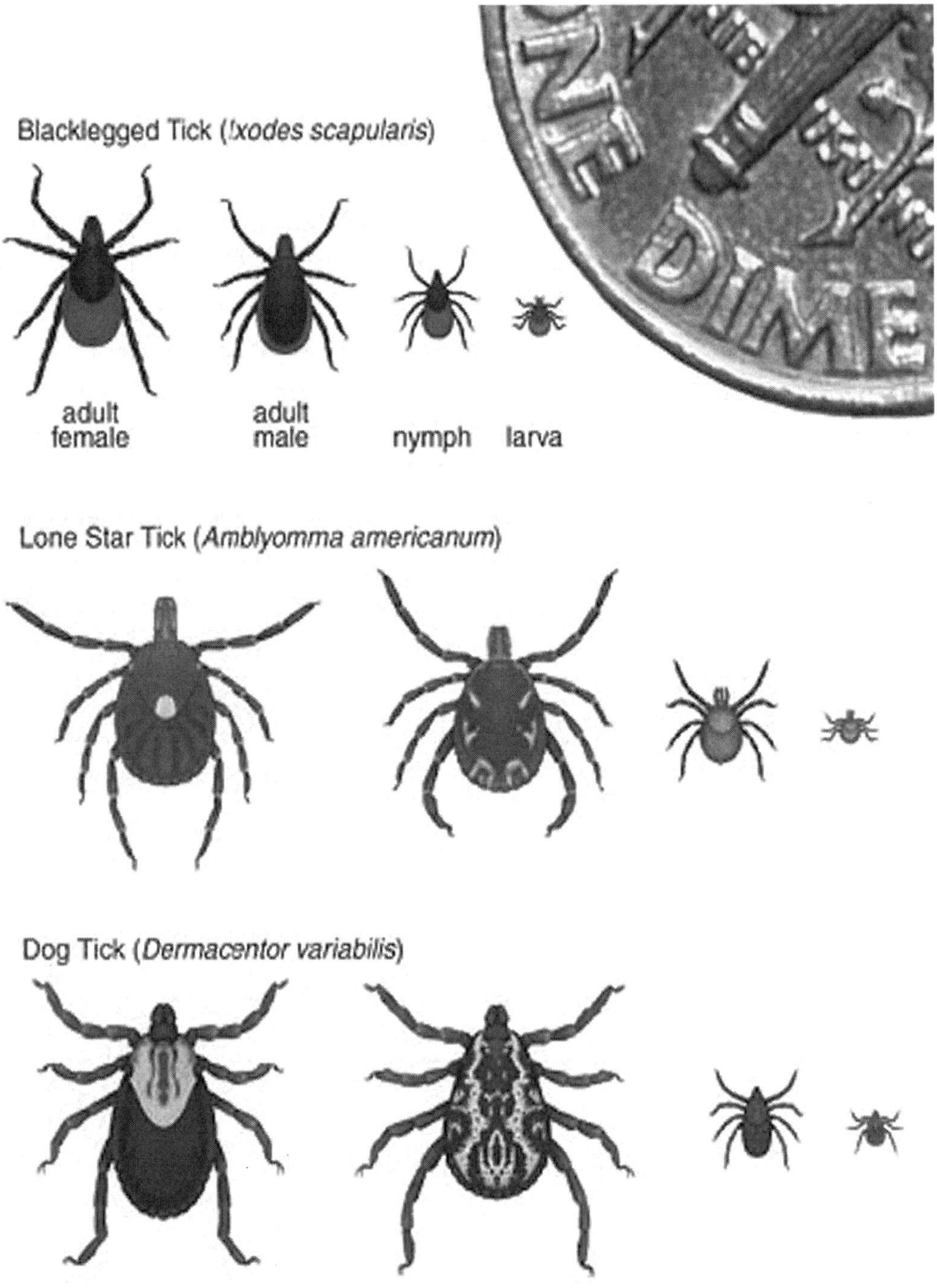

Comparisons of *Ixodes scapularis* (black legged tick), *Amblyomma americanum* (lone star tick), and *Dermacentor variabilis* (American dog tick), by life stages. Ticks shown in relative size to one another and to that of American dime. CDC photo.

How a Tick Feeds

The photos below show a close up of a typical tick's mouth parts. Contrary to what some may believe, a tick doesn't bite and then release like an insect such as a mosquito or a fly. A tick is an insect which attaches itself to the skin, feeds to engorgement, and then drops off.

It accesses the skin using its barbed mouth parts, called *chelicerae.* It uses its *hypostome* to penetrate the skin where it injects anti-coagulants and other substances, including a pain-reliever into the host so that the bite is painless. It then burrows its mouthparts into the skin and attaches itself with a secreted cement-like substance which makes it difficult to remove while it begins feeding from the tiny hole it has made under the skin. Adult ticks are harder to remove because their mouth parts are longer and are burrowed more deeply under the skin's surface than that of younger nymphs. As such, localized skin reactions can be larger with an embedded adult tick than that which might occur with a nymph. The entire process of attachment can take a half hour to an hour, or even longer, depending on the tick.

Borrelia burgdorferi, the spirochete causing Lyme lives in the midgut of the tick, so when the tick begins to feed, the spirochetes move into the tick's salivary glands. They are then transported through the action of feeding, and can be injected into the host animal or human as soon as a tick begins to feed. Although no one knows precisely the amount of time that must elapse before Lyme disease is transmitted, it could theoretically be transmitted as soon as the tick begins a meal – so assuming a non-engorged tick hasn't passed on Lyme or other tick-borne infections due to a short duration of attachment, is foolish thinking.

Below left: A close up of a typical tick's mouth parts, as indicated by the arrow. The mouth part appears at first glance, to be the insect's head. Photo courtesy CDC.

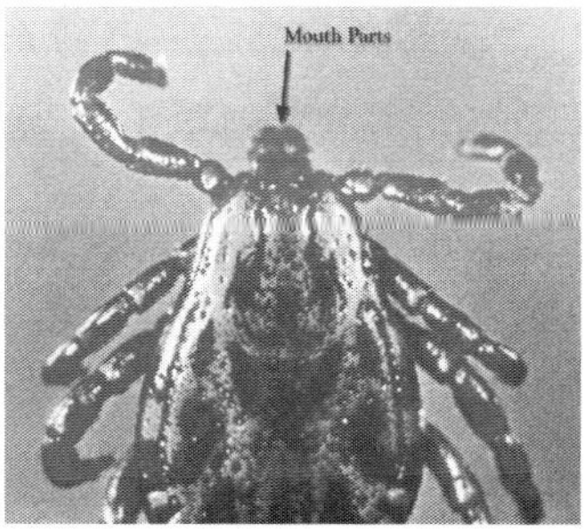

Right: A closeup of the tick's mouth. Photo courtesy of the CDC.

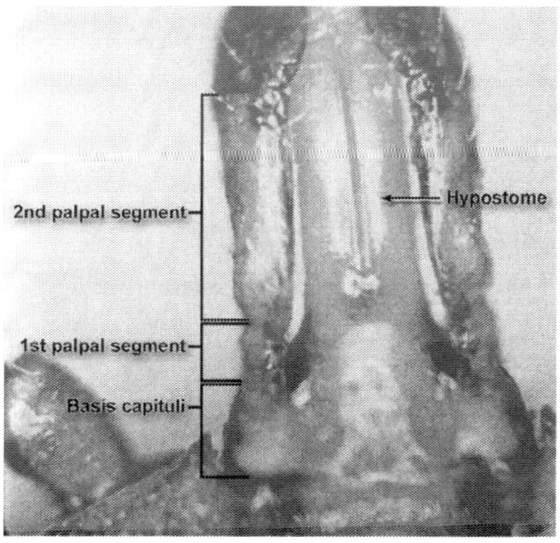

Tick Life Cycle

The typical life cycle of a tick includes 4 stages: the egg stage, the larval stage where the insect is about the size of a pinhead and has 6 legs; the nymph stage where it has 8 legs and is slightly larger, about the size of the period at the end of this sentence; and the even larger adult. Each stage requires adequate feeding from a host animal in order to obtain a blood meal to grow.

At the nymph stage, ticks typically begin feeding on larger hosts, including humans. The nymph and larval ticks must attach to a host, engorge, and then drop off and molt into the next stage. In order to obtain a ride on a passing animal, ticks will climb to the highest part of vegetation and display a behavior referred to as "questing."[17] This waving of the forelegs to and fro is how it finds its victim. There is no evidence to suggest that ticks drop out of trees, except anecdotal evidence whereby this author has seen it happen on two occasions. The adult tick will also feed on an animal or human in the third of the three-step feeding process.

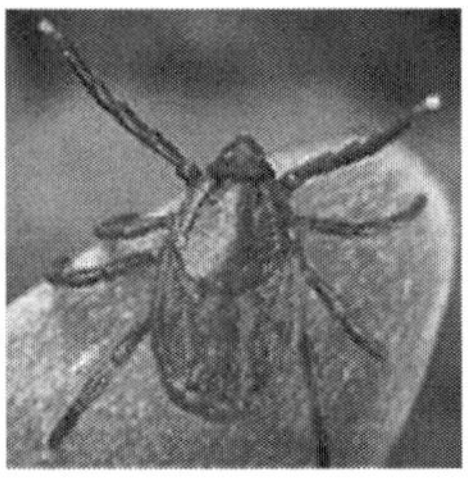

Adult *Rhipicephalus sanguineus* (brown dog tick) "questing." CDC photo.

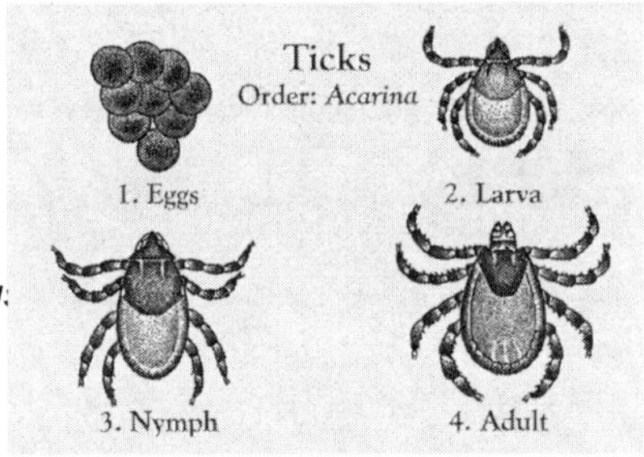

Male adult ticks occasionally feed on host blood, but are more interested in finding a mate on their host, and will sometimes even feed upon a female tick. Adult females will feed for up to a week before dropping off to lay between 3,000 and 18,000 eggs. Hard-bodied females will then die (soft-bodied ticks will lay many batches of eggs before dying).

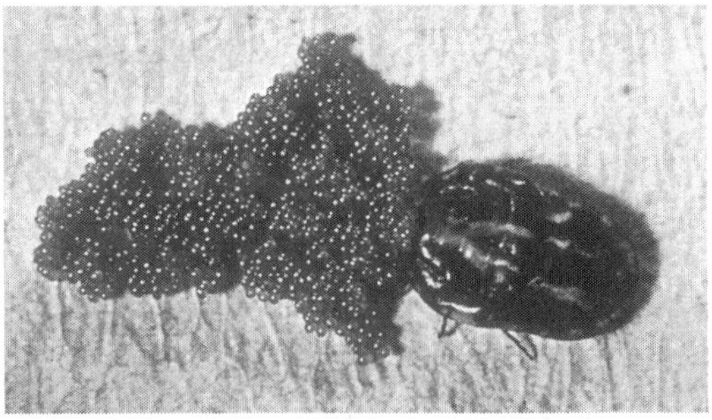

Female *Ixodes* tick laying eggs. She will subsequently die. CDC photo.

Tick Removal

The question of Lyme disease should always be taken very seriously. If you find a tick attached to yourself or a loved one, you must remove it properly, as soon as possible. The correct method of tick removal is felt to be by using a pair of tweezers. Never burn the tick with a lit match or smother it in any substance, as that will cause the tick to burp up the contents of its mid-gut into your blood, and the mid-gut (and saliva) is where the Bb spirochetes live and from where they are transmitted.

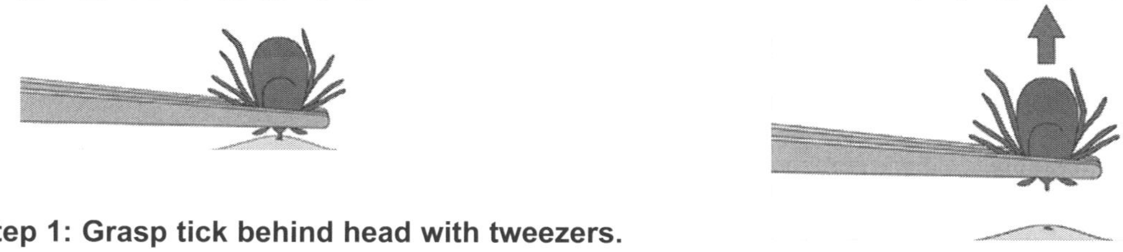

Step 1: Grasp tick behind head with tweezers.
Step 2: Pull tick gently out of the skin. CDC photos.

Grasp the tick just behind its head with a tweezers and gently but firmly pull it out of the skin. After removing the tick, disinfect the bite area and put the tick in a freezer bag in case you wish to send it out for testing, and see your physician promptly.

Prompt and proper diagnosis and treatment is of the utmost importance. If the disease is caught at onset and treated with antibiotics, the chances for recovery appear excellent. The key is in early detection and prompt treatment however. If people know they have been bitten by a tick, they *should not sit around for 30 days and wait for symptoms to appear*. It may be better to see a physician and obtain prophylactic treatment *in case of disease* than it is to wait for the organism to disseminate throughout the brain, central nervous system and other areas of the body, at which point, eradication will be most challenging if at all possible.

Prevention

The best way to avoid tick-borne illness is prevention. When traveling out of doors, camping, hiking, or walking in grass, leaves, or woods, tuck your pants legs into your socks. Wear long-sleeved, light-colored clothing and cover your head. Walk in the center of pathways and avoid brushing up against foliage. Do not sit or lay in leaves or tall grass. Perform frequent checks of yourself and others in your company. Take turns checking each other for ticks, especially in hard-to-reach areas like the scalp and back of the body.

Before you go out, you can spray your clothing with a product containing DEET. Some repellents are for skin, and some are for clothing. Read the manufacturer's label, and be careful when using on small children. There are some Permethrin-embedded products and special protective clothing available, some with and without chemicals. *Rynoskin* is chemical-free outerwear, guaranteed to protect you from ticks, and other biting insects. It is designed to be worn under clothing, but is lightweight, comfortable, breathable and moves freely when worn. It is made of an impenetrable fabric that provides complete protection from tick bites. The suits are affordable and ideal for most outdoor sports and activities.

Another helpful idea to use when you return from your outing, is to put your clothing into a clothes dryer and turn it on a high heat setting for at least a half hour, which will kill most ticks. Ticks can survive in a washing machine cycle! Be sure to check your pets when they have been outdoors as well. Dogs, cats, horses, and farm animals may contract Lyme disease and co-infections and transmit ticks to humans. If you find a tick attached to you or your pet, you can use a tweezers or a specialized tool that will remove ticks easily and safely.

There are ways to protect your family at home by utilizing landscaping techniques to build a barrier between tick environments and your property. There are also products that can reduce tick populations on deer that live in your area, but some of these products are expensive and take awhile to become effective. Nevertheless, bait stations are available to lure deer with corn, which (when the deer feed), coat the animals' head, neck and antlers with an insecticide. According to the U.S. Army, bait stations such as the 4-Poster Deer Treatment Bait Station or the Max Force Tick Management System, can eliminate up to 90% of ticks in a given area if used correctly. The limitations of bait stations are that they take time to implement and eradicate ticks, which have a 2-year life cycle.

When we think of our home environment, one of the last things we typically concern ourselves with is tick infestation, either in our yard or inside the home. And yet many areas are so endemic with ticks that people's homes are literally infested with them. The only alternatives for some of these people is to bomb their homes with insecticides. Many people relocate their families due to ticks.

Seasonally disinfecting the home, routinely checking pets (and children) for ticks upon leaving the yard are also good methods of prevention. Building tick barriers in and around your yard to reduce the possibility of tick exposure also helps. Keep feeding stations for birds and other small animals away from areas where pets and children may play. Erect deer fences to keep larger animals out of your yard if that is a problem in your area. Creating a tick-free zone in residential landscape is easy to do.

In the community at large, it is important to consider tick management programs including the culling of over populations of deer and elimination of rodents as effective ways to hold down tick populations. For more information on prevention techniques and removal tools, please visit: the CDC at *www.cdc.gov*, LDA at *www.lymediseaseassociation.org*, the American Camp Association: *www.acacamps.org*; Rynoskin Products at: *www.rynoskin.com* and The Tick Tool at *www.theticktool.com*.

Research for this book led me to discover some information about some bait systems mentioned previously that I thought worth sharing. Of course readers must make their own decisions on product purchases and use. The Maxforce Tick Management System was developed by Montvale-based Bayer Environmental Science, which launched it under a CDC license, so one might assume that the CDC makes a little money from the sales of the product.

The "4-Poster" Deer Treatment Bait Station was invented by the U.S. Department of Agriculture and is licensed to manufacturer C. R. Daniels Inc. of Ellicott City, MD and the American Lyme Disease Foundation (aldf.com), which receives a royalty on sales.[18-20]

The ALDF is a web site listing some members of the IDSA. IDSA members Dr. Durland Fish is on the foundation's board of directors, while doctors Alan Steere, Gary Wormser, and Eugene Shapiro are listed as National Scientific Advisors to the ALDF – and each of these gentlemen were co-authors of one or more versions of the IDSA Lyme Disease diagnostic and treatment guidelines.

These are guidelines which have stirred controversy among doctors and patients, and guidelines which many say have caused patients to remain undiagnosed and often completely untreated; not treated "appropriately" as the guidelines might suggest.[18,21-24]

Of course there is nothing wrong with anyone collecting royalties unless there is a conflict of interest, and I am not stating that any IDSA members have either of these. But readers might wish to know that some individuals might stand to profit from Lyme-related "product" royalties, and these may be individuals who may have also written medical guidelines which appear to minimize Lyme disease risk and pathology and/or recommend the constraint of certain diagnostic and treatment practices.

It is known in the Lyme community that some of these same individuals hold patents and/or may also collect royalties on diagnostic kits and/or vaccine components for these same illnesses. It is thought by many that some of these individuals may be assisting in the slow-playing of an epidemic. It is also known that some of these individuals may be compensated scientific advisors and/or speakers for insurance and/or pharmaceutical companies and other organizations...and therein we may indeed find various conflicts of interest.

❖ ❖ ❖

Lyme Disease

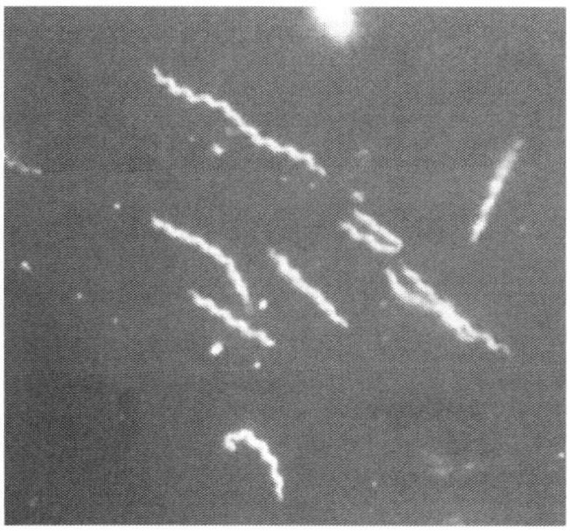

Borrelia burgdorferi **(Bb), under darkfield microscopy, magnified 400x, reveals corkscrew shaped spirochetes causing Lyme disease. CDC photo.**

Borrelia burgdorferi (Bb), also called *B. burgdorferi sensu lato* (latin for "broad sense,") is the scientific name of the spiral-shaped, gram-negative spirochete which causes Lyme disease. According to the CDC and NIH, at present, there are approximately 37 identified species[25] from the over 300 genotypes of *Borrelia* that can cause Lyme disease. Although *B. burgdorferi* sensu lato is present all over the world, most species have a limited geographical distribution.[26]

Dr. William (Willie) Burgdorfer was the scientist who reportedly identified this spiral-shaped organism in 1981, and it was named after him when he was looking for *rickettsia* (the rocky mountain spotted fever organism) in New York ticks. In fact, Burgdorfer tells us that the first discovery of human pathogenic spirochetes was actually credited in 1868 to Dr. Otto Obermeirer, a German physician who detected in relapsing fever patients, thread-like microorganisms similar to water spirochetes (*spirochete plicatilis*), which were first discovered in 1835 by German naturalist/zoologist Dr. Christian Gottfried Ehrenberg. Bb was the first infectious agent shown to be transmitted by an arthropod vector (tick) in that century.[27,28]

From 1857 to 1910, a number of scientists made discoveries that would confirm the link between relapsing fever and the bite of blood-sucking arthropods. As early as 1857 however, it was known that East African relapsing fever was transmitted by the bite of the African soft-shelled, or argasid tick, *Ornithodoros moubata.* A pathologist named Arthur Dawson renamed the East African relapsing fever spirochete *Borrelia duttonii.*[28]

Cases of Lyme disease were noted since the 1940's in Glastonbury

CT. Outbreaks of Lyme disease in the U.S., may have begun at the end of World War II during Soviet fur shipments, by traveling on Lyme-infested rodents that had been infected through Nazi research experiments.[29] The disease was detected in the U.S. by Navy doctors who reported their findings in 1976 of a cluster of patients near the New London submarine base in Groton, Connecticut. Lyme disease did not have an official name at that time however. In the book by author Michael Christopher Carroll, *Lab 257,*[3] Carroll cites Plum Island and its federal government germ laboratory activities, as the potential epicenter of many diseases, including Lyme disease, which were released into the states, either through accident, migrating flocks, or deliberate intent – the truth of which we may never know for certain but the evidence published certainly points in some sinister directions.

The person most credited with bringing the illness that is now named Lyme disease into the public spotlight was Polly Murray, an American housewife living with her family along the southern Connecticut River Valley. Polly and her family were sick during the 1960's and 1970's with odd illnesses that for years, no physicians could explain. She discovered that others in her geographic area were suffering similar symptoms as her family. After completing research at the Yale library, she and Judith Mensch, another housewife with ill family members, urged Yale Medical School researchers to study the situation. In 1975, Dr. Allen C. Steere and his colleagues identified the mystery illness as "Lyme disease," and it was so named after the town where it was found – a name remaining to this day. Working with Dr. Steere were associates such as Dr. Eugene Shapiro, Dr. Robert Schoen, and Dr. Stephen Malawista. Eventually in 1983, Yale University Medical School held its first symposium on Lyme disease and scientists from the U.S. and Europe attended to share knowledge of tick-borne illnesses.[30,31] Since that time, University researchers (Yale, Harvard, etc.) have been heavily involved in tick-borne illness studies and some of the politics and controversy that surrounds this illness, as well.

From the 1980's until present day, Lyme disease has continued to spread outward (by whatever means) from this east coastal region, postulated as through flocks of migratory birds, ticks and other vectors such as mosquitoes, deer and small animals and human modes of transmission that we are only beginning to understand.

Bb spirochetes present with many different forms within the human host, such as spirochetal, spheroplast (l-form), cystic forms, blebs, and granules, making them difficult to eradicate from the body.[33] *Borrelia* are pleomorphic or polymorphic spirochetes, (having two or more forms during a life cycle, the names are interchangeable). *Borrelia* are able to change form as necessary in order to survive various habitat changes within their host animals, including humans.

In addition to arthropod vectors (ticks) as modes of transmission, it is possible that Bb is spread through the bite of insects like mosquitoes or biting flies. In addition, researchers at the University of Wisconsin have reported that Bb can infect milk from dairy cattle, causing contamination. Bb can also be transmitted orally to animals. The Sacramento California blood bank believes that Lyme disease can be spread by blood transfusions, which is echoed by the CDC in Atlanta, Georgia, which holds data indicating that Bb can survive the blood processing techniques used for U.S. blood transfusions.[33] In fact, in the U.S., if you report that you have Lyme disease or have had active symptoms within the previous 90 days, your blood donation will probably not, (and should not), be accepted. Some studies are beginning to show evidence that active tick-borne illness may be sexually transmissible, and that it also passes from mother to infants while in utero, and in breast milk. This helps to explain why whole families are suffering from Lyme disease, especially those with infants who are born with congenital Lyme, and for those individuals who do not spend time outdoors where they might be otherwise exposed.

Lyme disease is called "the great imitator" due to its symptoms being similar to other, more well known illnesses. These symptoms are often baffling to those who are not Lyme-literate medical doctors (LLMDs). Their inexperience with Lyme leads them to misdiagnose patients with other diseases such as Multiple Sclerosis, Alzheimer's, Parkinson's, Chronic Fatigue Syndrome, Attention Deficit Disorder, Lupus, Asthma, and even psychiatric illness, when they really have Lyme. This is not to say that Lyme does or does not play a part in any of these illnesses, it is just to suggest that misdiagnoses can and do occur. In fact, Pathologist Alan MacDonald of St. Catherine of Siena in Smithtown, NY, performed studies using brain tissues from deceased Alzheimer's patients, obtained from the McLean Hospital Brain Bank of Harvard University. His study showed DNA evidence of *Borrelia burgdorferi* in 7 out of 10 of the patient tissue samples examined.[34,35]

Early Lyme Disease (Stage I)

Lyme in its early stages exhibits some distinctive symptoms, although not all patients infected by a tick bite are affected in the same manner, and with the same symptoms. One of the most characteristic symptoms of Lyme disease, is a circular, rash called *Erythema migrans* (EM). The rash is commonly called a bull's eye rash due to a distinctive red ring, with a central clearing portion. Unfortunately the tell-tale EM rash is only experienced in approximately 40% of Lyme patients, although the CDC sets that number considerably higher, at 80%.[36] The absence of this key symptom makes a diagnosis of Lyme difficult for the clinician since the accompanying symptoms may be vague and misleading.

The EM rash appears approximately 4 days after the tick bite, and should be treated immediately, before the illness has a chance to spread, and while it is most successfully treated. At this time, serologic tests such as an ELISA, IFA or Western Blot, are not expected to become positive for several weeks. It would be a good idea to treat at this time and not wait for some test result to come back – do not miss this chance to treat Lyme disease in its earliest stage![37]

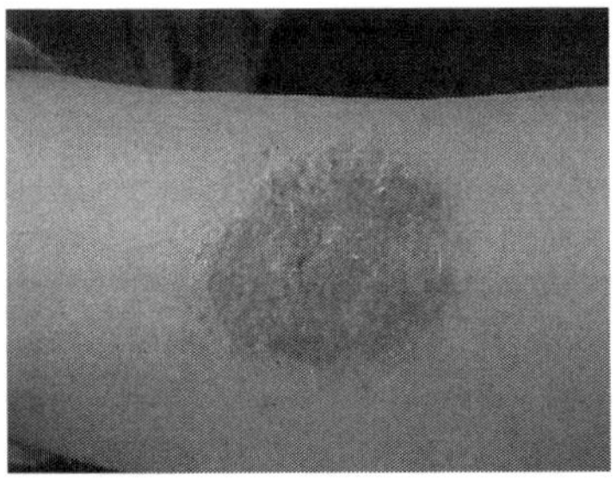

Erythema migrans rash on forearm. Photo courtesy of a support group member at www.sewill.org

Sadly, even when a patient has an EM rash, physicians can easily overlook, mistake, or even attempt to minimize what they see because they simply do not know what it is. Worse yet, some physicians wait for the rash to clear to see if additional symptoms appear before testing or treating for Lyme (30 days or more). The Infectious Disease Society of America (IDSA) states that the *"routine use of antimicrobial prophylaxis or serologic testing is not recommended."*[22] As a patient, I would have to ask why not? If the earliest stages of Lyme disease are *when the illness is most easily treated*, what motivation would anyone have to wait or refuse to treat a potential Lyme patient at exposure?

In my case, living in Wisconsin at the time of a tick-bite, (and an endemic area), my EM rash, was prominently displayed on my back.

And yet it was not recognized by either of the first 2 physicians I visited at onset of my illness in 1992, even after I directly asked them both if my rash could mean Lyme disease. I find their failure particularly ironic because the first reported case of EM rash in the United States was made in 1970 by a Dr. Scrimenti, a Wisconsin Dermatologist – and the second physician I saw was in fact, also a dermatologist in (Milwaukee), Wisconsin.[38]

Weeks after displaying my initial EM rash, I revisited the dermatologist, again asking if it was possible that I could have Lyme disease. At that visit, my body had multiple EM rashes (about 30 on my trunk, neck and back), and the Dermatologist gave me a bottle of what looked to be calamine lotion, and well wishes, but nothing more. Multiple EM rashes appear in only about 10% of Lyme patients[37], and here I had displayed 2 obvious symptoms of Lyme disease, and nobody recognized them, not even after I said I suspected Lyme.

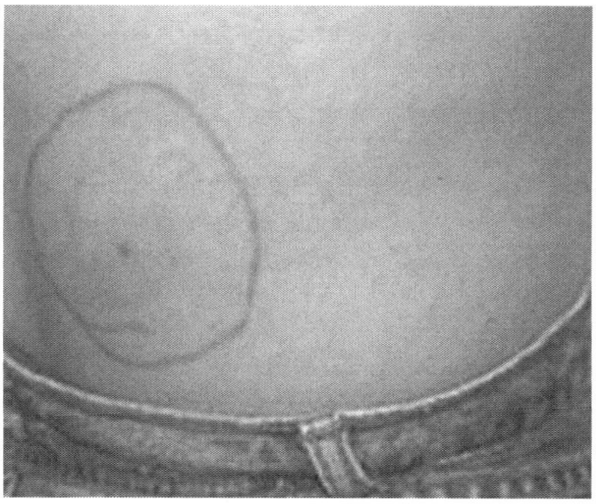

Erythema migrans rash on abdomen (circled for clarity). Note center bite mark, clearing center and then outer expanding ring. Photo courtesy of support group member at www.sewill.org

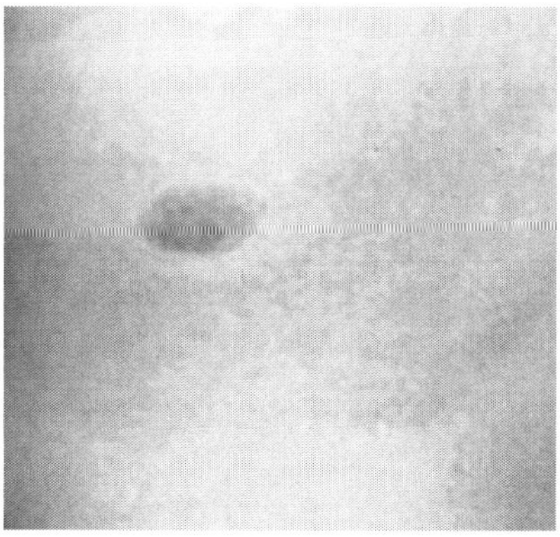

Large Erythema migrans rash on patient's back. Note large size of "bulls-eye" rash. Photo courtesy of support group member at www.sewill.org

When patients are bitten by a Lyme-infected tick, within hours to days they may manifest a combination of some or all of these symptoms:

- Characteristic bull's-eye rash (often expanding over days)
- Other irregular rash or rashes (sometimes multiple)
- Mild or severe headaches
- Flu-like symptoms
- Nausea/vomiting
- Fevers/chills
- Migrating pains or swelling joints
- Joint stiffening, shin splints
- Burning in hands or feet, sore balls of feet or heels
- Muscle pains or cramps, which migrate
- Extreme fatigue
- Increased motion sickness, dizziness, wooziness
- Sudden mood swings or depression
- Sleep disorders or hallucinations

Early Disseminated Lyme Disease (Stage II)

Early Disseminated (Stage II) Lyme disease is an illness that *should be diagnosed by clinical symptoms as well as augmented by laboratory testing*. Because ticks frequently carry additional infectious diseases (co-infections), patients should be carefully screened for these. Lyme disease and co-infections are systemic, not localized infections. The sooner an infected person receives treatment, the better their chance for complete recovery. If Lyme is undetected however, it will progress to a more disseminated form that includes symptoms such as:

- Bell's palsy (facial paralysis and drooping)
- Arthritic pains and loss of mobility
- Neurological impairments
- Buzzing sounds or ringing of the ears, deafness
- Poor balance and coordination, difficulty walking
- Irritability, depression or suicidal thinking
- Paranoia, delusions, chronic depression
- Hypersensitivities / new or increased allergies
- Meningitis, cranial neuritis or encephalitis
- Lesions in the white matter of the brain
- Seizures or strokes

- Hair loss
- Swollen glands, sore throat, chronic dry cough
- Paralysis or numbness
- Gastritis, abdominal cramping
- Irritable bladder/bowel, cystitis
- Visual and auditory hallucinations
- Cognitive difficulties, confusion, dementia, memory problems
- Disorientation, going to the wrong place, reading difficulties
- Visual disturbances, blindness, other ocular involvement
- Swelling around the eyes, eye pain
- Twitching of the facial muscles or other muscles
- Chest pains/difficulty breathing/shortness of breath
- Cardiovascular problems such as arrhythmias or heart blocks
- Problems with speech, or difficulty swallowing
- Incontinence where there was no problem before
- Menstrual problems, pelvic pain, testicular pain
- Sexual dysfunction/diminished libido
- Obsessive/compulsive behaviors
- Personality disorders/bi-polar like behavior

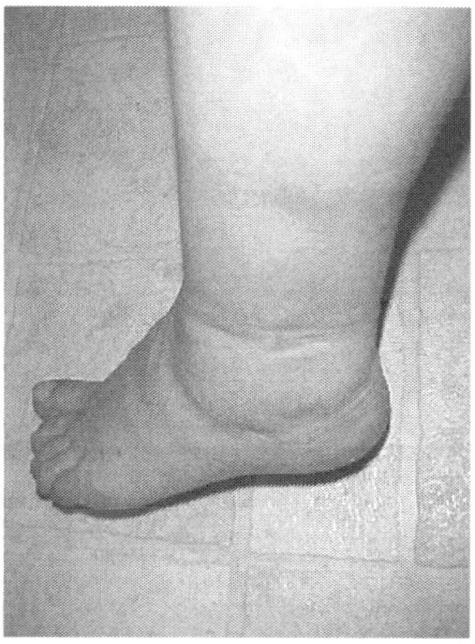

Patient with swollen ankle and calf due to Lyme disease. Note that the patient is not obese. Bartonella co-infection can also cause swelling in the extremities. Photo courtesy of a support group member at www.sewill.org

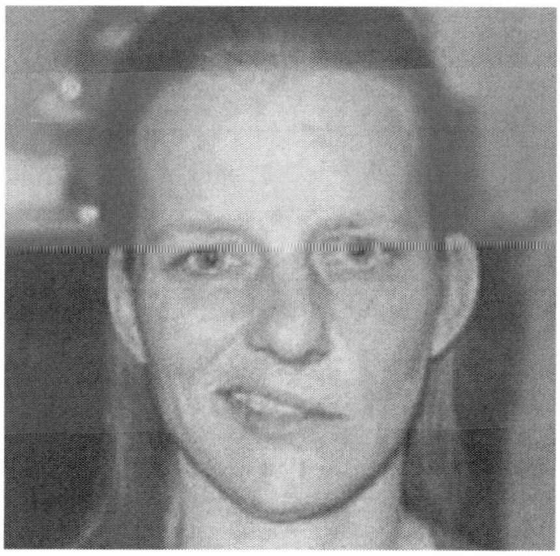

Facial paralysis on patient's left and central portions of face (Bell's palsy) due to multiple cranial nerve involvement, about 4 weeks after initial presentation occurred. Note the (now subtle) external ear, cheek and jaw swelling, and droopy eyelid on affected side. Sense of taste, smell and hearing were involved. Photo courtesy of the author.

Once the rash and initial symptoms have passed, patients progress to what is considered to be the second stage of Lyme disease. At this point, Bell's palsy and other neurological symptoms may begin to appear. Dissemination of the disease into the central nervous system can occur just days or weeks after skin infection, and neurological problems affect approximately 40% of the infected population. The latency period for Lyme disease, like syphilis, may be months to years before symptoms of late infection occur. The length of time before symptoms appear varies in each individual, and is affected by such things as stress, surgeries, the immunological states and the number of infectious agents present. In the author's case, Bell's Palsy did not appear until 8 years after initial infection.

Chronic Lyme Disease (Stage III)

In the third, (tertiary or disseminated) stage of Lyme, encephalomyelitis, radiculoneuropathies, and encephalopathy, long-term arthritis, and neurologic disorders can and do occur, and symptoms will become chronic in nature. There is often organ involvement and eyesight or hearing may be affected, and some patients lose these senses entirely. This stage is also referred to as "chronic" Lyme disease. Some physicians and scientists believe this stage is simply an autoimmune reaction to Lyme disease that has been "properly treated," and label this phase as "post-Lyme syndrome." While some will disagree, the research points to the fact that Bb survives in the body for extended periods even with treatment, and as a result, there may also be an autoimmune component to this stage of the disease, besides the fact that the spirochetes survive "standard" treatment, persisting in the body for many months to many years, as active or subclinical infection.

Disseminated Lyme disease can cause a host of psychiatric problems such as bipolar-like disorders, panic attacks, schizophrenia, dementia, paranoia, major depression, anorexia nervosa, attention deficit, and obsessive-compulsive disorders. Depression is fairly common, and affects up to 66% of patients, with suicide rates as high as 35%! Psychiatrists need to include Lyme disease in a differential diagnosis of persons having atypical psychiatric presentations if they live in, or have traveled to, endemic areas.[39]

Differing opinions exist about the treatment of chronic Lyme disease, although intravenous and long-term oral antibiotics as well as "alternative" therapies have proven effective for many of these patients. The most important thing to remember for chronic Lyme cases is that re-treatment may be necessary until symptoms are completely gone, and for those with chronic illness, that time period should remain open-ended in order to serve the patients best. For some patients, this may mean months or years of treatment before symptoms resolve.

Acrodermatitis chronica atrophicans (ACA) is a late, cutaneous (skin) manifestation of Lyme disease. It is characterized by erythro-cyanotic skin lesions (red/blue from under oxygenation) that are slow to heal and typically involve the limbs, fingers, ears or any extremity location. The lesions are insidious, slow to evolve, and have periods of inflammation and atrophy. Over time, generalized thinning of the skin occurs giving it a thin, transparent look and veins can be seen. The inflammatory phase can last for months or years, and ACA does not heal without treatment. *Borrelia* was determined to be the cause of this condition in 1984 when spirochetes were cultured from a skin lesion in a patient with this condition.[40]

Lyme During Pregnancy

Lyme disease infection during pregnancy has its own share of controversy. While individual case reports may suggest an association between maternal Borrelia infection and adverse pregnancy outcomes, not enough definitive studies have been performed to give an overall view of the clinical picture. Some studies have shown possible transmission of Lyme and HGE (human granulocytic ehrlichiosis) to infants while in utero, sometimes causing stillbirths.[41,42] In fact, with reference to the spirochetal cousin *syphilis*, up to half of all stillbirths may be caused by infection.[42] In a 1997 study of 105 pregnant women who were followed to delivery after exposure to Lyme and presentation of EM rashes, (trimester exposure varied), 93 of the patients gave birth to healthy children. The remaining 12 patients included 2 spontaneous abortions, 1 missed abortion at 9 weeks, one spontaneous abortion (10 weeks) and 6 women had pre-term births. Congential abnormalities were found in 4 of the children including syndactyly (fused fingers or toes), and urological abnormalities. In an earlier study in 1996, 58 pregnant women were treated for borreliosis, with successful outcomes in 51 women. One child born at term was found to have urologic abnormalities 7 months later. One pregnancy ended with a missed abortion, and 5 ended with pre-term birth. One of the pre-term infants had heart abnormalities.[43,44] One of the authors of the previous two studies, Dr. Franc Strle, was also a co-author of the IDSA guidelines.

According to the CDC's Weekly publication, *MMWR* in June of 1985, transplacental transmission of Bb was documented in a pregnant woman with Lyme disease who did not receive antibiotic therapy. Her infant was delivered with a congenital heart defect. In addition, the CDC recognized that fetal death, premature births, blindness and developmental delays in children were occurring for mothers who had Lyme disease while pregnant.[45] At the moment, the CDC has this to say about Lyme disease in pregnancy – there have been reports that Bb has been found in stillborns, and in infants who were born with severe abnormalities. The CDC recommends that pregnant women who have Lyme disease be treated promptly with antibiotics. Further, the CDC recommends that women who are nursing and who are suspected of having Lyme infection, to stop nursing until they have received "a complete course of antibiotic therapy."[46] I would ask how to determine what is a full course, since there is, at present, no definitive test to determine whether a patient has been cured of Lyme disease.

Pediatric Lyme

We see from the CDC chart below that people typically affected most from Lyme are children and adults over age 50.

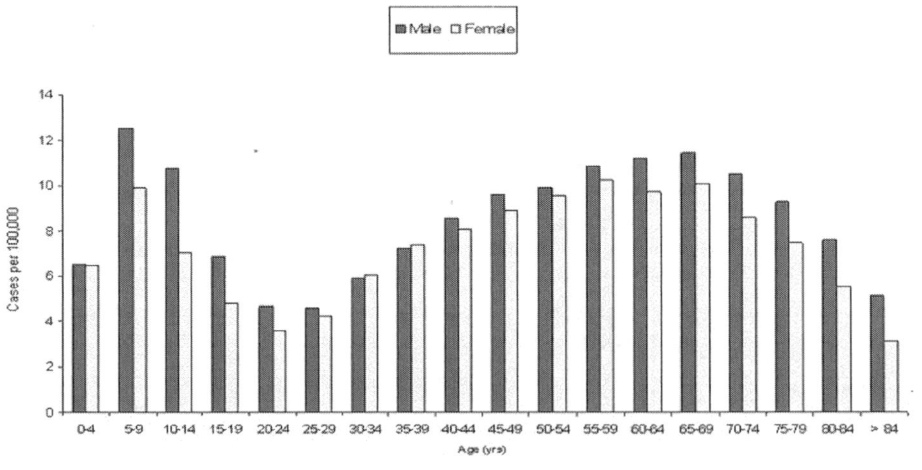

The above chart shows the average annual incidents reported for Lyme Disease in the U.S. by sex and age of its victims from 1992-2004. CDC photo.

Children are affected by Lyme disease in ways which differ from the adult population, and the school environment holds an opportunity to help diagnose students exhibiting variations in their normal behavior. Lyme disease manifests in many ways which may be observed by teachers, principals, guidance counselors or even the school nurse. Children and adolescents who have been infected with tick-borne illnesses will display the following symptoms:

- Fatigue, lethargy, falling asleep in class or hyperactivity
- Mood swings, depression, anxiety, suicidal thoughts or actions
- Withdrawal from peers
- Difficulty with concentration or memory, attention disorders
- Tardiness, or early morning absences
- Erratic academic performance, declining grades
- Behavioral problems, overt hostility
- Speaking and writing difficulties
- Headaches, stomach aches
- Joint pain or twitching
- Dizziness, disorientation
- Vision problems, sensitivity to light, sound or stimulus
- Severe PMS symptoms

Teachers don't need to know how to diagnose Lyme, the ins and outs of laboratory testing, or even which antibiotics are necessary to treat Lyme disease, but they do need to be aware of the signs and symptoms of tick-borne illness. Children who are falling asleep in class, are easily distracted, inattentive or argumentative, can be exhibiting signs of Lyme disease. Guidance offices can track declining grades and attendance, and nurses can see a pattern of ill health in students visiting them only if they are aware of the symptoms of this illness.

If children with Lyme and co-infections are attending school, the environment needs to be supportive of the child's abilities and limitations. Children suffering symptoms of Lyme disease often become isolated from their peers, and teachers are in a unique position to support these children, as well as teach educational curriculum to inform their classmates about Lyme disease. If teachers are unaware of tick-borne illness and the symptoms they present in children, they may unfairly label children with disciplinary problems when in fact those children are merely ill with infectious diseases. This mislabeling can have a lasting negative impact on children in school, both because their self-esteem suffers, and because they do not feel supported when they are trying their best but failing to reach academic goals.[47]

Adolescents need to be carefully evaluated when clearly showing a pattern of depressed thinking in creative writing projects, through internet posts, negatively themed artwork, negative or depressed answers on homework or essay questions, and other clear signs of "cries for help," even if the adolescents are dismissive or in a state of denial about their own behavior. Puberty and drugs are not the only issues causing depression and suicidal ideology – Lyme's affects on the adolescent brain are very real.

For some families with Lyme-infected children, home schooling is an option allowing uninterrupted education of an ill child, without subjecting the individual to school prejudices such as refusal to accommodate special needs, teasing from peers, and other issues. Home schooling is different from home-bound education, wherein schools send tutors to present coursework and homework assignments to those who cannot attend school. Home schooling, "unschooling" or "home-education" is distinctly different because it is geared toward learning in a self-paced environment, with the freedom to pursue interests that are compatible with health issues requiring flexibility, as well as the student's personal interests. Home schooling is legal in all 50 of the United States, although state requirements vary, sometimes even between districts. Check for a local home schooling group near you for more information about this option to continue education for your Lyme-afflicted child.

Geriatric Lyme

Other groups of individuals often affected by Lyme disease are the elderly. While the elderly are typically prone to many illnesses due to aging, common illnesses are beginning to be reclassified, as links to *Borrelia burgdorferi* are being discovered. One illness typically associated with the elderly, and which has been shown to have a link with Bb, is Alzheimer's disease.[48,49]

Symptoms in elderly patients with Lyme disease are compounded by the aging process. The "normal" aging process typically provides limitations to flexibility and mobility, as well as a decline in overall bodily function, (eyesight, hearing, immunology, cognitive thinking). Lyme disease exacerbates these symptoms, and the elderly are often in a difficult position due to retirement, limited resources and mobility, which complicates treatment.

Physicians who lack compassion are often quick to dismiss senior citizens when they complain about pain or discomfort, often writing these symptoms off as a casualty of aging. Joint pains, dizziness, heart problems and dementia or confusion are rarely considered abnormal in the elderly patient. And elderly patients with Lyme disease and cognitive impairments need an advocate for their health more than their non-Lyme infected peers. Often the elderly parent is separated from his or her family by geographical location. Visits and family gatherings are not commonplace, and family members who do not spend a large amount of quality time with their elderly family members may not notice the subtle changes in personality or behavior because of this lack of involvement in their lives. The information about an elderly patient's lifestyle, work history and daily activities can be critical for an accurate diagnosis, but physicians do not always ask the elderly patient's relatives for assistance in obtaining this information, even when the patient cannot provide this information personally.

Additionally, senior citizens do not often have access to computer technologies and other resources which would enable them to obtain information on Lyme disease, and must rely solely on their doctor's ability and education. This puts them at a distinct disadvantage, because often their education and experience with emerging infectious diseases is limited. Medications used to treat Lyme disease may complicate existing health problems, and/or interact with other necessary medications, so considerable effort may be required to medicate these patients properly. Physicians who specialize in elderly care do not always know how to treat Lyme disease, so collaborative efforts between healthcare providers is essential. In addition, nursing homes and centers dealing with our aging population could do much more to become better acquainted with Lyme disease in their elderly patients, especially in endemic areas.

Ticks on Tourism and Outdoor Sports

For people who travel, exposure to ticks in various parts of the world is a concern, especially in areas known to be endemic for tick-borne illnesses. When visiting a new area, people often have picnics, take hikes, camp, nature walk, fish, hunt or boat. And many individuals are involved with landscaping, forestry, wildlife and park management. Each of these areas of activity carry a risk for tick exposure, and it is important to practice prevention techniques whenever one is out of doors, no matter where that might be. Cabins, tents and campers are critical areas that people may be exposed to ticks, and care should be taken to inspect and disinfect these areas on a regular basis, especially concerning sleeping areas. Sleeping out of doors, on the ground, in sleeping bags or even on cots, especially in endemic areas, can be very risky. Additionally, sitting or laying on or in wet leaves, stone walls and damp grass or near wooded areas should be avoided. Use common sense when moving wood from wood piles, and inspect yourself and your clothing for ticks after carrying firewood into your home or cabin.

White-tailed deer, which are not involved in the life cycle of the spirochete, are the preferred host of adult *I. scapularis* ticks, and they seem to be critical for their survival.[50] Since deer and other mammals are tick vectors, those who hunt wild game are at particular risk for exposure to tick-borne illnesses. Take precautionary measures for personal protection but don't forget to disinfect hunting blinds, stands, and other outdoor clothing and even gear that remains outside, where it is tick-accessible. Handling tick-infested carcasses for both hunters and taxidermists alike can also expose individuals to ticks and tick-borne illnesses. Ticks do not survive long outside of a warm, moist environment, and hunters need to be aware that ticks can detach from a recently dead carcass and quickly relocate onto a human host should they come into direct contact with one. So take extra precaution when handling or transporting wild game.

Last, handling, processing or even eating uncooked or under cooked meats like venison, can possibly expose you to *Borrelia* spirochetes. Bb is temperature-sensitive (104°F) and by all accounts, does not easily survive the heat of cooking, so be sure to cook all game meats thoroughly before eating them, and do not eat them raw. One example of good precautionary measures comes from a Stewartville Minnesota man who processes deer meat from Minnesota and parts of Wisconsin. He removes his clothing after each shift, places the items into a plastic bag, checks himself for ticks and showers immediately, especially now that he has symptoms of Lyme disease. He noted he has handled many deer which were infested with literally "hundreds" of ticks, and calls the situation regarding tick-infested deer in his area, "scary."[51]

Lyme Disease – A Global Problem

Lyme borreliosis is the most prevalent and widespread vector-borne human infection in the northern hemisphere, according to the Centers for Disease Control (CDC).[52] The CDC reported 166,868 cases of Lyme disease in the United States between 1994-2003. Voluntary reporting yields on average only about 20,000 new cases of Lyme each year. Experts estimate that actual annual numbers of unreported Lyme infection are 10 times this, or 200,000 in the U.S. alone, with perhaps 1 billion globally.[53] This is not only possible but highly probable because many patients do not know they are infected, or they know they are ill, but have been improperly diagnosed with another disease. If this is true, then Lyme cases are severely under reported in the U.S., and probably elsewhere. Lyme disease has been found in all 50 United States, Canada, Europe, and most other parts of the world.

Lyme disease surveillance data is reported to the CDC through the National Electronic Telecommunication System for Surveillance, a computerized database of public health records for diseases that are required to be reported. But that is only for regions that are required to report, and for illnesses meeting mandatory reporting criteria. From 1992-1998, Lyme disease data collected included the county and state of residence, age and sex of the victim, and onset date. Statistics were gathered and statistical data was developed from this information.[54] Maps showing Lyme disease risk are offered on the CDC web site, but they are quite out-of-date and appear to minimize disease prevalence.

In my case, reportable information was collected with gross inaccuracy. A copy of the form completed by my physician in 2004, (the time of my diagnosis), reports only the county in which the *physician was treating*, and said nothing about the county in which I was currently living, nor the county where I was originally infected, a dozen years earlier. Further, it did not list the correct year of infection. Since states do not mandate the format that Lyme data is reported, statistics are only generally accurate, as in my case, above.

There are other problems. For example, if a patient contracted Lyme in state A and then moved to state B where they were diagnosed, the physician could have reported the patient's current state of residence, not the state where the infection occurred. Of course many patients travel and do not know when or where they were first bitten. Then there is the problem of patients who are misdiagnosed for years. If I had not found my treating physician, I might still be misdiagnosed and never reported as having Lyme. So we can see how inaccuracies in reporting would skew the number of new cases being reported and their locations as well. Surveillance data is merely a general idea of transmission and infection rates, and by nature of the data collection methods used, are only somewhat accurate.

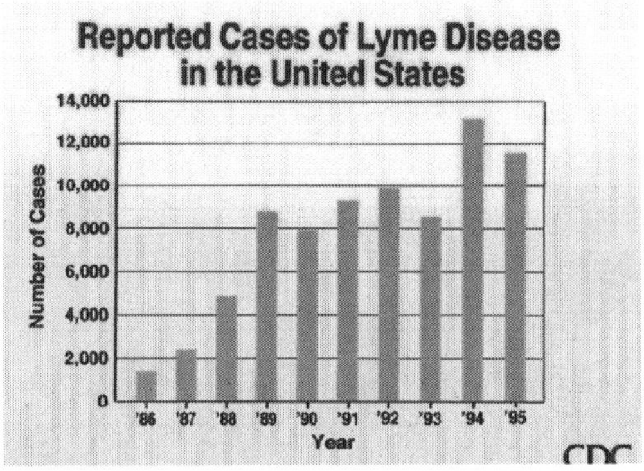

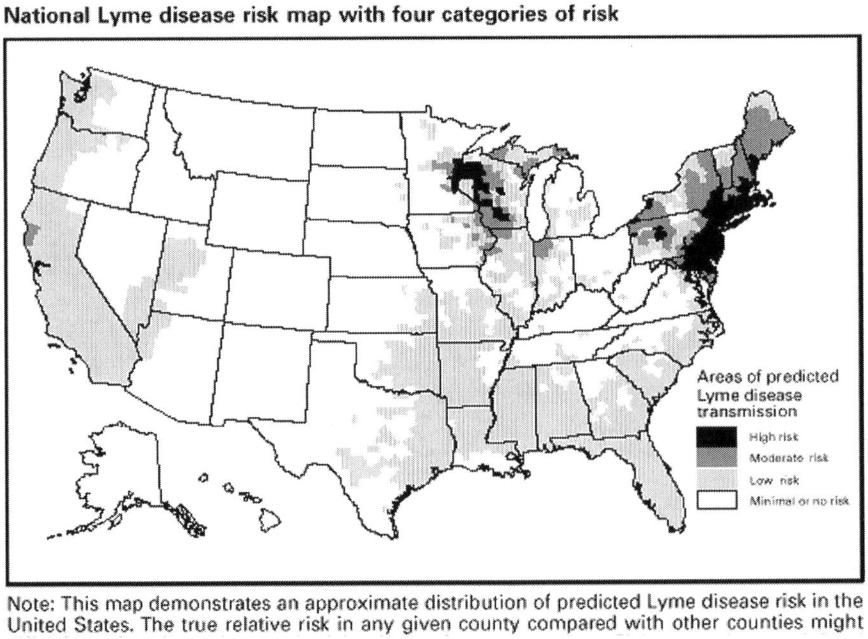

Above: This CDC Lyme risk map is from 1999. The areas in white say "minimal or no risk," but Lyme has been reported in 50 U.S. states and of course, the spread of Lyme has continued since 1999. CDC photo.

FIGURE 2. Incidence* of Lyme disease, by county of residence — United States, 2002

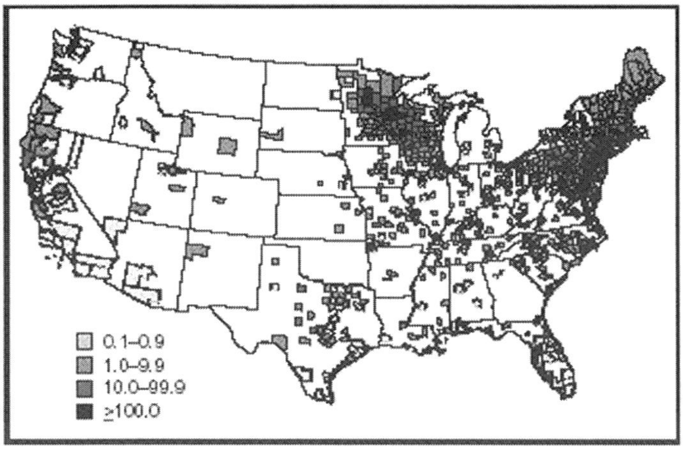

* Per 100,000 population.

Left: This CDC Lyme risk map is from 2002. CDC photo. There is already an increase of reported cases. Lyme disease has continued to spread all over the U.S., Canada, and in other countries.

Below, Incidence of Lyme disease by county of residence in the United States, in 2005. CDC photo.

Reported cases of Lyme disease—United States, 2005

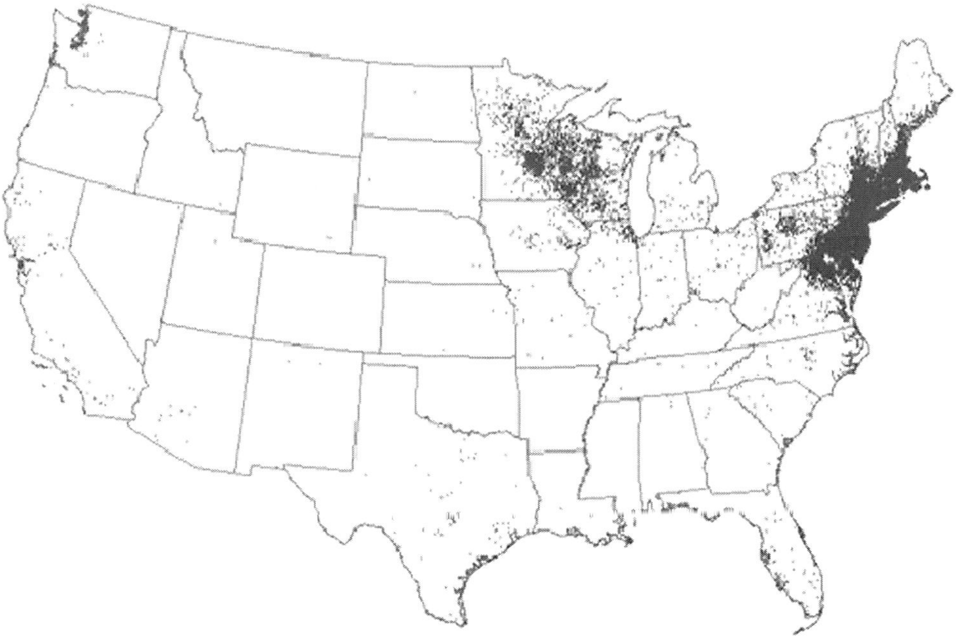

1 dot placed randomly within county of residence for each reported case

Below: The number of cases of Lyme Disease reported by year as of 2005. It is curious that the number of Lyme disease cases (on the maps) appear to be shrinking each year when the opposite is true, case numbers are rising (per the charts). CDC photos.

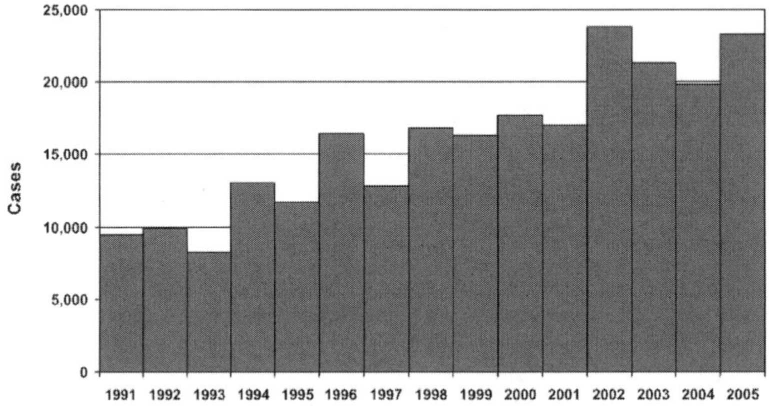

In 2005, 23,305 cases of Lyme were reported yielding a national average of 7.9 cases for every 100,000 persons. In 10 states, the average was 31.6 cases per 100,000 persons. CDC photo.

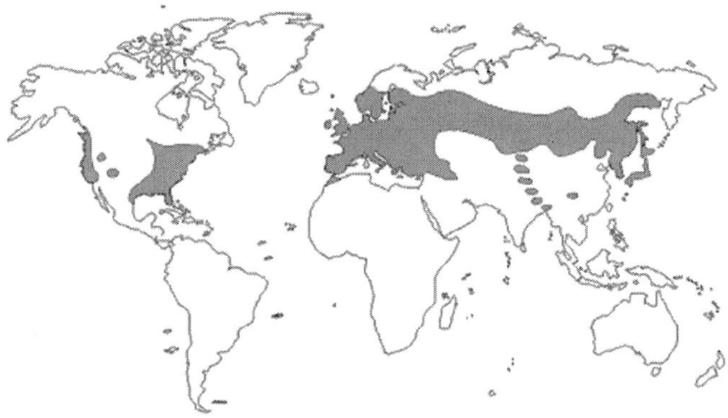

Above is the latest CDC image of the prevalence of Lyme disease globally that this author could locate. Obviously it is not an accurate reflection of the current problem, but rather this map shows prevalence according to approximate *reported case numbers*, according to the CDC. Cases of Lyme disease have been reported on 6 continents, including what is not shown here, in Africa, South America, parts of Asia, North America, and Australia. *Borrelia burgdorferi* has been found in migratory and non-migratory birds and animals on all 7 continents.

Tick Infections Are Everywhere

Within the United States, we find both hard- and soft-bodied tick species. *Ixodes scapularis* and *I. pacificus* are the main Lyme transmitting tick vectors in the United States, and *I. ricinus* and *I. persulcatus* ticks are the main vectors in Europe and Asia, respectively.[55]

Relapsing fever infections are primarily transmitted by the fast-feeding, soft-bodied, or Argasid ticks, while Lyme disease is primarily transmitted by the slower-feeding, prostriate hard-bodied ticks like *Ixodes*.[56] Among the hard-bodied species reported in the United States as biting humans, we find:

- *Amblyomma americanum,*(lone star tick)
- *Amblyomma cajenneunse,* (cayenne tick)
- *Amblyomma inornatum,* (rabbit tick)
- *Amblyomma maculatum,* (Gulf coast tick)
- *Amblyomma tuberculatum,* (gopher, tortoise tick)
- *Boophilis annulatus,* (cattle tick)
- *Dermacentor albipictus* ("winter" tick – moose/elk/deer)
- *Dermacentor andersoni*, (rocky mountain wood tick)
- *Dermacentor occidentalis,* (pacific coast tick)
- *Dermacentor variabilis,* (dog and wood ticks) widely distributed
- *Haemaphysalis leporispalustris,* (rabbit tick)
- *Ixodes brunneus,* (bird tick)
- *Ixodes cookei,* (coyote/fox/skunk/woodchuck tick)
- *Ixodes dentatus,* (rabbit tick)
- *Ixodes pacificus,*(black-legged tick) west coast
- *Ixodes scapularis,*(deer tick) east, south and mid-west
- *Rhipicephalus sanguineus,* (brown dog tick) widely distributed

The soft-bodied ticks are less prevalent, but are still abundant across the globe. Those found within the United States and reported as biting humans are:

- *Argas miniatus,* (fowl tick)
- *Ornithodoros kelleyi,* (bat tick)
- *Ornithodoros stageri,* (bat tick)
- *Ornithodoros turicata,* (relapsing fever tick)
- *Otobius megnini,* (spinose ear tick)[57]

Many soft-bodied ticks like *Ornithodoros* have soft leather-looking bodies when not engorged, and resemble a raisin in appearance.[58]

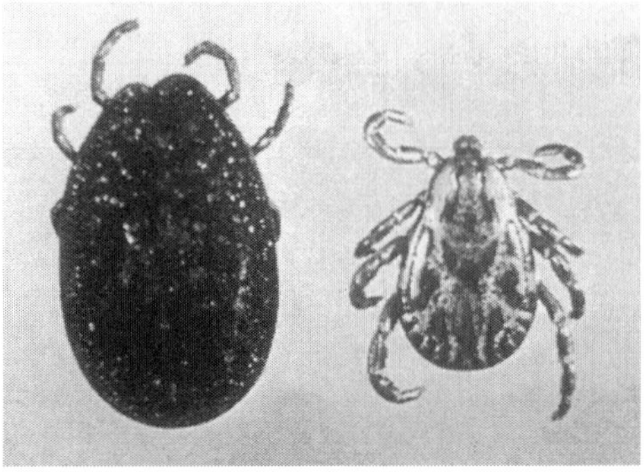

Left in the photo, two North American Ticks. *Argasidae* "soft" bodied ticks, and right in the photo, *Ixodidae* "hard" bodied ticks. CDC photo.

The global picture for tick-borne illness is presently somewhat vague. The CDC tells us that Lyme disease is found in broad areas of Europe, in "temperate" forested areas. Relapsing fever is found in "focal areas" of Greece, Italy, Portugal and Spain with "sporadic" cases elsewhere.[59] The case numbers for Lyme infection are very vague abroad, and I would assume that is either because they simply do not have the data collected, or the information is being withheld, with the former the probable scenario.

Maps on the CDC web site, as stated before, are too old, but also do not reflect the spread of tick-borne illnesses abroad, so I have not included any here. In fact, I could not track down any *decent* maps relating to tick-borne illness except for those on the CDCs web site, though I only performed a limited search. Nevertheless, if we study the rate of voluntarily reported cases in other parts of the world with the understanding that overall numbers are probably inaccurate and under reported, we catch but a glimpse of Lyme disease as the global, emergent infectious disease it truly is.

Since the most commonly known mode of transmission for Lyme is the tick, and ticks are able to feed year-round in temperate climates; and roughly from May through December in colder climates, we can determine that the spread of tick-borne illness has global potential. And there are other vectors for Lyme transmission we are not addressing here, besides the many species of ticks that transmit these illnesses.

Let's briefly examine the presence of ticks in countries outside of the United States. Our Canadian neighbors are reported as routinely finding hard-bodied tick species *Ixodes scapularis* (east and central regions), and *Ixodes pacificus* and *Ixodes Angustus* (western regions).[60] They also have the soft-bodied tick *Ornithodoros hermsii.*

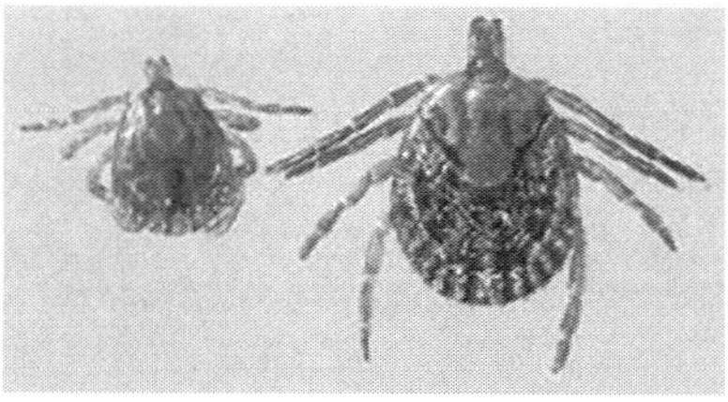

Adult male (left) and female (right) *Amblyomma cajenneunse* (cayenne ticks). Courtesy CDC/J. Occi, Forestry Images, Athens, GA.

In Cuba, Lyme disease had not been reported as of 2004, but in the last two decades, *Amblyomma cajenneses* ticks have been found in the Cuban village of Las Terrazas, Pinar del Río. Tick bites were widespread, and many children were hospitalized without a confirmatory diagnosis. The symptoms that these victims displayed were similar to the hallmark characteristics of Lyme disease. *Erythema chronicum migrans* (ECM or EM) skin rashes, fevers, fatigue, headache and malaise, painful muscles and joints, and meningitis, cardiac problems and neuropathies were reported.[61] In 1969, *A. cajenneses* ticks were found in Mexico, Panama, Columbia and Brazil.[62]

In 1993 in South America, a case of Lyme was reportedly transmitted by a tick bite. The victim was living in a Jaguare slum (Sao Paulo), and she showed the characteristic EM rash, and other symptoms. An ELISA test was performed from whole, sonicated antigens from the *Dr. Allen C. Steere* laboratory, and it showed a high IgM titer (1:1600). Because the high IgM persisted for 2 months, she was treated with tetracycline at 2g/day for 10 days. She was also positive by CDC testing standards with 5 bands present.[63]

In Africa there is the soft-shelled, or fast-feeding argasid tick, which is known as *Ornithodoros moubata.*[64] A few clinical cases of Lyme borreliosis have been reported in North Africa.[65] South Africa has *Amblyomma hebraeum,* and *Rhipicephalus simus* is in Kenya. India has the tick species *Haemaphysalis spinigera* which transmits Kyasanur forest disease (KFD), and was first identified in 1957 in Karnataka State, although a similar virus was also found in Saudi Arabia.[66] In Nepal we find *Dermacentor auratus,* and Greece has *Hyaloma marginatum.*

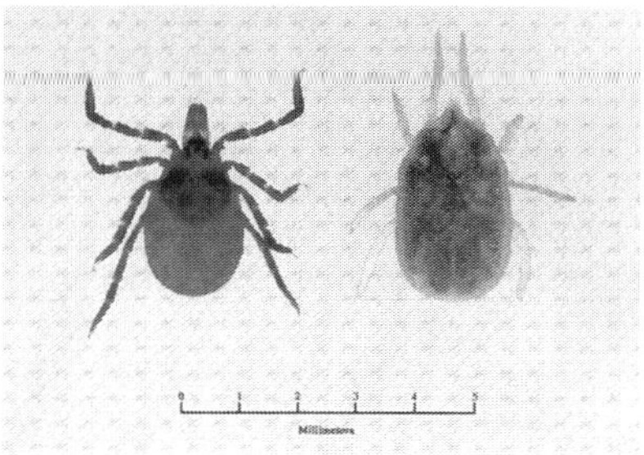

Dorsal view of female *Ixodes scapularis*, the vector of *B. burgdorferi*. (Left) in photo. Female *Ornithodoros hermsi* (right in photo: family Argasidae, soft-bodied ticks), vectors of *Bb*. CDC photo.

In Australia we find the species *I. holocyclus*. In 1984 Lyme disease was reported in Australia, where none of the established vectors were known to exist.[67] The most common tick in the northern hemisphere (but unknown in Australia), that bites humans, is *I. Persulcatus*.[68]

Annual Lyme incidence rates that are voluntarily reported throughout European countries range from 16 in 100,000 cases (France), to 80 in 100,000 (Sweden), to 120 in 100,000 in Slovenia. The EM skin rash, a classic symptom of Lyme disease, was first described in Sweden in 1909. Thousands of cases of Lyme disease have been reported from at least 19 countries on 5 continents, although Bb has been found on 7 continents in mammals.[69]

Lyme disease surveillance in Wales and England began in 1986, based upon the voluntary reporting of serologically confirmed cases by laboratories to the Public Health Laboratory Service (PHLS) Communicable Disease Surveillance Centre (CDSC).[70] Both the prevalence of *B. burgdorferi*-infected ticks and the incidence of Lyme borreliosis abroad are highest in eastern Europe and decrease westward across the continent, including the British Isles.[71]

In 2005, data reported to the UK's Health Protection Agency (HPA), indicated that the number of case reports of Lyme borreliosis in England and Wales were similar to previous years. In 595 patients tested that year, approximately 46% were aged 40-64 years, and 10% were children under 15 years of age. *Erythema migrans* rashes were reported by 42% of patients, and neurological disease was identified in 62% of patients, of which nearly half had facial palsy. Arthritis was identified in 5 patients who had acquired tick-borne illness overseas. In 2005, travel-associated infection rates were similar to the year prior, with 18% of cases known to have been contracted abroad, mostly in the USA, France, Germany, Scandinavia, and other European countries.[72]

Another vector that can transmit Bb infection to humans in Europe is the sheep tick, *I. ricinus, also called the "castor bean" tick, because of its resemblance to a castor bean.*[73,74]

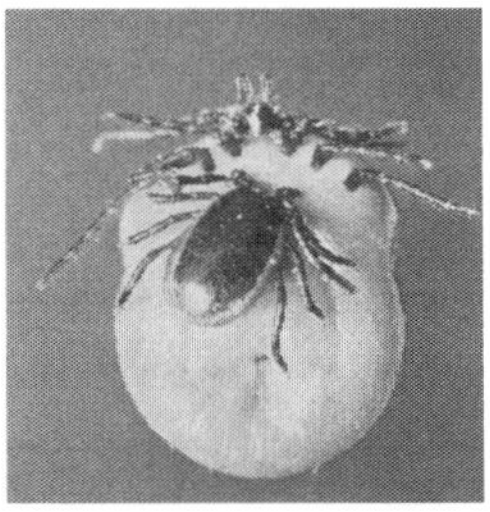

Male *I. ricinus* (smaller) copulating with female tick (larger). CDC/WHO photo.

Approximately 60% of infections indigenous to the UK were acquired in the southern counties of England. These areas are known to harbor Lyme borreliosis ticks and include Salisbury Plain, Exmoor, New Forest, Thetford Forest, Yorkshire Moors, Lake District, and Scottish Highlands and Islands.[75] *Borrelia spielmanii* was found in 1996 in a patient in Slovenia. This species has also been found to occur in Hungary, Germany and the Netherlands.[76]

Bb was first isolated in *I. ricinus* ticks in Trieste, Italy in 1977, but other strains (*B. burgdorferi sensu stricto, B. garinii* and *B. afzelii*), have been isolated from humans, intermediate hosts, and ticks. Other reported cases of Lyme disease in Italy were in Liguria in 1983 and in 1987. The latter patients were also from Trieste Karst and the Eastern Ligurian Coast.[77,78] The exact number of Lyme cases in Italy is unknown as it was not a notifiable disease until 1990. Through current data, we find that 1,324 cases were observed between 1983-1996. The majority of ticks (89%) biting humans in Italy are *I. ricinus,* though we also find the presence of *I. hexagonus, I. ventalloi,* and *Rhipicephalus sanguineus.*

In fact, the sheep tick *(Ixodes ricinus)* is the most common hard tick species in western Europe and carries *B. burgdorferi* as well as Encephalitis, Anaplasmosis, Ehrlichiosis, Bartonella and Babesia.[79] In 1996, Kruszewska et al. reported *I. ricinus* ticks from a park in Walz, Poland.[80] In a study in the Netherlands, *I. ricinus* ticks harboring *Bartonella* were removed from Roe deer. In areas of Europe known to have tick-borne illness, some cases of *Human Granulocytic Anaplasmosis* (HGA) have also been reported, including during one study in northeastern Italy.[81,82]

In Russia in 1950-1970, large-scale efforts to control the taiga tick (*Ixodes persulcatus*), were carried out,[83] but tick-borne illnesses in this area go back to the 1940's.[84] In 2000, a number of methods for tick control and/or eradication occurring during the nineteenth century were reviewed. Case studies of these types of programs in the United States, Australia, Africa, Puerto Rico and the Caribbean were analyzed for identifiable factors, and to collect information and offer practical suggestions for future tick control methods.[85] In 2007, the chief health officer of the Chelyabinsk region (Oblast) signed a document implementing urgent measures for prophylactic treatment of tick-borne encephalitis. In the South Urals, the first tick bites of the season were recorded in March, after the first spring thaws. In 2006, approximately 18,000 South Urals inhabitants suffered tick bites, with a total of 126 cases of encephalitis and 260 cases of Lyme disease recorded in that area.[86]

In 1991, in the Alashian region of Inner Mongolia, *Rickettsia sibirica* was found in *Hyalomma asiaticum* ticks collected there. Since that time, *H. truncatum* and *H. excavatum* species of ticks have spread *R. sibirica* to other countries, including South Africa, Greece, France and Portugal. The first case of *rickettsia* infection reported in France was in 1996 in March, an atypical time of year for this infection, and cases in Greece and Portugal occurred in winter months as well. In Portugal, a patient who was initially diagnosed with Mediterranean spotted fever (MSF), was discovered to have *Rickettsia sibirica*.[87]

From 1987-1996 a study showed that residents of 22 Chinese provinces had high antibody titers for *B. burgdorferi*. Studies there concluded that Lyme was endemic in 17 provinces. *Ixodes persulcatus* played a key role in transmitting *B. burgdorferi* to humans in northern China. *Ixodes granulatus* and *Ixodidae acarina* were proposed as principal vectors in the southern region. Asia has the taiga tick, *I. persulcatus*, that predominantly transmits Bb to humans.[88]

In Japan, in 1994, the first case of human infection by the co-infection *Anaplasma phagocytophilum* was reported, and transmitted by *Ixodes persulcatus* and *I. ovatus* ticks. The severity of this co-infection ranges from mild to severe, although severe illness is more frequently reported. The number of illness with this co-infection has risen in the United States. In Europe, the first human cases of this disease were described in 1997, and it is believed that *A. phagocytophilum* is distributed through Europe and portions of the Middle East and Asia.[89]

In Scotland, problems with the accuracy of laboratory diagnostics for detecting Lyme disease, led to an audit. Before the audit of samples taken from 2003-2004, a significant number of patients had clinical symptoms of Lyme disease but were seronegative or equivocal by a Scottish Western Blot test. When current practices were compared to American and European standards however, the Western Blot scoring system was revised. Previously tested serum samples were compared to these adjusted standards and they were found to be weak positives or even stronger. Approximately 80% of these samples had come from patients who had clinical symptoms of early Lyme disease.[90,91] The use of Scottish strains of *B. afzelii* and *B. burgdorferi* sensu stricto to provide "local" antigens for the IgG Western Blot tests, improved the diagnostic ability of the testing for patients in Scotland.[92]

It is noteworthy that isolates recovered from China are different from those found in North America,[93] Europe, Australia, Africa, or other parts of the world. Of note is the practice of standard U.S. laboratories which routinely utilize a small number of specific Lyme isolates in their diagnostic tests, which affects the accuracy of these tests.[94]

Lyme "Co-infections"

What is a co-infection? A "co-infection" is one or more infectious diseases that are transmitted to humans during a tick bite. Some of the more common co-infections are listed here. However, ticks do not always transmit Lyme disease. Ticks not infected by Lyme can and do transmit multiple infectious diseases besides Lyme. Additionally, humans may become infected by these same diseases through other modes of transmission, such as other insect bites, cat licks or scratches, handling or consuming infected deer meat, and even coming into contact with the saliva or fecal matter of *Borrelia* or otherwise infected animals.

One thing is certain however, and that is if you are infected with Lyme disease and have one or more co-infections along with a Lyme infection, it is likely you will become much sicker, and treatment will be more difficult than with either Lyme disease or co-infections alone. This author thinks that the term "co-infection" is actually somewhat misleading, and seems to denote an infection somehow "less" important or "less" harmful than Lyme disease. Nothing could be further from the truth. And in the very near future, I predict that we will begin to see emerging infectious diseases now known as "co-infections," taking their rightful place as primary infectious diseases. No longer will Babesia, Bartonella or Ehrlichiosis be referred to as "co-infections," indeed they will be *additional* infections, as they are serious, life-threatening agents all to themselves. In keeping with current trends, here are some of the more common co-infections found in Lyme-infected ticks, which affect people world wide.

Ehrlichiosis/Anaplasmosis

Human Monocytic Ehrlichiosis (HME), and Human Granulocytic Ehrlichiosis (HGE) are 2 emerging infectious diseases first described in 1987 and 1994 respectively, when found in patients from Wisconsin and Minnesota and later, Illinois. HME is caused by *Ehrlichia* *chaffeensis,* and HGE is caused by *E. phagocytophila.* These diseases are transmitted primarily by the lone star tick, *(Amblyomma americanum)*, whose habitat is *traditionally* the southeastern and south central regions of the United States, but is found elsewhere in the world. Ehrlichiosis is transmitted by other tick species as well. [95-98]

The first cases of HME and HGE were found in Europe in the 1990s. Evidence of both illnesses has been found in Sweden, Norway, Mali, and Africa. Evidence of HME and HGE was found during a survey in 1994-1997 in Israel. A case of *E. canis* infection was found in South America (Venezuela).[99]

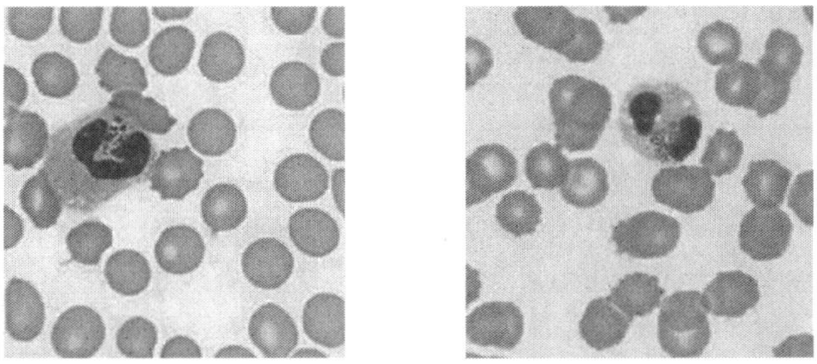

The cytoplasmic inclusions seen in the white blood cells above indicate *Ehrlichiosis*. CDC photos.

Symptoms of Ehrlichiosis are similar to Lyme disease, making it difficult to distinguish between the two. The CDC reports symptoms of Ehrlichiosis as fever, headache, general malaise, muscle aches, nausea/vomiting, diarrhea, cough, joint pain, mental confusion and occasionally, rash. They reported that approximately 60% of pediatric patients infected with the form *E. chaffeensis* (one of the more severe forms), exhibit a rash, (considered rare in adults).[99]

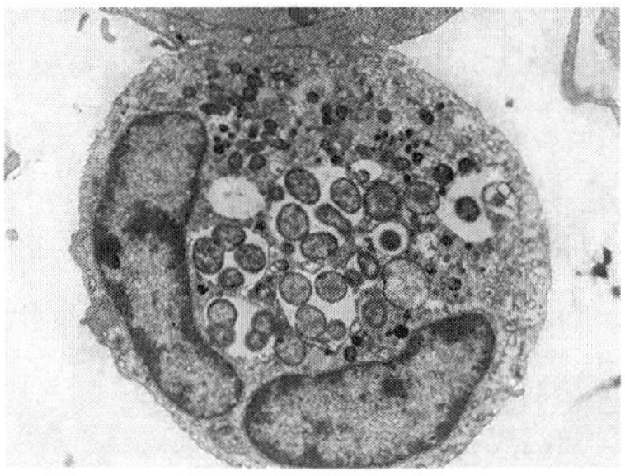

***Anaplasma phagocytophilum* by transmission electron microscopy in HL-60 cell culture. (Courtesy of V. Popov; original magnification ×21,960). CDC photo.**

Laboratory tests will show leucopenia (decrease in white blood cells), thrombocytopenia (abnormal decrease in blood platelets), and elevated liver enzymes. Severe illness can cause prolonged fever, renal failure, disseminated intravascular coagulopathy (problems with blood clotting), meningoencephalitis (inflammation of the brain and spinal cord and their coverings), respiratory distress syndrome, seizures, coma or death.[100] The agent of HGE, *Ehrlichia phagocytophila* was recently reclassified as *Anaplasma phagocytophilum* or Human Granulocytic Anaplasmosis (HGA), or more simply, Anaplasma.[101]

Bartonella

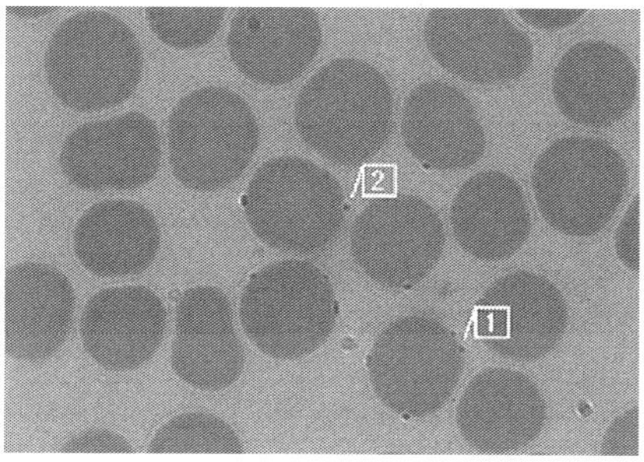

Tiny bartonella adherent to the erythrocyte cells indicated with arrows. Photo provided by Dr. Steven Fry, Fry Clinical Laboratory, Scottsdale, AZ.

Bartonella has at least 8 known forms which can affect humans[102]. Bartonella is the etiological agent causing Bacillary Angiomatosis (BA), septicemia, trench fever, lymphadenopathy (chronically swollen lymph nodes), peliosis (bleeding) of the spleen or liver and endocarditis (inflammation of the membrane that lines the heart). *B. henselae* was first reported in 1990, and the organism was later isolated from a patient with HIV and described as a new species in 1992.[103]

Bartonella henselae is often referred to as Cat Scratch Disease[104] because it is commonly found in cats and can be transmitted by bites, scratches or licks. Other known vectors are flea bites, biting flies, and feline fecal matter.[105] Bartonella is also transmitted by *Ixodes* tick bites and is often transmitted as a co-infection. Cat Scratch disease (CSD) was first described in 1950, but it was not until 1992 that Bartonella henselae, which was formerly called *rochalimaea*, was formally identified as the agent of CSD.[106,107]

Bartonella *quintana* is known as "trench fever," and is another possible co-infection that is tick-transmissible and also found in body lice. It is prevalent among homeless persons in the United States and Europe.[108] Symptoms of Bartonella are fatigue, swollen lymph nodes, encephalopathy, headaches, irritability, cognitive dysfunction, rashes, visual changes, numbness, tingling, aggression, sudden fits of rage, obsessive compulsive symptoms, depression, panic attacks and sometimes hallucinations.

Babesia

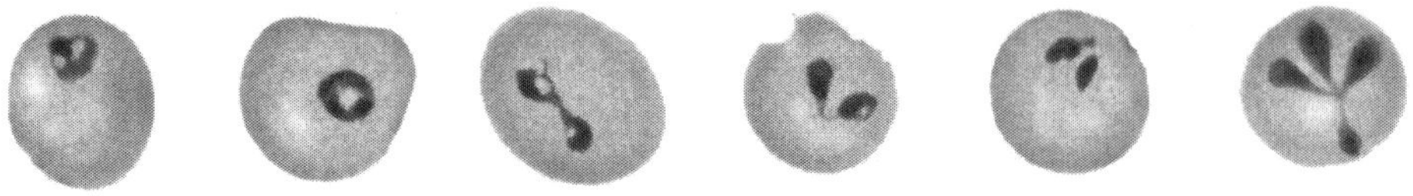

Photomicrographs of *Babesia*-infected erythrocytes on a Giemsa-stained smear of peripheral blood. CDC photo.

Babesia is an infectious disease that resembles malaria. In 2000, there were only 4 known types of Babesia, *B. microti, B. divergens, B. bovis* and *B. equi.* At present, there are approximately 14 known types, the most common of which is *microti.* Babesia is a highly variable illness with symptoms ranging from severe illness to no symptoms at all. In fact, in about one-third of people infected with Babesia, the infection is silent, and that status can change to active infection at any time. Moreover, because Babesia symptoms closely mimic those of Lyme disease, the physician can easily overlook this important and sometimes deadly, infection.[109]

At present, blood donor supplies do not screen for Babesia, and if they did, they may be surprised to find it present in many of its samples. In 2002, more than 40 cases of *B. microti* infection in the United States that were acquired through blood transfusions or platelet donations were reported. Physicians in Georgia acknowledge that cases of post-transfusion illness should include Babesia infection in the differential. In addition, some effective means of preventing Babesia transmission in donated blood products is needed.[110] In fact, Babesia is not even listed on the CDC's web site as a 2007 nationally reportable disease within the United States.

You are at a higher risk for Babesia if you have Lyme disease. In addition, even if you test negatively on Babesia testing, suspect Babesia nevertheless if you have symptoms such as the following:

- High fevers
- Listlessness / Mental dullness
- Sweats or chills
- Headaches / Fatigue
- Decreased appetite or weight loss

- Daytime sleepiness or excessive sleep (more than 8.5 hours/day)
- Muscle aches/joint pains
- Depression/anxiety/panic
- Nausea/vomiting
- Cough/shortness of breath
- Air hunger or unsatisfying deep breathing
- Dark urine
- Enlarged liver or spleen
- Yellow hue on eyes, hands and skin (jaundice)
- Enlarged lymph nodes (also in Lyme and Bartonella)
- Significant memory changes
- Profound psychiatric illness
- Difficulty organizing
- Balance deficits or dizziness
- Waves of generalized itching
- Random stabbing pains, or chest wall pains
- Sensitivity to light
- You have received blood from another person[111]

There are excellent reference materials for physicians and laypersons available on Babesia and Babesia treatments, such as written by Dr. James Schaller, available at www.personalconsult.com.

Rickettsia – Rocky Mountain Spotted Fever

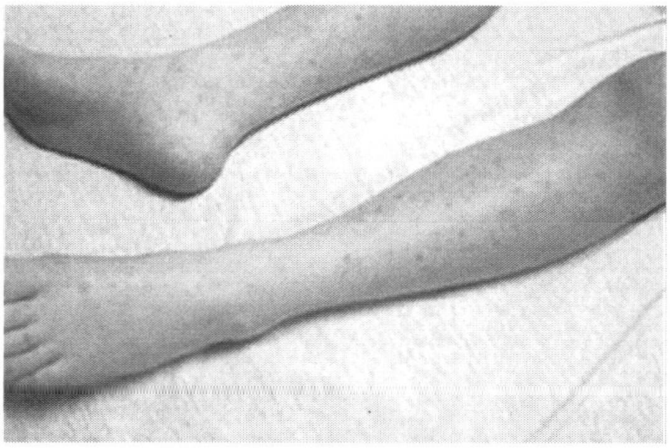

Rash on legs and feet of patient with Rocky Mountain Spotted Fever. CDC photo.

Rocky Mountain Spotted Fever, is an acute, potentially fatal infectious disease which is caused by the organism named *rickettsia*. Vector transmission is known to occur by dog and wood ticks. The name Rocky Mountain Spotted Fever came about in the Rocky mountain region of the United States in 1873. In 1906, Howard Taylor Ricketts, an American Pathologist, discovered that the disease could be transmitted to humans by a bite of a particular kind of tick.

The organism causing this illness was named after him. In 1908 he proved that Rocky Mountain Spotted Fever was not only carried by ticks, but that it was also found within their eggs.[112]

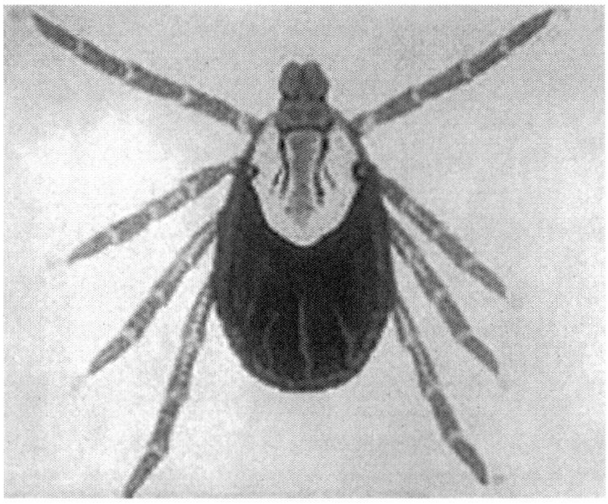

Left: Rocky Mountain Wood Tick, which can transmit RMSF, and other infections. CDC photo.

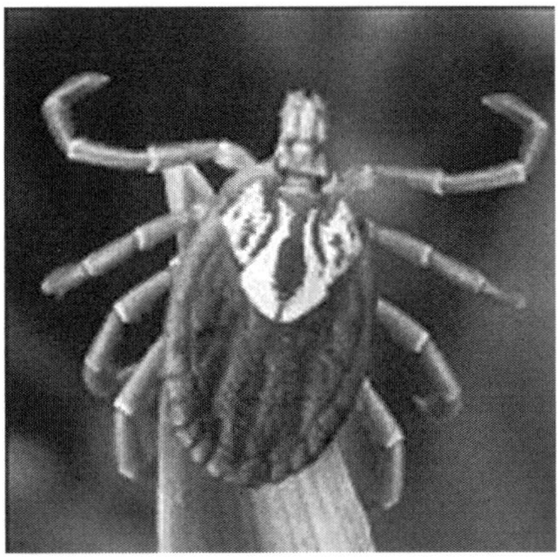

Right: Adult Gulf Coast Tick. CDC photo.

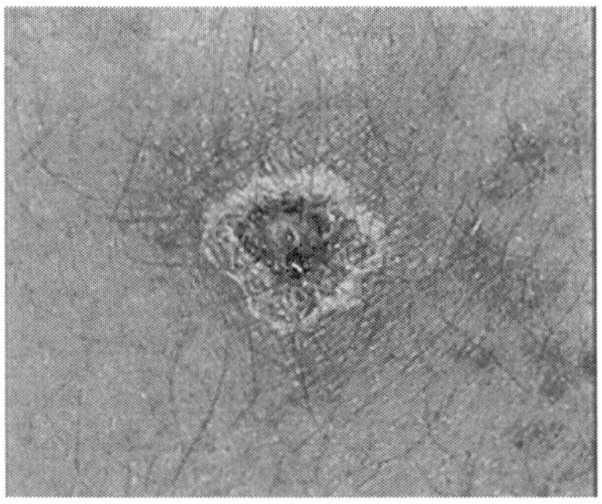

Ulcerating lesion associated with *Rickettsia parkeri* infection. Photo CDC/C.A. Ohl, Wake Forest University School of Medicine, Winston-Salem, NC.

According to the National Institutes of Health, symptoms of RMSF are fever, chills, severe headaches, confusion and muscle pains, and a spreading rash beginning on extremities and spreading to the body. Patients can also experience nausea/vomiting, excessive thirst, diarrhea, anorexia, hallucinations, and sensitivity to light. In 2004, a total of 13 cases of Rocky Mountain Spotted Fever were reported in Arizona. An emerging *Rickettsial* infection identified as *Rickettsia parkeri,* has been observed in U.S. ticks. It was found in a patient living in the southeastern coastal region in 2002. *Rickettsia parkeri* is found in the Gulf Coast tick, from the same region. This illness has a similar clinical presentation as African tick-bite fever (ATBF), and Mediterranean spotted fever (MSF), with headache, fever, eschars (ulcerating lesions) in about 50% of patients, and regional lymphadenopathy, and was found in an American patient with no travel history.[113]

Tick-borne rickettsial diseases occur worldwide. International travel to destinations such as the southern Mediterranean, Central and South America, Costa Rica, Columbia, Mexico, Panama, Africa, Asia and the Middle east, might result in tick exposure and individuals should check themselves carefully each day for ticks. African tick-bite fever is caused by the organism *R. africae*, with an estimated incidence of 5% among international travelers and relief workers. *R. conorii* causes Mediterranean spotted fever and is endemic in the Mediterranean basin, Middle East, and parts of Africa and India.[113]

Tick-Borne Relapsing Fever

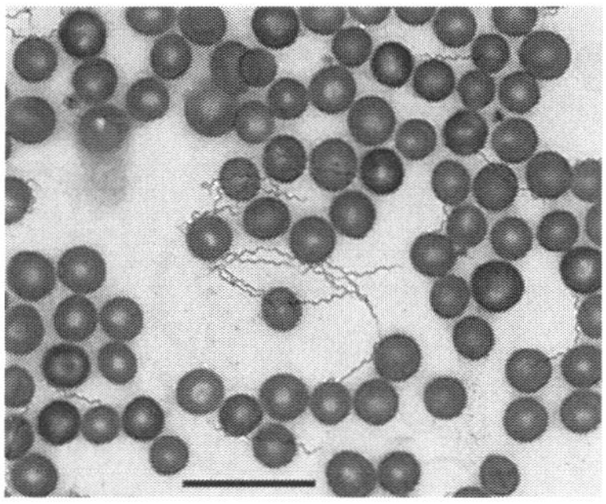

Right: *Borrelia hermsii* in a thin smear of mouse blood stained with Wright-Giemsa stain. Note the presence of spirochetes. CDC photo

Tick-borne Relapsing Fever is a disease caused by at least 15 different *Borrelia* species. It is transmitted by the body louse, but also *Borrelia recurrentis, B. hermsii, B. turicatae, B. parkeri and B. duttonii.* Relapsing fever is marked by relapsing episodes of fever, and is usually transmitted by a soft-bodied tick like *Ornithodoros,* which typically feed on rodents but will feed on humans when there is a lack of other sources. Soft-bodied ticks usually feed at night and drop off after a period of a few minutes to a half hour, and do not remain attached, so most victims are unaware that they have been bitten. Many people become ill after sleeping in cabins that are infested with spirochete-infected ticks.[114,115] Following a tick bite, spirochetes will enter the skin and then the blood stream where they will reside in the central nervous system, bone marrow, and organs such as the spleen, lungs, liver and kidneys. Neurological symptoms are reported in about 30% of the patients, and can include meningitis, neurologic deficits, seizures and even coma. Treatment with antibiotics commonly causes a Jarisch-Herxheimer reaction.[116]

Symptoms of Relapsing Fever include a sudden, high fever, chills, headache, body aches and sweating. Sometimes nausea, vomiting, loss of appetite (anorexia), intolerance of bright light (photophobia), neck and eye pain, dry cough, confusion and dizziness occur. Symptoms typically surface between 3 to 7 days after infection. Symptoms persist for a period of about a week, which is followed by a period of 7-14 days of few or no symptoms, then symptoms reappear in the same manner, for several cycles. Relapsing fever can be transmitted to an unborn child in a woman who is pregnant.[117] If contracted during pregnancy, relapsing fever has a high risk of fetal loss (up to 50%), so treatment is critical during pregnancy.

Incidence of relapsing fever in the U.S. is located primarily in the western states (west of the Mississippi) but is endemic in higher elevations and coniferous forests, including the U.S. and southern British Columbia, Canada.[118] It was first identified in the U.S. in 1915 in Colorado, though the first case was recorded in 1905 in New York by a traveler to Texas. It has since been reported in 14 western and southern states but it has also been reported in Ohio. It was nearly removed from the nationally notifiable conditions list in 1987, but 11 states are still required to report the disease. In addition it is found in the plateau region of Mexico, Central and South America. Abroad, relapsing fever is found in northeastern Africa (Ethiopia) , the Mediterranean, and Asia. Relapsing fever is a serious illness, but if treated, has a mortality rate of less than 5%.[119,120]

Tick Paralysis

According to the CDC, Tick Paralysis is a "rare" disease, that is characterized by flaccid paralysis. It is often confused with other neurologic disorders or diseases like (Guillain-Barré Syndrome, or botulism). Tick Paralysis is thought to be caused by a toxin in tick saliva that is transferred during feeding. Symptoms usually occur between 4-7 days of tick feeding. The ascending paralysis progresses over hours or days, sensory loss does not usually occur and there is an absence of pain. Tick Paralysis is reported to be short-lived. If a tick is not removed and the paralysis continues, the mortality rate from respiratory paralysis is approximately 10%. Cases of Tick Paralysis have been reported world-wide, but most cases occur in the western regions of Canada and the United States. The species most often associated with this illness are *D. andersoni* (Rocky Mt. wood tick), and *Dermacentor variabilis* (American dog tick).[121]

"Masters" Disease or STARI (Southern Tick-Associated Rash Illness)

Masters Disease is also known as Southern Tick Associated Rash Illness (STARI) and is believed to be caused by *Borrelia lonestari,* and transmitted by the Lone-Star tick. Masters Disease was detected in a Missouri patient in 1991. The lone star ticks have been found from Oklahoma down to Texas, and eastward across southern states, along the Atlantic coastline as far north as Maine. Symptoms of Masters Disease include a red expanding rash around the bite site, (similar to a Lyme EM rash), which usually appears within 7-10 days following tick bite, and can expand to 8cm (3") or more. Additional symptoms may be fatigue, fevers, headache and muscle and joint pains. According to the CDC, it has not been linked to neurological symptoms and is reported to resolve following antibiotic treatments.[71]

Right: Adult female (*Amblyomma americanum*) Lone Star Tick, which transmits RMSF, Masters disease and other diseases, is so-named for the white Spot on its scutum (back). CDC photo

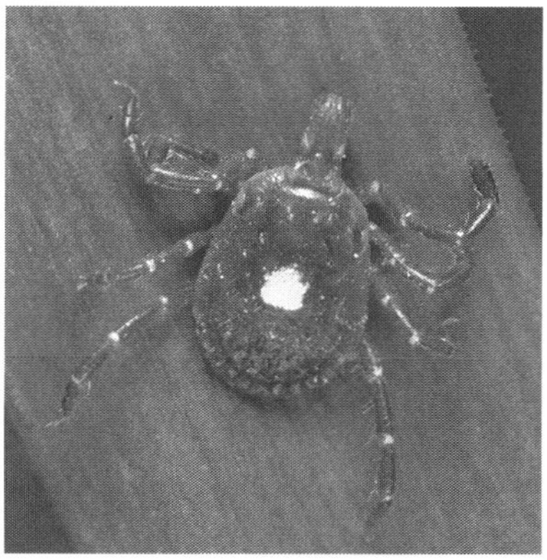

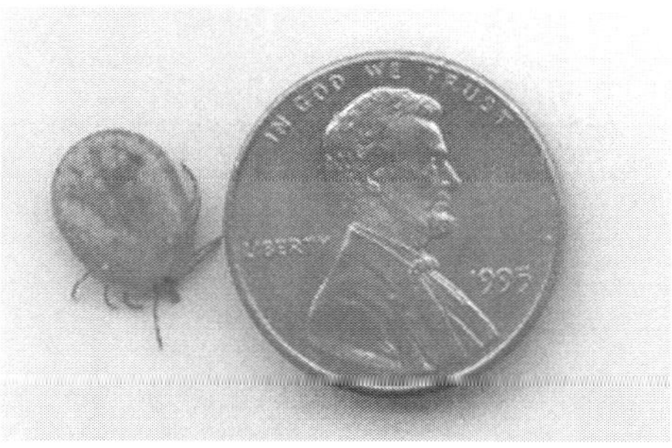

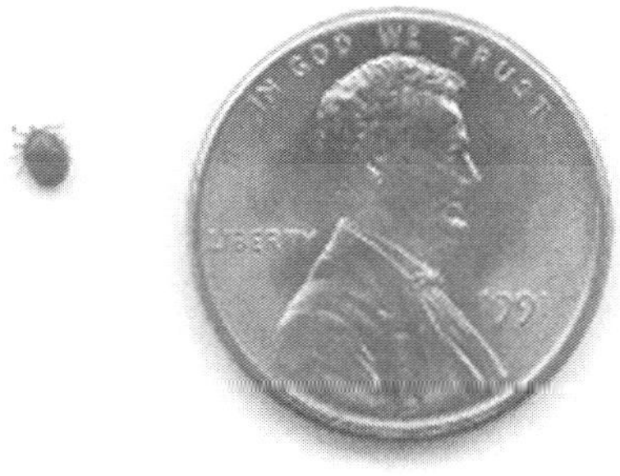

Fully engorged Lone Star ticks (*Amblyomma americanum*) Adult female – top left; Nymph – top right. The white dot on the scutum identifies this tick as a Lone Star tick. In all engorged ticks the scutum does not expand and is a good place to start for identification. Photos reprinted with permission of Marc G. Golightly, Ph.D., Stony Brook University School of Medicine, NY.

CDC image showing prevalence of lone star ticks in the U.S. Redrawn and updated from Hair and Bowman, 1986.

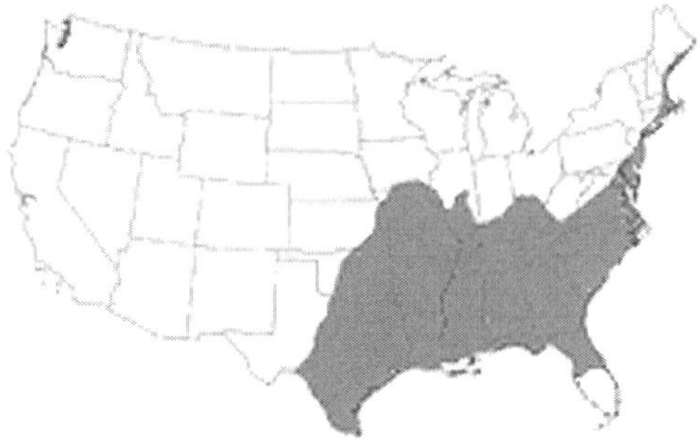

Tularemia – "Rabbit Fever" or "Deer Fly Fever"

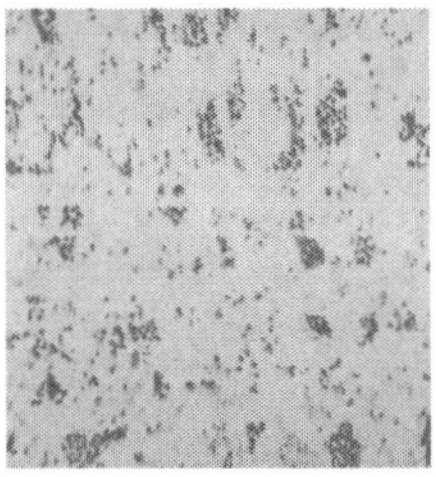

Photomicrograph of Tularemia (*Francisella tularensis*) using methylene blue stain. CDC photo courtesy of P.B. Smith

Tularemia is also known as "rabbit fever" and "deer fly fever" and is caused by a gram-negative bacterium called *Francisella tularensis*. It was first noted in 1911 in California. The CDC removed the disease as a nationally reportable one in 1994, but reinstated the practice in 2000 due to its potential as a bioterrorism agent.[123] Tularemia has been reportedly found in all states except for Hawaii.

In the United States, most people are infected with Tularemia by the bite of a tick, deer fly, or other infected animal, particularly rabbits. Outbreaks of pneumonic Tularemia, especially if it occurs in an area of low incidence, should prompt concerns of possible bio-terrorism because it is especially virulent after being aerosolized.[124]

Thumb with tularemia ulcer. Photo by CDC, courtesy of Dr. Sellers, Emory U.

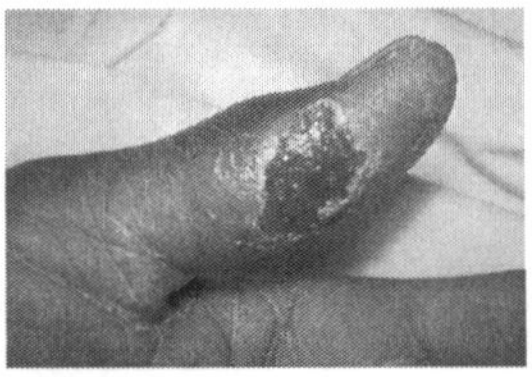

In the 1950s, the U.S. Army developed a live vaccine of *F. tularensis* from a live strain provided by the Soviet Union.[125] Symptoms of this

illness depend upon the type of Tularemia contracted, as there are half a dozen forms. Symptoms include sudden fever, chills, muscle/joint pain, swollen or painful eyes or lymph glands, headaches, diarrhea, progressive weakness, sore throat, dry cough. The inhaled form can cause chest pain, bloody sputum and difficulty breathing or stopped breathing. Other symptoms can include ulcers on the skin or mouth. Tularemia is actively being studied as a bio-warfare agent in laboratories in the United States and around the world.

Mycoplasma

Mycoplasma has about 200 species of which most do no harm, and only 4 or 5 are pathogenic. *Mycoplasma fermentans* (*incognitus* strain) is an apparently man-made organism that is a mutation of the *Brucella* bacterium (probably from the nucleus), which was combined with a *visna* virus (a *lentivirus* or slow virus), and then extracted. Mycoplasma was basically harmless until 1942 when biological warfare research was conducted which resulted in the creation of this deadly infectious form of mycoplasma. This form was converted into a crystalline form so as to be "weaponized."

Since World War II, there has been a marked increase in the prevalence of all types of neurological and systemic degenerative diseases, such as previously unheard of diseases like chronic fatigue and AIDS.[126] According to the Armed Forces Institute of Pathology's senior researcher, Dr. Shyh-Ching Lo, mycoplasma can cause many different illnesses like Cancer, Chronic Fatigue Syndrome, Multiple Sclerosis, Wegener's disease, Type I Diabetes, Crohn's disease, Parkinson's disease, Alzheimer's, Rheumatoid Arthritis and even AIDS. I guess he would know, being an Army Pathologist, and also the individual holding a patent on the organism: (Lo, Shyh-Ching Potomac, MD. **Pathogenic mycoplasma**. U.S. Patent 5,242,820. Issued Sept. 7, 1993).[127]

Even the National Institutes of Health's own Dr. Charles Engel admitted in 2000 that he was "now of the view that the probable cause of Chronic Fatigue Syndrome, and Fibromyalgia is the Mycoplasma."[128] Dr. Richard Horowitz, board-certified Internal Medicine doctor who specializes in Lyme disease, stated that in his clinical practice, out of 645 of his Lyme disease patients screened between 1999 and 2004, approximately 14% of them had mycoplasma as a co-infection. Lyme patients with co-infections, including mycoplasma, are much sicker than patients having Lyme alone.[129]

In 2002, mycoplasma contamination of the licensed *anthrax* vaccines administered to military personnel was blamed as a possible cause for Persian Gulf illness (Gulf War Syndrome). Anthrax Vaccine Adsorbed (AVA, BioPort Corp., Lansing, MI) is the licensed anthrax vaccine that was administered to about 150,000 U.S. military personnel during the Gulf War. More recently, it was used as part of a comprehensive vaccination policy for the Department of Defense (DOD) service members.[130] Mycoplasmas seem to be sensitive to the medication doxycycline.

"Morgellons Disease"
Tick-borne Illness or "Delusional Parasitosis?"

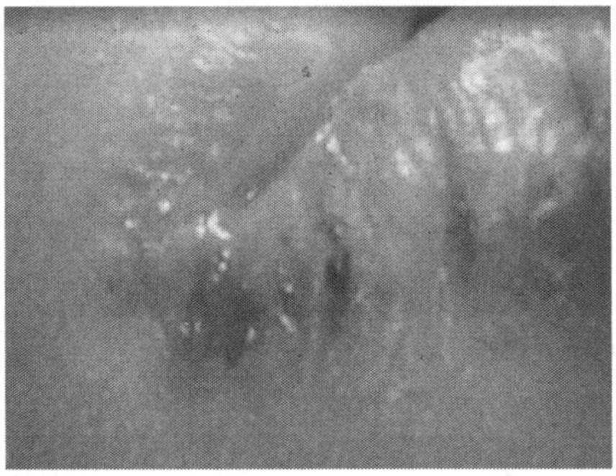

Morgellons lesion on the lip. Courtesy Morgellons Foundation, reprinted with permission.

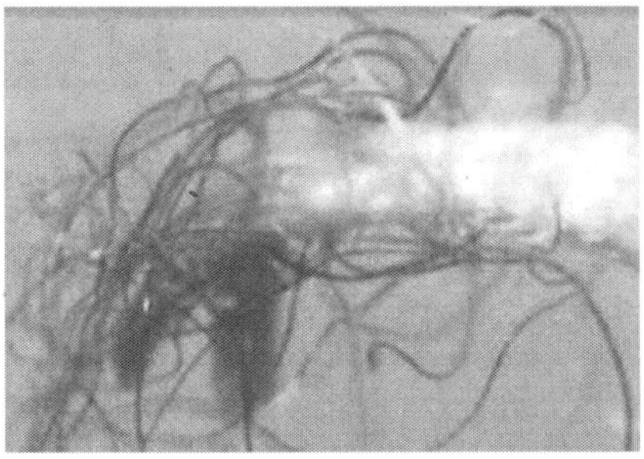

Morgellons tissue fragment with fibrous "hairs." Courtesy Morgellons Foundation, reprinted with permission

Morgellons disease was first dubbed as such in 2001 by a mother, Mary Leitao, whose 2-year old son developed a set of odd symptoms. She noticed what looked like a dandelion fluff emerging from a sore under her toddler's lip. He would develop more sores later, and after at least 8 physicians examined him, Mary tried an infectious disease specialist at Johns Hopkins University, but was denied. Instead it was suggested her son's case was one of "Munchausen's By Proxy," a rare psychiatric syndrome where a parent or someone else pretends that an illness exists in someone else, when it does not, to gain attention.

Frustrated, it is said that Mary picked a name from an obscure 17th century French medical article describing an illness similar to her son's. Mary would later found the Morgellons Research Foundation and the following year, people from all over the world were reporting similar symptoms. At present there are around 9,500 registered families on this site.[131]

The cause of Morgellons is unknown at this time, though some feel it to be a tick-borne illness, but there appears to be multiple causes. The illness is mainly concentrated in California, Texas and Florida, although it has been reported in all 50 United States. Cluster areas in California have been noted in San Francisco, San Jose, San Diego and Los Angeles; and in Texas, near Houston, Austin, Dallas and Round Rock. Overseas, the foundation has received reports of infection from New Zealand, South Africa, Japan, Indonesia, the Philippines and Australia. European clusters have been reported in the Netherlands, Ireland, Denmark, Italy, Spain, France, Germany and England.[132]

Victims of this disorder report non-healing skin lesions that are often accompanied by pain or intense itching, and may be self-generated due to itching. Skin lesions may appear hive- or pimple-like, and may have a white center. The lesions may also appear as linear excoriations from "picking." Lesions, (even without picking) appear and progress to open wounds that heal very slowly, with discolored skin, or seal over with a thick, gelatinous outer layer. Scarring can persist after healing. The patients report "moving" sensations, that seem to occur on or under the skin tissues. Patients describe intermittent "stinging" or "biting" sensations. Any area of the body may be involved including the scalp, nasal passages, ear canal or face.

Patients reportedly see "filaments" on the skin lesions that at times extrude from skin which appears intact. Fibrous filaments may be white, blue, red or black in color. Size is near microscopic but may be seen under 10-30X power. In ultraviolet light, fibers may fluoresce. Filaments have consistently been documented by physicians using a hand-held commercial microscope. Granules in the shape and size of sand grains, may be white or black in color and may appear on or in skin or clothing. Acute changes to skin texture and pigment occur, as patients will have thickened or thinned irregularly textured hyperpigmentation patterns. Overgrowth or hyper-growth of skin tags, nevi, microangioma, lipomas, and callus formations are common.

Musculoskeletal effects are usually present which manifest as pain in joints, (fingers, shoulders, knees), tendons, muscles and connective tissues. Visual changes, headaches and vertebral pain are common, and premature degeneration of discs and vertebrae may be observed. Emotional and cognitive dysfunction can occur. Examples of frontal lobe processing interference (logical thinking, short-term memory, attention deficit) are apparent and measurable by standard psychometric test batteries. Emotional problems similar to bipolar disorder occur, as well as intermittent episodes of obsession, or loss of boundary control.

Additionally, neurological disorders such as peripheral neuropathies, abnormal reflexes, neuropathic pains and brain control abnormalities (motor function, circadian rhythm, body temperature, respiratory drive) have been noted. Symptoms may affect the gastrointestinal system, similar to IBS or Chron's disease. Limitations due to pain and discomfort are significant enough to interfere with daily activities. There are a number of common laboratory abnormalities that can be found in Morgellons patients. Please see *www.morgellons.com* for more information on these laboratory findings.[132]

Many physicians have unfairly labeled Morgellons patients with "delusional parasitosis," for lack of a better diagnosis.[133,134] We must question why medical professionals unfairly place blame on the patient simply because medical science fails to offer an immediate solution. Instead, physicians choose to believe that the patient is imagining their illness until proven scientifically otherwise, even for an illness that is well documented, with thousands of patients world-wide.

[Note: This chapter discusses only a small fraction of the numerous infectious diseases transmissible by ticks to humans; and some of the ones more commonly found. When screening for tick-borne illness, it is helpful to request lab tests using ***regional isolates*** *applicable to your area of the country. Contact your physician or local support group for information on laboratory testing for tick-borne illnesses or see the contact information later on in this book. It is also important to note that routine laboratory tests are not very accurate for many infectious diseases and diagnoses should be made based on clinical findings, not lab tests alone.]*

The "All In Your Head" Philosophy on Herxing and Munchausen's

The Herxheimer Phenomenon

Have you heard of a *Jarisch-Herxheimer* reaction? I never had until I began medical treatment for Lyme disease. A herxheimer reaction, or "herx," is believed to be a reaction caused by organisms that are dying off and releasing toxic chemicals (endotoxins) into the body faster than the body can dispose of them. The phenomenon was first described by two Austrian brothers who were dermatologists. Adolf Jarisch Herxheimer (1860-1902) worked in Vienna, and Karl Herxheimer (1862-1942) worked in Frankfort, Germany.[135,136] Both physicians were offering treatments for syphilitic lesions of the skin. They noticed that patients would respond to treatment with a temporary worsening of the inflammation of their lesions, and display symptoms such as fever, perspiration, night sweats, nausea and vomiting, before healing. They observed that those who had the most intense reactions tended to have the most rapid and complete healing.

The problem with a herxheimer effect is that when it is happening, it is difficult to tell if a patient is having a herx reaction to die-off or a drug toxicity problem. The patient should always contact their treating physician if there is any change in their symptoms to discuss the possibility of drug interactions, toxicity, allergic reactions or the herxheimer effect. Some people undergoing Lyme disease treatment will experience a herx at some point during the treatment process, whether they are using antibiotics or herbal therapies. The strength and duration of a herx is dependent on illness severity and treatments, and usually occurs within days of beginning treatment and again at the fourth week, and is variable in length from hours to days. It can flare every 4 weeks during treatment due to the destruction of spirochetes and the release of antigens and toxins. The flares seem to reflect the organism's cell growth cycle, which occurs about once a month. Antibiotics can only kill Bb during the growth phase, so therapy should continue for at least one full cycle. Symptoms flares should lessen with ongoing treatment as the viral loads are lowered.[137]

"You have to get worse before you get better" is a common phrase, with the end result being an ill patient who is made to temporarily feel even more ill. For the most part, the Lyme patient will feel as if they have suddenly contracted the flu, and symptoms may feel discouraging to the patient. A brief worsening of symptoms should always be monitored by your physician, especially if it involves cardiac symptoms, or difficulty breathing – but may simply be an indication that your current treatment is *working*.

A herx is considered to be a healing crisis, a detox reaction or die-off syndrome. It is a model of the human cytokine cascade, which are small secreted proteins that mediate and regulate immunity, inflammation and the formation of blood (hematopoiesis), when responding to an immune stimulus.[138] Research has lead to the belief that a herx reaction is triggered by cell wall deficient or polymorphic L-form microbes. *B. burgdorferi* has cell wall deficient and L-forms, and is polymorphic. Herxheimer reactions were originally observed in patients receiving mercury treatments for syphilis but have also been reported in Rheumatoid Arthritis, Lyme and relapsing fever patients when treated with appropriate antibiotics. It does not appear in normal, healthy individuals.[139]

Some of the more common symptoms associated with a herx reaction are:

- Chills, or cold extremities
- Headache
- Joint and muscle pains
- Body aches
- Sore throat
- General malaise or "flu" symptoms
- Sweating or chills
- Nausea
- Bloating
- Photosensitivity
- Increased heart rate
- Itching, hives or rashes (may seem like allergic reaction)
- Mental confusion
- Bone pain
- Anxiety and panic attacks
- Depression.[140,141]

It sounds much like typical Lyme symptoms, doesn't it? There are things that are suspected to intensify the symptoms of a herx, and may need to be avoided. *Check with your physician if unsure of symptoms during treatment.*

- Fear, anxiety, worry
- Hormonal imbalances
- Anti-virals, anti-bacterials, anti-fungals, anti-parasitics
- Chronic illnesses and depressed immune function
- High doses of vitamins, and chelation therapy
- Cold temperatures
- Fatigue or exhaustion
- Heavy foods
- Clotting agents
- Air pollution or ozone
- Excessive exercise
- Enzymes, (bromelain, pancreatin, etc.)[142]

The treatments for a herx reaction vary. One thought involves improving blood flow in order to clear toxins more quickly; attempt to neutralize the toxins, or both. There are many different methods employed to treat a herx. Some of those may include the following, (as collected from patients and doctors over the past 2 years). *Again, consult your doctor before trying anything listed herein.*

- 2 Tbsp lemon juice (organic) or one half of a lemon rind
- Lemon juice and olive oil drink (may use water or grape juice)
- Herbal liver/gallbladder cleanse
- 1 Tbsp cold pressed extra virgin olive oil (with water or juice)
- Hot baths or hot tub
- Steam bath or dry sauna
- Infrared hot house treatments
- Antihistamines
- Anti-inflammatories or NSAIDS (non-steroidal anti-inflammatories)
- Aspirin
- Therma-Flu or equivalent
- Control panic attacks, anxiety and worry (constricts blood vessels)
- Enemas, colonics (to reduce ammonia levels)
- Blood thinners or the kitchen spice tumeric
- Flavanoids (widens blood vessels)
- Aerobic oxygen supplementation

- Bentonite clay or diatomaceous earth, usually in a bath
- Lymphatic massage
- Cleansing bath (1 cup salt, 1 cup soda, 1 cup epsom salts, 1 cup aloe vera added to hot bath water. Remain in and keep water hot for 1-1/2 hours all the while consuming about 2 quarts of warm water.)

Remember, a herx effect may be an indicator that your treatment may be working, and is relatively short-lived, (hours to a week or 10 days). If you do not improve following a herx event, then the process may not have been a herx. With a herxheimer event, the key is that the patient will become *more ill*, then recover to a *higher plateau of wellness* some time afterward. Always consult with your physician for advice, especially if you have, or think you may be having any type of reaction, as serious reactions to medications and treatments can occur, which may be confused with a herxheimer reaction. If your physician has never heard of a Herxheimer reaction, ask him or her to research the topic because it is not "all in your head," though some patients have been accused of fabricating herxheimer symptoms.

[This section was informational only, for the purpose of review and discussion. It is not intended to replace or represent medical opinion or discussion with your physician. The author is not a medical expert or physician. Always seek the advice of your treating physician or other expert before following any suggestions, treatments or advice for any other sources, including this book.]

Munchausen's and Munchausen's By Proxy

The term "Munchausen's disease" has been thrown around over the years, and actually refers to a rather uncommon psychiatric illness where someone exaggerates or fabricates an illness or symptoms that they otherwise do not have, in order to gain medical attention or notoriety. In cases where otherwise healthy children are involved in the scenario, (typically pre-schoolers), the syndrome is termed "Munchausen's By Proxy Syndrome," MBP, or MBPS.

MBPS was named after Baron von Munchausen, an eighteenth-century German dignitary who was known for telling outlandish tales. MBPS is also called Factitious Disorder by Proxy, and is listed in the American Psychiatric Association's *Diagnostic and Statistical Manual of Mental Disorders* (Fourth Edition, Text Revision), which is also called a DSM-IV-TR, or in short, DSM-IV.[143]

In *rare* actual cases of MBP, the perpetrator claims illness of another person, or actually causes another person to become ill. The necessity to gain sympathy and attention, combined with the need for the perpetrator to convincingly deceive medical professionals, is felt to be the behavior pattern in these psychiatrically disturbed individuals. Munchausen's and MBPS behaviors are considered a severe form of child abuse or neglect, and are statistically very *rare.*

What is frightening is that in the arena of Lyme disease, the terms Munchausen's and MBP are being utilized in greater numbers in recent years by physicians who cannot quantitatively measure a Lyme patient's illness. When a patient or a parent of a potential Lyme patient enters the doctor's office, the doctor attempts to diagnose their illness. When laboratory results return negative showing "nothing" wrong, the doctor becomes frustrated and often tells the patient "its all in your head." And yet the patient continues to describe symptoms they or their children are experiencing, but for which no medical "proof" seems to exist. (Sometimes even with medical evidence these illnesses are dimissed). Instead, these patients are labeled with psychiatric disorders, including Munchausen's and MBP, simply because the physician is unable to convince the patient that they are not ill – when they *are indeed sick.* The physician then sometimes unfairly labels these patients with one or other of these disorders, without any basis for that diagnosis other than a refusal by the patient to accept the doctor's "diagnosis."

Further, occasionally social services are called on behalf of the physician when parents repeatedly attempt to obtain what they believe is proper medical attention for their children or themselves, or even sometimes when they merely have a heated discussion about illness within the physician's office. Many doctors don't like their patients "questioning" their medical expertise. To complicate matters, social services has no expert knowledge of the politics of Lyme disease; problems with testing, diagnosis, and treatment inaccuracies. Caseworkers must make assumptions based upon conjecture, and ill-drawn conclusions; typically in favor of "protecting" children from potential situations of "abuse," whether there is any evidence of abuse, or not. Parents are accused of "treating" their children in ways deemed by social services as "unacceptable" or "abusive" when in reality, it is not the parents treating children, it is their physicians! And yet parents are paying a high price for questioning or disagreeing with their physicians. That price often includes the removal of their parental and custodial rights.

I have heard of this happening with Lyme disease and other illness, (in addition to my own family), especially in the realm of post-divorce and child custody matters, or on occasion, because of patient activism in the arena of Lyme disease. In post-divorce matters, one parent will pit the children against the other parent, (usually against the parent who is ill), in an effort to control the outcome of divorce and custody matters. In the patient advocate role, sadly, the price of doing nothing more than protesting or attempting to raise awareness in an arena fraught with political controversy, is sometimes much higher than anticipated. Some advocates have lost personal credence and custody of their children, merely for daring to stand firmly against a body of medical opinion.

Doctors, social services and the family court systems seem blindly unaware of the chronic nature or symptoms of Lyme disease, and a parent impaired by this illness may appear angry, irrational, irresponsible, moody or even hostile. Patients may lack impulse control on a large or even a subtle, level. Further, the lack of a diagnosis, expert witnesses, and/or documented "evidence" in the form of positive laboratory testing which clearly spell out a diagnosis, forces courts to blindly agree with social services and the parties to an action who are claiming that Lyme patients are *not ill* but that they are fabricating illness, or worse, that the ill patient who seems to be fabricating their illness, must somehow be "mentally" ill.

Lyme patients then are forced to endure lengthy court battles, are sometimes falsely arrested, and are forced to afford up to hundreds of thousands of dollars to pay for attorney fees, expert medical witnesses and so forth, while simultaneously trying to obtain medical diagnoses and treatment for themselves and/or their children. **This is a heinous situation for families who are affected by Lyme disease and is caused by those ignorant of chronic or hidden illness, and/or those who would attempt to silence these patients perhaps due to personal agenda.**

By nature of the Lyme disease process, these patients will find it very difficult to control their anger at being falsely accused of child abuse, mental illness, and the inexplicable loss of their custody rights and children. They will rightly become frustrated with an ignorant and abusive ex-spouse, or uneducated legal system. Their subsequent responses toward these accusations and actions by parties rampantly determined to remove children without evidence will undoubtedly be misjudged and held very harshly against them – simply because they are *ill* and no one wishes to investigate matters properly or wants to believe they or their children are physically ill and nothing more.

I wrote about a situation like this from my own personal experiences after spending nearly a decade in a family court system, fighting to return custody of my own children in a system that told me I "didn't look sick" when I had no working diagnosis. It held me in contempt for being unable to work due to the disabling effects of Lyme disease, and accused me of having a "flat" facial expression and a face "full of rage." A social worker gauged my emotional well-being and parenting skills with these harsh comments, instead of seeing my facial expressions as evidence of nerve damage from facial paralysis which I told her about. She completely and entirely dismissed my physical illness and accused me of "mental" problems, instead, making comments such as "don't you think I can see what's going on here," and "I have more experience in 'these kinds of cases' than anyone else in the county." Funny, because after later admitted to botching the investigation of our case when on the witness stand, (but not before she recommended my children be removed from my care), the female social worker suddenly immediately retired.

My book describes how families are torn apart by a court system ignorant of Lyme disease and its symptoms, and how families are easily manipulated by ex-spouses with a private agenda. That book is called, *The Singing Forest, a Journey Through Lyme Disease.* More information is available about this story at the end of this book for those desiring to learn more about some of the legal aspects of the discrimination of the chronically ill and disabled.

Another aspect of Munchausen's By Proxy is that when children *are* ill with Lyme disease, often physicians cannot verify these illnesses through available diagnostic tests, so parents have no concrete evidence in hand to prove illness in the family courts. At best, a judge will regard positive Lyme Western Blots and other diagnostic tests (as in our case), as nothing more than "a test" which means "no diagnosis," even if the test results are positive. The court does not feel it is capable of determining a diagnosis on the basis of one test, and that is true, however when it is rendering judgment whereby test results are involved, its responsibility should be to validate the tests in question, and not be dismissive of them, as was the case in our family court trial. The judge didn't understand what he was viewing, and therefore, simply ignored key evidence.

Not unless there is an *actual diagnosis plainly spelled out upon the same piece of paper as the test result which must say 'diagnosis,'* will judges take note of a medical ill. As a result, individuals like my children will be left standing all alone, unable to get treatment for a disease that will progressively disable them, in a court system which refuses to consider the fact that these patients may be legitimately ill. Discretionary judgement has flown out the window for "fact-finding" and "rules of evidence." The system is fallible and clearly doesn't work. In the divorce arena as above, parents like myself who desire to treat their ill children (and I *have* proof of exposure to Lyme disease in the form of laboratory testing for them), often have their hands tied most tightly by the very systems that are supposed to protect our children in the first place.

Finally, if a physician or other professional truly believes they are looking at a case of Munchausen's or MBP, then further, *careful* investigation needs to be done including medical and psychological testing of *all parties involved,* ***before*** accusations or judgments are made leading to court or social services involvement, and before families are torn apart through ignorance and rash action, (especially to fulfill social service "quotas," and yes we have heard about those). The stakes are far too high for patients and their children if the former are falsely accused. This includes but is not limited to losing a crucial opportunity for proper diagnosis and treatment of illness, and/or losing custodial rights to our children, and a chance for the family unit to remain intact. Incidentally, **there is no effective treatment to ever cure the harm that a loss like false accusations, and the deliberate, unjust and grossly immoral separation of children from their parents after false accusations, creates.** The only recourse we have as victims of this process, is to work to raise awareness to prevent that situation from ever happening again. We must educate those responsible for decision-making in social services, the justice system, and in healthcare, and we must change the laws to protect families from this kind of legal manipulation and injustice. There simply is no other way.

Lyme Testing – What is the Confusion?

Regardless of any specific guidelines which may be imposed by medical societies and accepted by the medical community at large, until specific and accurate testing is readily available, the diagnosis of Lyme disease for most patients remains a *clinical* one. The Infectious Disease Society of America (IDSA) seems to agree with this statement, although its recently published guidelines[144] seem to suggest under which circumstances Lyme may be diagnosed and/or treated. Lyme diagnosis should *never* be excluded on the basis of lab results, nor on the direction of singularly set criteria, but should remain the rightfully confidential and personal choices made between doctor and patient. In a clinical diagnosis, the patient's complete medical history, presence of rash or other symptoms, and exposure to ticks or other vector transmissions should always be considered. In fact, the IDSA guidelines appear to agree that the EM rash is the only manifestation of Lyme disease (in the U.S.) that is distinctive enough so that clinical diagnosis is possible even in the absence of laboratory confirmation.[144]

Compounding current Lyme issues are challenges over the accuracy of laboratory tests, problems with test interpretation, difficulty culturing spirochetes within samples, and the organism's ability to change forms (pleomorphism). These and other issues often prevent doctors from definitively capturing both the elusive spirochetes that plague humans, and obtaining valid information to make an accurate diagnosis. Often patients are presented lab tests which (by admission from their manufacturers) are inaccurate.[145,146] Physicians wrongly assume these tests are 100% accurate, then tell a patient they "don't have Lyme disease" based upon one negative result. To dismiss patient concerns about symptoms by refusing to test due to personal opinion about the presence of infectious disease in a particular geographic area is also a serious disservice to the patient.

As an example, I removed an engorged tick from my back in 1992, which was quickly followed by a bull's-eye rash, fevers, flu symptoms, and other constitutional and physical symptoms, and I was told for 12-1/2 years by many doctors that I did *not* have Lyme disease. Several doctors even told me there was "no" Lyme disease in this part of the United States (Wisconsin). Despite my symptoms, distinct rash and personal research that convinced me that I probably had Lyme disease (and this was in the days before the internet was what it is today), each doctor I saw for *years*, told me I *did not, and could not have Lyme.* And what is astounding to me is that *not one single doctor* would agree to even *test* me for Lyme disease for an *entire decade*; and I live in an endemic area.

Finally in 2002, I managed to convince a physician to test me, and he performed a Lyme titer, which basically looks for Bb antibodies in the blood. But things can skew the results of a titer, rendering it useless. The available body of medical research teaches us that a course of antibiotics before the test, or any previous antibiotics taken during onset of infection may affect results, or the test could have been taken before a body has a chance to make antibodies. Also, Bb may not be present in the blood, especially some time after infection where it migrates to tissues, cells, organs, the brain and central nervous system.

Well, my Lyme titer came back negative, which just meant no antibodies were detected; meaning any number of things, including the fact that my blood sample had no free antibodies to attach to the antigens in the test kit, and thus a very high viral load. Instead, my doctor took that one test result to mean that I simply *did not have Lyme disease.*

In my case, he couldn't have been more wrong. Instead, he got angry with me and accused me of being a hypochondriac, wasting his time, and needing a therapist. It would take me 2-1/2 more years before I would find a doctor able to diagnose me properly, supplemented by additional laboratory testing. All told, it took nearly 100 doctors over the course of 12-1/2 years, (including a fruitless 10-day visit at Mayo clinic), and all this patient had to show for that time wasted was serious physical disability, partial paralysis, cognitive dysfunction and a myriad of "diagnoses," all of which were horribly inaccurate. Simple laboratory testing at the onset of my illness might have shown antibodies to Lyme disease and saved me many years of disability. My doctors simply refused to do it.

Finally in 2004, I was correctly diagnosed with Lyme by a positive Western Blot test, followed by many lab tests from several "standard" laboratories, (and some highly specialized ones). Some of these tests revealed infection, and some revealed nothing at all, because they were performed at routine laboratories using CDC *surveillance* criteria. Some of my co-infections were photographed from peripheral blood samples and stained in such a manner as to facilitate the viewing of these actually quite fascinating looking microorganisms. I found it quite difficult to argue with photographic evidence and would believe photographic evidence and presenting symptoms over lab tests results which might seem to indicate otherwise through low cut-off numbers, or other restrictive criteria. Experiencing the symptoms is one thing, but seeing the actual organisms causing those symptoms, truly is believing, because lab tests can be inaccurate. But the microscope doesn't *create* the organisms, it merely *displays* them. **And you can't catch these "viruses" from internet research!**

The ELISA

The CDC (Centers for Disease Control) and the IDSA (Infectious Diseases Society of America) guidelines suggest a 2-test approach using an enzyme-linked immunosorbent assay (ELISA) or an immunofluorescent assay (IFA), followed by a Western Immunoblot (Western Blot or WB) to screen Lyme patients. ILADS (International Lyme and Associated Diseases) physicians and others refute this approach, stating that these tests lack sensitivity and specificity and fail to diagnose as many as up to 90% of Lyme patients because in part, there is no distinction between infection stages, whether acute, chronic or resolved.[147] The CDC says specimens proving negative by the EIA/IFA approach *should not be tested further*. Those equivocal or positive should be followed by the WB.[148] The IDSA guidelines also appear to say this.

The CDC's recommendation of a 2-test approach comes directly from IDSA researcher Dr. Allen C. Steere's study, published in the *Journal of Infectious Disease* in 1993.[148] But the ELISA test, which the IDSA and CDC call the "preferred" or "recommended" testing method, routinely misses Lyme disease cases due to insensitivity, and ability to be affected adversely by antibiotic treatments. One problem with this 2-test system is that the ELISA has too many "false negatives" and "false positives" to act as an accurate diagnostic tool.

Studies were conducted by the group that was responsible for Lyme disease proficiency testing for the College of American Pathologists (CAP). They concluded that the current ELISA assays for Lyme disease did not have adequate sensitivity to be part of the 2-tiered approach of the CDC/ASPHLD definition.[149]

Dr. Alan Barbour, who applied for U.S. patent #5,582,990, filed just 3 weeks before he voted as a member of the diagnostic/surveillance criteria-establishing committee in Dearborn, Michigan, (October 1994),[145,150] had this to say about the ELISA in his patent application. *"Conventional diagnostic tests for Lyme disease have used whole spirochetal sonic extracts as test antigens in ELISA to detect antibodies to* B. burgdorferi, *but this test yields* unsatisfactory low diagnostic sensitivity *(20 to 60%) during the early stage of infection, possibly due to a slow and late-appearing antibody response and to the inclusion of irrelevant cross-reacting antigens in the whole-cell preparations."*[151]

In his book titled *Lyme Disease. The Cause, the Cure, the Controversy,* Dr. Barbour had this to say about the ELISA test on page 88: *"Even so, tests are not the end-all or be-all for diagnosis. To ensure the best medical care, laboratory tests should complement, not replace, the results from the history and the physical examination."*[152] He also said there is danger in physicians becoming "overly dependent" upon the use of laboratory testing to make their diagnoses.

Western Blot Made Easy

The Western Blot or Immunoblot test name originated from the laboratory of George Stark at Stanford. The name was given to the technique by W. Neal Burnette, and is a play on the name "Southern blot," a technique used for DNA detection which was developed earlier by Edwin Southern.[153]

The Western Blot (WB) test maps the antibodies that our immune system makes to *antigens* (substances that stimulate the production of antibodies, like Bb). The blot test utilizes isolates to detect the presence of them, and reports them by weight in measured units called *kilo Daltons* (kDa). These kDa measured units are commonly referred to as Lyme "bands." Each band is assigned a specific number to correspond with a different *piece* or *protein* belonging to the Lyme spirochete.

The WB looks for "free," unbound antibodies that our bodies make to the spirochete (*antigens*), and records what it finds as being present (positive), or not (negative). If a negative result is recorded, it represents a negative result as *no antibodies were detected in that particular sample.* It could mean that all available antibodies are already bound to some other antigen, and thus are not free to bind with the antigens within the test. There are also other variables in testing. A result can also register as *equivocal*, which means that a *very weak positive* may have been detected, but that amount was insufficient to cause a strong positive test result.[154] Some tests do not report equivocal results, or in some studies, equivocal results were counted as "negative" when they could in fact, have been weak positives, simply because the detection of antibodies were at or below the established numerical cut-off point. So antibodies may have been detected, but the test was deemed negative since the number or value was below that which was previously set by the lab. It doesn't mean that no antibodies were detected, it means simply that the test's positive limits were not necessarily satisfactorily reached, and all tests have limitations.

What are IgM and IgG?

IgM stands for Immunoglobulin M, which are the body's first antibodies to be produced in great quantities, in response to infection. It is a large antibody (larger than IgG), with 10 antigen binding sites, but it cannot bind that many simultaneously. When IgM antibodies are present in large numbers, it is because there is active infection, whether new or reactivated. Many chronic Lyme patients (whether treated or not), still have measurable IgM antibodies decades after initial infection. As infections are treated, IgM antibody numbers should decline.[155]

IgG stands for Immunoglobulin G, a small antibody having 2 antigen binding sites. It is the most abundant immunoglobulin in the body, about equally distributed between the blood and body tissues. It is the only antibody that can pass through the human placenta. IgG antibodies are produced later during the course of infection, and may still be present after an acute infection clears.[156] IgG is not always detectable in chronic Lyme patients or in the early part of the disease process.

Lyme Bands and Interpretation

Some bands on the Western Blot test do not specifically belong to the Bb spirochete. An example is the "41" band, which is specific for *many* organisms with flagella (tails), including Bb, the Lyme spirochete. Therefore a WB showing *only* the non-specific 41-band as positive, is *not considered a true positive result*,[157] only positive for *some* type of organism having flagella. Any *non-Lyme-specific* antigens may *cross-react* in testing to give a positive result, and these cross-reactive bands are often referred to as "junk" bands.

These are the known Bb genus-specific Western Blot bands: 18, 22, 23-25 (considered the same), 31, 34, 37, 39, 83, and 93.

The presence of only ONE of these Bb genus-specific bands should be considered as laboratory evidence of Bb antibodies. If you have even ONE of these bands testing as positive, you have been exposed to Bb, and that evidence *should* be enough to help confirm a clinical diagnosis of Lyme disease, but routinely is not.[154,158]

Out of a possible 25 bands used for Lyme testing, (including so-called "junk" bands), 11 total bands were selected by the CDC as reportable for IgG and IgM testing purposes.[158] The CDC's *surveillance* criteria includes "junk" bands in their testing and some of these may cross-react and cause a "false positive" reading.[154]

Bands able to cause a "false-positive" on CDC definition dependent diagnostic tests as they are not Bb-specific: 28, 41, 45, 58, and 66.

If you consider *only* Bb genus-specific antibody bands, there can be no such thing as a "false positive" test result. In fact, because of the inclusion of these "junk" bands, **you can actually have a CDC surveillance "positive" IgG Lyme test result with the 5 total antibodies they require, without having any Bb genus-specific antibodies present![154] Only in this manner can you be falsely positive.**

Due to the potential for false positive results, the CDC *surveillance* criteria is inappropriate for screening patients and should not be utilized as structured. Rather it should be revised to include only Bb-specific bands. *This should then eliminate false positives during testing.*

Instead, physicians should carefully examine *Bb genus-specific antibodies* (bands) and the tests which report them. They should take care to exclude "junk" bands from their interpretation of test results. This necessitates the reporting of *all* test bands, (not just those CDC-reportable) appearing within a Western Blot test, something that specialty laboratories, like IGeneX labs, provide. This makes it easier for doctors to interpret test results properly, and to *focus on the genus-specific antibody bands, not the surveillance criteria bands.* If physicians used this one rule of thumb alone, significantly more patients would be classified as Lyme "positive" than currently are. Of course this does not mean we ignore the patient history and tick exposure, but reporting all Bb-relative bands further facilitates physician accuracy in diagnosis.

The CDC considers an **IgM** test positive if 2 of the following 3 bands are present: 24, 39, and 41. Only 24 and 39 are Bb-specific. Band 41 includes the Bb flagella, but may cross-react due to the presence of flagella from other organisms. It is interesting that the CDC surveillance criteria for the IgM test includes only 2 known antibody bands. We know that within the body, any other Bb-bands, when detected, would have been IgG antibodies at one time, so it is highly questionable as to why the CDC criteria would omit important Bb-specific bands from their criteria.[154]

For CDC **IgG** criteria, the only known Bb genus-specific antibodies included in their criteria are 18 and 93. They exclude others in their total of 10 required.[154,158] Again, why would the CDC exclude *genus-specific antibodies* from a test that should utilize them for detection?

The CDC considers an **IgG** test positive if 5 of the following 10 bands are present: 18, 21, 28, 30, 39, 41, 45, 58, 66, and 93.[158] Again, 8 of these are not specific for Bb, so you can actually have a *false positive CDC* test containing the 5 required number of bands, *without any Bb-specific bands present! Once again, this is the true definition of a false-positive test.*

Remember the CDC criteria includes "junk" bands, and this faulty criteria **eliminates much of the Lyme-exposed population.** In a way, excluding patients with Lyme-specific bands just because they don't follow CDC definitions, is nearly the same as saying someone is a only "little bit" pregnant, because only a little bit of pregnancy hormones are detected. We all know that in time, the pregnancy becomes more than a "little bit" obvious, much in the same manner as excluded positive Lyme bands and their associated symptoms become impossible for the patients, and their doctors, to ignore.

The CDC recommends that when a WB is used during the first 4 weeks of disease, to use both IgG and IgM Western Blot tests.[159] But the problem with that line of thinking is that some people don't make antibodies within that short a timeframe, and others will *never* make antibodies at all. Some patient's antibodies are tied up and not detected because there aren't any free antibodies floating around, and only after antibiotic treatments might some of these patients seroconvert from negative to positive. Additionally, antibiotics can interfere with the body's ability to make antibodies, and *Borrelia* spirochetes are "smart" organisms which chemically suppress our immune systems into thinking they are not present, when in fact they are. This can easily prevent antibodies from being made. More testing is not necessarily better, or more accurate in this case; and timing may be everything in diagnostic testing.

It has been suggested by at least one Lyme diagnostic kit manufacturer, *MarDx*, which concluded in its own technical report abstract on Lyme Western Blotting in reference to their IgM and IgG western blot tests, that *"These tests must not be used on first stage EM patients (4 weeks after onset) or patients known to have had Tick-borne Relapsing Fever."*[160,161] And yet the first month following infection is of course a critical time period whereby patients should be treated at least prophylactically if they have been exposed to Lyme disease. This is the time period where it remains localized and has not yet disseminated to other parts of the body, the central nervous system and the brain.

This creates a "catch-22" when patients aren't diagnosed by virtue of their clinical history, tick exposure, and by using supportive lab tests, if the tests can't rule out a disease they cannot detect. Criteria are too narrowly defined to be practical, and some doctors take a "wait and see" approach. Others (including the IDSA guidelines) contraindicate routine prophylactic treatment. Doctors tell patients they "don't have" Lyme on the basis of one negative laboratory test result. We can easily see how patients develop disseminated Lyme disease due to misdiagnosis, especially if tests are performed too early after initial infection.

Different laboratories and the CDC also set their "positive" test result criteria differently. And any Bb-specific band registering as "positive" on a Western Blot, should still be considered positive, even if it does not meet CDC surveillance "standards." A body infected with Bb at some point may make these Lyme-specific antibodies, (or not) and we should pay attention if any appear during testing. Remember, Bb is the only organism that can force the body to make its genus-specific antibodies.[154]

The CDC cautions that a positive IgM test result in and of itself (without a companion IgG), is "not enough" for persons having illness more than 1 month in duration because positive results in those patients would be considered a "false-positive."[155] But remember, we have seen why the CDC is concerned about "false positives" and now we know there can really be no such thing in tests which do not follow CDC "surveillance" guidelines, if one includes only Lyme-specific bands.

Other laboratories using Western Blot testing report the kDa bands in different ways. The best laboratory results report **all kDa bands present**, not just CDC definitions. As explained above, patients can, and should request that *all* bands be reported on their test results, to aid their clinician in a diagnosis. It is a good idea to use a lab approved by federal CLIA standards (Clinical Laboratory Improvement Amendments of 1988). CLIA certification requires all testing laboratories to register with the Centers for Medicare and Medicaid Services, and adhere to strict quality control, quality assurance, record keeping, personnel and other standards.[162]

IGeneX Inc. Western Blot Interpretation

IGeneX, Inc., is a California clinical laboratory founded in 1983. It was purchased from 3M Diagnostics Systems (3MDS, Santa Clara, CA) and BioWhittaker, Inc., (Walkersville, MD) in 1991. The reference laboratory invented an important, patented Lyme urine antigen test, and played a key role in the development of this assay. In fact, some of the 3M research team members who helped develop this assay, came to work at IGeneX labs.[163] IGeneX is a tick-borne illness only lab, internationally known for its excellence and holds licenses in every U.S. state that allows, and is CLIA- and Medicare-approved.

IGeneX utilizes sophisticated tests that are *more sensitive* and *better designed* than those used by most routine national labs. IGeneX obtained pedigreed strains of Bb from individuals having early, mid- and late-stage Lyme disease. Additionally, IGeneX Western blots have reactivity against many Bb strains. These include *B. afzelli* and *B. gaiinii* (European strains), *B. japonica* (Japanese strain) and sub-strains from Colorado, Texas and Missouri. Current Western blot testing from some other labs (including those recommended by the CDC) on the other hand, utilize strains from patients having *only* early Lyme disease,[164] and do not have such reactivity, making them possibly less accurate and less sensitive than IGeneX tests, (for example), as a screening tool.

I found that the innovative scientists at IGeneX designed their Western Blot test results upon principles published in the *Journal of Clinical Microbiology* 1989 (revised 3/29/05). The data that is provided on IGeneX Western Blot tests is helpful to the physician in arriving at, or ruling out a diagnosis of Lyme disease because they voluntarily report all reactive bands, not just those required by the CDC/ASPHLD surveillance criteria.

Because of their excellence in testing, more and more patients who have returned negative Lyme and co-infection panels from routine labs are retesting and obtaining helpful diagnostic clues through the use of these more sensitive and specific tests. Because of this, IGeneX and other laboratories which reveal Lyme disease and tick-borne illness in greater numbers than the CDC-supported labs, are under serious political attack from special interest groups and others. Rather than investigate the practical use of these more sensitive tests for the benefit of the patients, some prefer to denigrate laboratories like IGeneX and make erroneous accusations of test "unreliability" and "inaccurate" reporting methods, even with tests which have proven to return higher numbers of positive results in patients having clinical symptoms, and perhaps will in time, prove to be superior in accuracy. Keep in mind that labs like IGeneX are the *competition* to the CDC, NIH, University spin-off companies and other laboratories, who make *competing* diagnostic tests. The most useful tactic of course would be to discredit the competition and promote one's own testing as *more accurate* or *more effective*, right? This is product marketing 101 – discredit the competition, get your buddies to promote your testing, and gain the lion's share of the market. I am not saying that this is definitely what is happening, but I am saying that it is something worth considering.

The media loves to pick on these specialty laboratories in an attempt to sweep Lyme patients "under the carpet" and/or promote their self-interested partners – especially those in the media who are sympathetic to the positions possibly held by certain Infectious Disease, or CDC personnel; and who perhaps might wish to conceal the truth about Lyme disease from the masses – that Lyme is *not* easily curable, and is often a *permanent infection.*

Time and again we will read of the same tired parties interviewing the same tired individuals who say the same tired things about this illness, despite emerging research and clinical experience which shouts loudly that these viewpoints may be wholly inaccurate. When we study the different societies and who their members are, we see a pattern of interconnectivity between a very small subset of personnel all seemingly working to try to silence Lyme patients, their doctors and the published research, or perhaps even to slow-play a known epidemic illness. Again this is perplexing unless you take into consideration the tremendous hypothetical idea that there may be conflicts of interest among these individuals, including but not limited to the holding of patents on Lyme-related technologies; payment by pharmaceutical or insurance companies to be their spokespersons; private and government research funding; and ownership of spin-off companies which produce Lyme diagnostic tests or vaccine components – which would make any individuals truly wealthy the longer and more effectively they can promote their own interests, if that was indeed what they were doing, and again we're talking hypothetically.

The problems concerning the discounting of laboratory tests is not solely the media's ball game. I have personally witnessed within my own court trials opposing counsel attempting to manipulate a ruling on the validity of my children's (and mine) IGeneX Western Blot test results, using excerpts from magazines such as *Forbes* and others – information which perhaps makes accusations against the use of IGeneX testing as an accurate diagnostic screening tool. Attorneys love to argue. That means that anything which they can utilize to support their arguments in a court of law, may be presented by an unscrupulous attorney attempting to dismiss a mother's concerns about her positive laboratory test results for herself, and her children. It is up to the discretion of the judge then, to decide if the media source is accurate, or even the be-all, end-all of authoritative measure. Fortunately, in our case of course, they were not, but the mere suggestion of allegations against a laboratory, even if completely unfounded, could be enough to raise doubt about a laboratory or test result within a court of law; especially one ignorant of Lyme disease and its swirling controversy.

Lumbar Puncture

Some doctors recommend lumbar puncture to be performed on patients who are suspected as having Lyme disease with neurological involvement. From a patient standpoint, lumbar puncture has proven disappointing as a reliable diagnostic tool. One reason is because of poor sensitivity in current testing. Additionally, not all Lyme patients have antibodies present in spinal fluid, either initially or over a longer period of time. Many patients must then endure this test only to be told that because their test results were negative, they "don't have" Lyme disease. Perhaps they do not *produce* antibodies, they have *no detectable antibodies* in a sample, or due to poor test sensitivity the antibodies present are simply undetected. And due to heavy physician reliance on test results when forming a diagnosis, these patients leave their physician wrongly informed that they "don't have" Lyme from one spinal test. Not only is this unfair to the patient, it often leads them to further despair and depression due to a continuing lack of credence (and diagnosis) for their illness. Of course the very real possibility exists that they do not have Lyme, but when the clinical symptoms, history, risk of exposure etc. fit the profile, and other illnesses have been ruled out, then what is left?[165,166]

Q-RIBb Testing for Lyme

According to their web site, Central Florida Research Inc., in Lake Alfred Florida, replaced the laboratory operations of Bowen Research and Training Institute, Inc. One of the new tests offered there is a test said to be more definitive than a Western Blot. It is called the Quantitative-Rapid Identification of *Borrelia burgdorferi* (Q-RIBb) test and uses a *Borrelia burgdorferi* fluorescent antibody to detect the antigen in blood samples, and is read by a Flow Cytometry process.[167] The laboratory accepts major insurance carriers and Medicare. They are also CLIA-approved and kits can be ordered by physicians in the US and abroad. According to their web site, colleagues Eleanor Fort (a medical laboratory technologist) and Dr. Jo Anne Whitaker, (a prominent medical researcher suffering from Lyme disease), developed the Q-RIBb test which is noteworthy for both its sensitivity, and the short amount of time required to perform the test. The test is reportedly unaffected by antibiotics taken by the patient.[168]

PCR and Urine Tests

Other tests have been evaluated for screening patients for Lyme disease. Some of these are polymerase chain reaction (PCR) tests, antigen capture tests and urine antigen tests. Each test has advantages and disadvantages, and may or may not be reliable due to a lack of standardization. PCR tests are performed on blood, urine, cerebral spinal fluid, joint fluid, tissue biopsies, breast milk, semen, lymph nodes and tick specimens that have had Bb DNA amplified so that it can be measured. The PCR is potentially very sensitive, but the sample utilized must contain at least one recoverable organism to amplify DNA, and pieces, or blebs of Bb antigen for the plasmid assay. IGeneX laboratory in California is one laboratory that has this type of PCR test available.[169]

Lyme Urine Antigen Testing (LUAT/DotBlot)

One of the diagnostic tests routinely used in NIAID's clinical studies on chronic Lyme disease is the Lyme Urinary Antigen Test (LUAT). The LUAT is an immunoassay used for direct detection of Lyme antigen in urine. Even though it has not been approved by the FDA as a "valid" diagnostic test for Lyme disease, it is widely used. According to the NIAID, independent quality control studies were performed by scientists, which concluded that the LUAT was unreliable because it yielded an unacceptably high percentage of false positive reactions.[170] IGeneX at this time offers the Lyme Dot-Blot Assay (LDA), which checks for 23-25, 31, 34, 39, and 93 kDa antigens in urine.[171]

The National Institutes of Health (NIH) also developed a patented assay for Lyme antigen in urine. This assay utilizes a gold-conjugated antibody for improved resolution under an electron microscope, but has not been commercialized for routine patient use by any clinical reference lab.[172] NIH collects data from their own tests using single-isolates from early Lyme patients as *designed* by them. The CDC posts mainly IDSA-supportive information on its web site, and does not promote so-called "specialty labs," like IGeneX.

During a study in 2001, two IDSA guidelines authors, Drs. Mark Klempner and Allen Steere dismissed IGeneX's urine antigen testing as "unreliable" as compared to serological testing.[173] But in response to this published study, in a letter to the editor of the *American Journal of Medicine*, where the study was published, IGenex doctors Boyd Stephens and Nick Harris indicated that the samples sent to their laboratory by New England Medical Center had been "improperly handled," and they "confirmed" that finding with the supervisor of the laboratory sending the samples to IGeneX at the time. The two men also expressed their concern over the use of the test results published by the authors of the study, because IGeneX concluded that the data was *unreliable and uninterpretable due to the samples being mishandled.*

IGeneX says they informed the laboratory that the tests could not be performed nor could they release the results. IGeneX claims that NEMC's laboratory manager said that because the testing had been paid for by an NIH (National Institutes of Health) grant, IGeneX could not refuse to perform it. NEMC did not send new samples and IGeneX performed the tests but attached a disclaimer to them.[173]

Further, offers to redo the tests at IGeneX's expense with a third-party evaluator were refused at "all levels" including by NEMC, and the NIH. The disclaimer about contamination was not revealed when the results of these tests were revealed a half year later at the Munich International Lyme Conference. According to IGeneX, the authors of this study have published results using samples "clearly stated" as contaminated, and IGeneX raises concerns that the study was published for peer review, using flawed data.[173]

As we look at the 2006 IDSA guidelines for the treatment of Lyme disease, we find this same study quoted as number 337 within the guidelines references.[174] **If this particular study was indeed made using flawed research, then the IDSA is publishing treatment guidelines citing <u>flawed research</u> to dictate treatment guidelines to the masses.** This could in effect, deny treatments to hundreds of thousands of patients unnecessarily. This might be construed as gross negligence (if accidental) or perhaps indifference or even deliberate scientific fraud (if intentional).

As a patient, one can't help but begin to question why independent American labs like IGeneX are under such harsh scrutiny from some of these sources. Perhaps the real reason behind others' attempts to discredit labs like IGeneX, stem from little more than interlaboratory conflicts such as in the example above. Instead of being acknowledged for their excellence in uncovering positive Lyme patient serology, IGeneX is routinely accused of returning too many "false positive" results. Perhaps they are finding real cases of undiagnosed Lyme disease using better criteria.

A Word About False Negatives

It is worth mentioning that researchers, test manufacturers, and some physicians are aware that Lyme patient's bodies do not necessarily make antibodies during the first month of infection. This can lead to "false negative" test results. There are many reasons why a false negative test can occur, which is simply a result showing that no Bb antibodies were detected in the sample. There are many reasons why Lyme diagnostic tests should be used as an *aid* to diagnostics; not as definitive all by themselves. Antibiotics have an antibacterial effect on the body, thus inhibiting the production of antibodies. The body could also have too high of a bacterial load so the patient's antibodies are already bound with as many antigens as possible, leaving too few free antibodies in the blood sample to be detected by the test.

Sometimes the sickest Lyme patients are those who have the highest viral loads and the least amount of free antibodies. Once their co-infections are cleared however, sometimes these patients begin to make antibodies to Bb which might be revealed in a new test, as fully positive. This is sometimes referred to as seroconversion. Further, Bb inhibits the immune process in our bodies, so some patients *never* make enough (or any) antibodies, and a WB test may *never* return positive on these patients, no matter when it is performed. Timing is everything in Lyme testing. Last, a negative test result in and of itself, does not mean Lyme disease is not present in the body, it only means that Bb antigens were not detected *in that one sample alone.*

What happens to patients who do not make antibodies – and what happens to patients when doctors ignore their symptoms delaying their diagnosis until years later? According to the conclusions drawn from reading the IDSA guidelines, (and echoed on the CDC web site), we should perhaps just ignore testing these individuals for fear of "false-positive" test results. According to many, the CDC/IDSA criteria seems so narrowly defined that *hardly any* Lyme patients can, or ever will, realistically qualify for them. That is one reason why laboratories like IGeneX and others are returning more positive tests than the CDC-condoned labs. It is because they are using *better* tests which are able to reveal Bb in those who have fallen through the very wide cracks of the CDC *surveillance* definitions (and IDSA guidelines).

The larger question to ask is why would the CDC state on their web site the following information if they did not mean it: *"This surveillance case definition was developed for national reporting of Lyme disease;* it is **NOT** appropriate **for clinical diagnosis**" (emphasis added).[175] And yet it might seem that the CDC and IDSA recommends that every Lyme physician and laboratory follow this *surveillance* criteria for diagnostic testing.

CDC and the IDSA

Let's take a look at what the CDC uses to interpret its test results and see if there is any obvious relationship between the IDSA. The CDC interprets its Western blot criteria based on only 2 studies, which it cites on its web site:[176]

1.) Immunoblot interpretation criteria for serodiagnosis of early Lyme disease, published in the ***Journal of Clinical Microbiology*** in 1995,[177] – and

2.) Western blotting in the serodiagnosis of Lyme disease, published in the *Journal of Infectious Diseases*, in 1993.[178] One of the authors of this study was Dr. Allen C. Steere, an author of the IDSA guidelines.

Incidentally, the *Journal of Clinical Microbiology* is an ASM publication (American Society Of Microbiology). Another ASM publication, *Clinical Microbiology Reviews* has Martin J. Blaser on its editorial board. Of course Blaser is a staunch supporter of the new IDSA guidelines, he was President of the IDSA when the guidelines were introduced, (and is now past President), and chairman of the Dept. of Medicine at NYU.[179,180] In addition, the *Journal of Infectious Diseases* (from #2 above), is published by the IDSA.

So we have studies performed and published by some IDSA members and their associates/societies, funded in part by the NIH/CDC, which is not necessarily a bad idea, in and of itself. But we have *surveillance* guidelines that are somehow magically morphing into recommended *[read: will be misinterpreted as mandatory by insurance providers and physicians]* guidelines by the IDSA. Then we have the IDSA staunchily defending their guidelines, with certain co-authors convincing their other organizational members (AAN) to sign on in support of these same guidelines.

Naturally the CDC promotes its paid researchers, which should be arguably legitimate, except that some IDSA members repeatedly dismiss competitor's laboratory testing and physician diagnostic methods while seeming to promote their preferred diagnostic testing methods. And some of these are perhaps promoted because they or the Universities which employ these individuals, hold some or all of the patents on some or all of the components of test kits, and/or provide substrates or components for those kits. If this is true, it would seem to present a certain, at least questionable, conflict of interest.

If other laboratories utilize different tests which are considered to be *competitive* and not complementary to those designed by the CDC/NIH, we can see how independent laboratories may appear "threatening" to those providing this competitive testing; especially when these "threatening" labs offer patients what appear to be *more accurate test results*. This idea becomes more solidified when we see the NIH and CDC funding studies on Lyme disease, and recognize that the much criticized independent laboratories (like IGeneX) and their test kits, are often not utilized within those studies except perhaps when they are utilized to attempt to discredit them. And to the best of my ability to locate them, competitor's products are not promoted on these government web sites, but IDSA recommendations are posted and promoted on these sites, even when we see that they may contain possibly "flawed" data...

Testing Outside the U.S.A.

Without diagnostic criteria of their own, our next door neighbors in Canada are following the United States CDC *surveillance* criteria, but are doing so to *diagnose* their Lyme patients, not as a surveillance tool, despite CDC warning that the criteria is not diagnostic.[181]

In February 2007, a letter was sent to Dr. Paul Sockett, the Director of Foodborne, Waterborne and Zoonotic Infections Divisions of the Centre for Infectious Disease Prevention and Control at the Public Health Agency of Canada. It referenced an earlier letter from March 2006, regarding the creation of Lyme disease guidelines, and the possibility of the group *www.Canlyme* (Canadian Lyme Disease Foundation) participating on the committee to facilitate this process. But the process of creating guidelines forged ahead without the involvement of *Canlyme*. On behalf of the board of directors, Jim M. Wilson, President of *Canlyme*, wrote the February 2007 letter to Sockett. Among other points, he requested an explanation of why the group was misled into believing it would be allowed to participate in the formation of the guidelines. He requested the issue to be reopened on behalf of the citizens. He also asked for the names of the authors and signators of the guidelines that were submitted for publishing. To date, the group had no reply from either the PHAC, Dr. David Butler-Jones, Chief PHO, Dr. Robert Clarke, Deputy Chief PHO, or Tony Clement, the Minister of Health.[182]

Another point well taken in the letter was that the American IDSA guidelines (which were the basis to form the Canadian set), are under current investigation with the Connecticut Attorney General's office for possible anti-trust practices. "Anti-trust" here means that the guidelines were allegedly written without outside participation, with implications affecting physician and patient rights and choices, as well as the effect on insurance company benefit payments. Wilson also mentioned that **Infectious Disease doctors across Canada have routinely phoned general practitioners warning them not to diagnose Lyme disease, but instead to refer patients to a Psychiatrist if Lyme is brought up during a patient visit.** Rather unfairly (as in the U.S.), Canadian doctors lecture their patients on how they could not "have" Lyme disease, and that doctors who diagnose and treat Lyme in Canada are "quacks."[182] It is a sad repetition of what American patients are hearing from their non-Lyme literate doctors.

On the Canadian Lyme web site, *www.canlyme.com*, patients can find quite a bit of information about the situation here in America, and they are rightly concerned, because what Americans do with regard to Lyme testing, Canada follows suit. But if citizens there are aware of the serious issues surrounding diagnostic and treatment guidelines in our country, why can't we see the same thing? Canadian Lyme patients are rightly upset because they cannot conceive of why the U.S. would allow a panel of researchers possibly wielding some unknown self-bequeathed authority, to define diagnostic and treatment criteria when those authors appear to have possible conflicts of interest. As it stands, Canadians are forced to use American laboratories in order to obtain more accurate test results, because the Canadian labs use the CDC's criteria, which as we understand misses many Lyme patients. As a result, some people in Canada who test negative in that country and get retested through American laboratories like IGeneX, Inc. in California, which uses tests with higher sensitivity and specificity; thus yielding a higher number of Lyme-positive patients.[183]

The Public Health Agency of Canada says that late-stage Lyme disease testing is "more accurate," but there is no real data to support that statement. Testing in any stage of Lyme infection is an inexact science at best, and there are many factors that can affect the outcome of any test as previously explained. As always, diagnosis of Lyme disease must be based on *clinical history* as well as exposure to tick-vectors, symptoms present and any testing that may prove supportive. Serological testing can only provide some measure of antibody response in the blood and only some of the time. In fact, much of the time, Bb hides in cells, organs and tissues; within the central nervous system, in the brain, and in places most serological testing can't detect them.[183]

Canadian citizens want and need fully-equipped testing laboratories designed to deal with Lyme disease, including a department of pathology. At least those who donate their remains could help researchers locate Bb in body tissues, and work towards better diagnostic tests. And Canadian citizens propose that they set their own diagnostic and testing guidelines instead of blindly following an adjoining country's Infectious Disease Society who did not seem to allow outside participation in the formation of those guidelines. Our neighbors offer a good suggestion – that a non-conflicted group of medical professionals and others draft medical guidelines and that oversight committees be used to police government bodies, universities, insurance and disability programs, medical societies and the like, especially those with strong ties to pharmaceutical companies. I couldn't agree more. Canadian citizens wanting to do something about getting better legislature to protect their physician and patient rights, should write their federal members of Parliament, or their Provincial government members and ask why more effort isn't being shown on behalf of Lyme patients. See *www.canlyme.com/parl.html*.[183] American citizens wanting to do the same should write their Congresspersons or the Connecticut Attorney General's office with their concerns.

Testing Laboratories

Here is contact information for some high-quality laboratories performing Western Blot and other kinds of Lyme and tick-borne illness testing, including the testing of ticks. Besides the laboratories listed below, in the U.S., you can check your state's Department of Health web site to see if they offer Lyme and tick testing.

Central Florida Research Laboratory
(formerly Bowen Laboratory)
Lake Alfred, Florida 1-863-956-3538
www.centralfloridaresearch.com
Performs Lyme and co-infection testing to anywhere in the world;

Europe through DHL or UPS. Does not perform tick testing.
Requires physician ordering of test kits.
Will not send test kits directly to patients.

IGeneX Inc., Palo Alto, California
1-800-832-3200
www.IGeneX.com
Performs Lyme & co-infection and tick testing to anywhere in the world. Will send test kits directly to patient or physician.

Medical Diagnostics Laboratories, Mt. Laurel, New Jersey
1-877-269-0090
www.mdlab.com
Performs Lyme & co-infection and tick testing to anywhere in the world.

NJ Labs, New Brunswick, New Jersey
(732) 249-0148
Performs Lyme & co-infection and tick testing to anywhere in the world.

Pass/Fail Mentality is Failing Patients

Regardless of where tick-borne illness occurs, it is important to utilize regional isolates for antigen detection in tests, even in different areas of the same country. The routine use of single or non-regional isolates may explain why patients with symptoms of Lyme disease may test seronegative in some laboratories and not others. If a test is not sensitive enough to detect a specific strain of *Borrelia,* it may be due to a lack of regional isolates.

Labs using multiple isolates (like IGeneX), explains why some tests are more sensitive, and why they yield higher numbers of positive results – results other labs are clearly missing. Labs using single isolates as standard practice (like some CDC-backed tests) for testing should take their cue from labs using this expanded diagnostic approach and embrace, rather than discount this forward-thinking methodology if they genuinely wish to help ill patients achieve proper diagnostics.

Because routine national laboratories use tests with less reliability and sensitivity, many people's Lyme disease fails to be detected, and instead, returns a "false negative" result. Thus the physician sees this test result upon which he or she relies, and tells the patient, "you do not have Lyme." Only the smart and aware physician accepts a negative result from the standpoint of having no *B. burgdorferi* detected *in that one sample*, and then forges ahead with a differential diagnosis based upon the physically presenting symptoms, patient medical history and history of tick exposure. The physician then would follow up with additional testing as deemed medically necessary, but does not wholly make the patient wait for the progression of additional symptoms to occur, nor a magically "positive" flashing red light with siren to appear on laboratory testing before reasonable symptomatic treatment can begin.

As Lyme patients, we know that many of us are not tested for our diseases until well after the initial phases of our illness have passed, and well after exposure and infection have occurred. Still we have a right to demand the highest quality testing we can obtain in order to be diagnosed simply, quickly and effectively.

The single routine national laboratory that tested this author's blood for Lyme disease detected absolutely no antibodies to Bb in that sample, but perhaps that was because that first test occurred 10 years after initial infection. Perhaps my body never made antibodies. Perhaps the infection had "cleared" you might say. There are some who might say, "this patient did not have Lyme." Yet only 2 years later, using more sensitive tests (IGeneX Western blots and others), this same patient not only showed *B. burgdorferi* antibodies present, but also *multiple co-infections* that were subsequently measured and photographically imaged by another clinical lab, and not IGeneX. Following those tests, doctors ordered additional testing from routine national labs, which still returned negative on LD and curiously only detected *one* co-infection, *Bartonella henselae*, and not the several other co-infections that were later detected. *Obviously someone's testing is not sensitive enough to pick up infections that ARE present, which can be readily photographed, and which respond to subsequent treatments.*

As a patient needing treatment, I place my bet on labs like those used at IGeneX, especially since a positive Western Blot revealed 2 years after a "negative" Lyme titer showed what I knew to be true all along, based on my increasing symptoms and disability. By 2005 I had been ill with Lyme and co-infections for at least 13 years. I would have continued into the oblivion of incapacitation had I not received

IV treatments shortly thereafter, which made a **significant** impact on my symptoms and disease course, though was not entirely curative.

My physicians eventually diagnosed Lyme disease and I received treatment despite never being fully CDC "positive," nor did either myself or my 2 children fall completley within CDC surveillance guidelines as outlined on their web site, by 1990, or even current standards. Our obvious symptoms and rashes appeared, were dismissed by doctors, and weren't diagnosed until 12-1/2 years later. I offer by example 3 individuals denied a diagnosis for a dozen years, until through persistence and proper laboratory testing, we received an accurate diagnosis. As progressively ill as I grew over a dozen years, without treatments I received in 2005, I can safely say that I might have been either institutionalized or deceased had I chosen to accept without question, my many misdiagnoses and the narrow, restrictive guideline recommendations of the CDC and the IDSA. Many patients are not as "lucky" as I was, and many of them die and/or are horribly debilitated with a quality of life that drives many to suicide.

When testing my blood and reviewing my present and ongoing symptoms, *B. burgdorferi* and multiple co-infections can *still be measured and/or photographed* in my peripheral blood, 15 years after I was bitten, despite these therapies. **This is a common scenario echoed in many Lyme patients across the globe**, whether they received "adequate" treatment, in whatever way "adequate treatment" is presently, though poorly defined by medical science. This is because Lyme disease is a complex illness that does *not* respond to pat-answer treatments for all cases. At this point in my life, I believe Bb to be *incurable* or *nearly incurable* in its chronic state, though viral loads can be lowered to such an extent that patients experience few or no symptoms, with the disease hiding subclinically silent in the background. Of course, I hope that I am proven wrong. In fact, the very least that most chronic Lyme sufferers are hoping for (and they will openly tell you this), is a chance to have half of their life restored – just half. We are so debilitated by our disease that we find a new appreciation in being able to do just *half* of what the "healthy" population is able to do. And we are so very grateful for any improvement whatsoever, that is how bad our life becomes.

Understandably the Lyme community is left with a bad taste in its mouth as patients are having difficulty finding quality laboratory testing in their area and Lyme-literate medical doctors (LLMDs) to obtain a diagnosis and treatment. Infectious Disease doctors and others who rely upon a single or CDC 2-tiered test result are turning their patients away with diagnoses that are at best, well-meaning but clueless, or at worst, humorous, insensitive, or insulting.

I challenge anyone to apply substantial research dollars and energy to the *cure for Lyme disease*, and not just provide band-aid philosophy funding or menial legislative changes designed by the insurance industry or pharmaceutical lobbyists, and their cohort advocates; but to study and provide an overt *cure.* And I challenge researchers, legislators and others to **accept now that chronic Lyme disease is real and to validate these patients and not dismiss us because we are dealing with real disease and we deserve better.**

Despite limited research that a handful of doctors or researchers might otherwise quote for their own interests, the body of scientific evidence combined with the "anecdotal" evidence (the clinical patients) is increasing exponentially, and holds the abundantly clear truth about Lyme disease. The patients will not be dismissed forever. Lyme disease is a persistent illness and you *will* have to deal with us at some point.

Lyme Patients Speak

In the course of preparing this book series, requests for stories went out over the internet to the United States, Canada and countries abroad. Many stories and emails were received from all sorts of people – all whom share a common illness, named Lyme disease. Their stories, though uniquely different in detail, share a common bond, one which should never have occurred. They all speak of a lack of credence for their symptoms and their inability to comprehend why physicians are ignoring them. Time and again their concerns were dismissed by physicians, family members and peers, often convincing the patients, at least for a time, that their illness was *"all in their head."*

In this day of medical science, diagnostic testing and gene mapping, one might be tempted to believe that medicine is infallible, reliable and definitive. Sadly, in the illness that is known as *Lyme disease*, this isn't the case. Denial, uncertainty, inaccurate testing methods, and political firestorms prevent patients from obtaining diagnoses, treatments and credibility. It is shameful and illogical when a patient can be treated for acne with long-term antibiotics; and cancer and terminally-ill patients are allowed to use "experimental" therapies…while Lyme patients are denied even basic antibiotics and treatments which are claimed to be "dangerous" or "unproven" according to a handful of people attempting to set global policy, and who seem to have other interests beside the patients, in mind.

The treating physician is often the first line of defense for these patients, and when insurance companies use pressure to prevent clinicians from diagnosing illnesses that are plainly visible, then health care for the population is in dire straits. When it is easier to obtain dangerous, psychotropic drugs for a diagnosis of "depression" when a patient has no signs or symptoms of such, simply because the physician doesn't have an answer, we have to ask what medical schools are teaching our doctors. When patients come to their doctors in hopes of ending chronic pain or bodily dysfunction and they are summarily turned away and told "not to worry," we have to wonder why we bother to visit them in the first place. Still the majority of physicians are sincere and earnest in their approach to patient care, and for those who willingly step outside the box of "mainstream" medicine, we applaud your courage.

There is one universal truth where it comes to patient care. Physicians who listen to their patients are generally rewarded with grateful people who try harder to get to their appointments, refer others to them, and work to get well. Meanwhile, it is the opinion of this author that physicians who readily dismiss their patients are not worth the paper their diplomas are printed on.

The Book I stories herein, are Lyme patient stories which attempt to illustrate what life is like when someone has to deal with Lyme disease in anything but its most acute form. Past the initial infection, when the organism has had a chance to disseminate into the body, this stage is commonly referred to as "chronic" Lyme disease. Opponents of the chronic Lyme "theory" who suggest that patients are "adequately" treated but that they go on to develop a "post-Lyme syndrome" will find that the stories in this book series leave us wanting explanations.

These individuals have clear symptom histories which, despite "adequate" treatment, never diminish, but steadily increase until one of many things happens. Either they receive repeated courses of long-term antibiotics (oral and/or IV); they receive combination antibiotic therapies; they attempt multiple so-called "alternative" treatments; or they go on to full-blown disability and are left without any ability to pursue long-term treatment. These patients and their families will be the first ones to report (along with their Lyme-treating physicians) that there is much more going on within their bodies than simply polymicrobial infection, or autoimmune response. The fact of the matter is that Lyme *borreliosis*, once inside the body, if it is not fully eradicated, can and does lie dormant and then reinfects or rather, continues to infect, patients when the immunological and environmental factors are favorable for a grand resurgence within the host organism.

In some of the stories, we can clearly see how the cognitive thinking and psychiatric behavior is altered, whether temporarily or permanently, by infectious disease attacking different portions of the brain. Perceptions become altered; what once seemed logical becomes illogical, and patients lose awareness of their surroundings and insight into their own behaviors. How others directly perceive these patients is a key factor in whether the ill patient's life is made easy, or more stressful. Interpersonal relations and communication become difficult when Lyme-infected. Family and friends must work to separate conflicting emotions and deal with the tasks at hand, like obtaining good medical care for their ill loved ones. The ability to overlook the ill person's shortcomings is mandatory when dealing with the chronic Lyme patient, for they often cannot help themselves; especially in the areas of fear, hostility, comprehension, or forgetfulness.

These are very honest and revealing stories about the chronic and neuropsychiatric aspects of Lyme disease, and we present them here for your analysis. These stories are true, detailed accountings of what these patients have been through, and are at times, emotional and powerful. Each patient tells their story in their own words, and hence each story has a unique feel. Please respect each persons' attempt to tell their story, and understand that these individuals are revealing themselves in order to teach others about the disease process.

Each person's journey with infectious disease is absolutely unique, which is why treatment options must remain open-ended and flexible. What works for one patient does miserably for another. This is the nature of the human body, and as such, the disease processes itself. Most of the individuals in Book I have *already spoken before some form of the media* about their illness. If not, I have presented them here because they clearly communicate important information. They are offered here for their strength of focus which has led their voices to become loud enough to be heard by many.

By joining collectively, the beginning of greater understanding may be brought to Lyme disease patients, and with that, better diagnostic and treatment options. For at this moment in time, (2007), treatment options are extremely narrow if they exist at all for many patients. Medical science simply *must do better* for patients, and it is our hope that through this book series of personal stories, the beginnings of understanding the nature of this illness can finally occur.

These patients not only face the issue of having to deal with chronic Lyme disease, but also they have had to deal with some of the "tougher" aspects of being ill. Family deaths, suicides, ignorance within the social and justice systems, and accusations of mental illness, "Munchausen's," (fabricating their own and their children's illnesses); custody issues and ignorance of medical professionals combine to weigh down the patient; exponentionally increasing their suffering. Some of these patients have been willing to try anything, and indeed have gone to other parts of the world in order to find a cure for Lyme disease.

Illness is multi-dimensional, as is the human animal. It is important that the mind/body/spirit connection be honored in all forms of medicine, though some forms of medicine seem to accommodate only one dimension – the physical body. Indeed, the emotional impact of illness upon the human psyche is complex and somewhat vague. And yet we have the power to reach into the black hole that is chronic and/or psychiatrically affecting illness and grasp the hand of the ill patient – with simple but effective tools like compassion and dedication which go far to support someone lost to a devastating illness such as neuropsychiatric Lyme disease.

If *one* patient is inspired with hope, or the knowledge that they are not alone after reading any of the stories herein, or if *one physician* learns to listen to his or her patient after reviewing same, then the suffering of these individuals, and the suffering of untold *thousands* will have been made a little easier to bear. It is our hope that the stories within this book series will become impactful teaching tools for patients, medical professionals and society members. We have ears, we need to listen, and not just hear. We have eyes, we need to see, and not just observe. We have minds, we need to use them to think outside the box, and not just memorize or repeat scientific rhetoric. We have the tools not only to diagnose, but to discern the truth and apply it to patient care. We have hearts, we need to exercise compassion toward our patients and family members; and stop telling them "It's All In Your Head."

❖ ❖ ❖

The Paradox of Lyme

Ryan Guerin, North Carolina

[Ryan's story is told posthumously by his family; and is narrated by his father]

Ryan Patrick Guerin was the youngest of four children. He was born in 1971 in Carmel, New York. He was a beautiful baby and by the time he attended first grade, he was developing a great interest for sports. He was a chubby little guy then, with curly hair and a great smile. Ryan was asthmatic almost from the time he was born, and was rushed to the emergency room on a number of occasions during his adolescent years. He was naturally very close to his mother, as were his siblings, as she spent a lot of time with them while they grew up. He looked forward to family gatherings, loved his dog, played baseball, and accepted going to the doctor's office once a week with his mom, for his allergy shot.

He was an above-average student during his elementary and middle school years, and enjoyed being in the cub scouts and playing sports both in school, and after school, around our neighborhood.

When Ryan was eleven years old, our first granddaughter was born. Needless to say, that tiny baby affected the family greatly, especially Ryan. All of a sudden most of the family's attention was now focused on our new addition. Also at this time we suffered the tragic death of his cousin. Looking back, while Ryan was growing up, he liked music very much. He dabbled in song writing as well as trying his hand at playing various instruments. In fact, he played the clarinet in the high school band.

As time went by, things seemed to settle down, except in hindsight I guess we took for granted that Ryan was also doing fine. Then when he was sixteen years old, Ryan and a friend ran away from home. We failed to recognize that he was not doing so well in school, and actually was beginning to get into trouble. Our two older sons set out to in search; and after four days, found both children in Virginia. I must say that family, friends and the power of prayer are powerful tools. We were so happy to have Ryan back home.

While Ryan was growing up, he liked music very much. He dabbled in song writing as well as trying his hand at playing various instruments. Ryan began to do well again in school. He was playing high school football and it seemed that he was looking forward to graduation and going to college. He achieved entry into Eastern Carolina State University (ECU), but as it turned out, he was not a successful college student. I guess partying was more important to him than academics. After a year and a half at ECU, Ryan dropped out and joined the U.S. Navy. The day he graduated from Navy boot camp in Orlando, Florida, we attended a church service on base at which he sang lead in the choir and led the congregation in song.

He was stationed aboard the Air Craft Carrier *Abraham Lincoln,* which was based in Alameda, California, and served in the Persian Gulf during the first Iraq War. While in the Navy, he taught himself to play the guitar and the piano. After four years of active service, he was honorably discharged and returned to civilian life, and once again we were happy to have him home.

We were all very surprised to hear how well he could play, and even more surprised to learn that he was writing songs. He actually cut a couple of disks (CDs) after coming out of the Navy. In hind sight, we see that God does have a plan because after all, it was while Ryan was in the Navy that he discovered that he had a drinking problem. The Navy placed him in a rehabilitation program which led to his journey with Alcoholics Anonymous, and he never drank against since that day in August, 1992.

After service, Ryan settled into civilian life, and after completing some courses in engineering, he was certified to operate unlimited tonnage air conditioning and heating systems. He was employed, as he progressed, at three different fortune 500 corporations as a Facilities Engineer.

During this time he fell in love with a girl, but he also became ill from Lyme disease. The illness was devastating. He was obviously diagnosed too late, although he began intravenous treatments. He was diagnosed with spinal meningitis at the same time. After a series of treatments, he began feeling better, and finally seemed to be "out of the woods." Unfortunately, he and his girlfriend broke up after that, which was devastating for him, although he seemed to recover well enough from that experience.

A friend and co-worker of Ryan's received a job offer from a North Carolina-based company and relocated here to the Charlotte area. Our older son Mike became interested in the area as well as Ryan, so they investigated the possibility of moving to North Carolina. My wife Vickie and I also explored the idea as we were planning to retire. After some serious thought, we decided to take the plunge. Once again, God's plan was in motion. During 2005, my wife and I, our four children, and all eight of our grandchildren moved from Putnam County, New York, to Mooresville, North Carolina. Only a miracle can explain how it all materialized.

Ryan accepted a position as a Project Manager with a fairly large corporation here in Charlotte. He purchased a condo on the fringe of Lake Norman, and also bought a boat which he enjoyed immensely. He loved his job, and he was sober and still very active in AA for the past thirteen years. Because of his loving and giving nature, he made many new friends at work. He was also very instrumental in helping many young people with substance abuse problems.

Then Lyme disease returned with a vengeance. He sought the help of the medical community, to no avail. Finally he heard about Dr. J in North Carolina. He began antibiotic treatment again, but this time through a picc line inserted near his heart.

He went on medical disability leave from work, and for a time Ryan thought he might be getting better. There was a time during this relapse when he could not even get off of his bed or sofa. My wife and I, as well as his brothers and sister, and nephews and nieces, would all bring him his meals; and friends were constantly looking in on him.

Just about the time he thought he was getting well, the Lyme attacked again, but this time it was worse than ever. He was brave and tried to hide the pain. He refrained as much as he could from taking pain medications because of his addictive nature, so he battled hard, even to the point of purchasing a small piece of property and struggling to be "normal."

But the pain was severe and disabling, and coupled with meningitis and encephalitis, it apparently left him with little hope. It's so mind-boggling how this insidious disease caused by a tiny tick, can cause such devastation.

His unquestioning faith in God and his unconditional love for others; his ongoing selflessness toward his family, friends and the addicted, is certainly a paradox inasmuch as Ryan chose to end his own life.

We are left with one main question, and that is **why?**

[Others easily come to mind.]

- Why isn't there more being done to research a *cure* for this insidious, almost evil disease?
- Why is there a 35% suicide rate associated with this disease?
- Why are concerned professionals being denied insurance in order to continue treatment for the affected?
- Why isn't the Congress of the United States passing laws to fund research for a cure?
- **Why does it seem like no authority really gives a damn?**
- Why did my 36-year old son have to die?

The paradox: Disease / Suicide v. Faith in God / Love of Man

– With love, the family of Ryan P. Guerin

❖ ❖ ❖

[Author note: the following story contains strong statements which are not necessarily the opinion of the author/editor or anyone else in this book. But in the interests of telling the patient stories objectively and from the Lyme patient's perspective, the contributor's opinion has been retained for the reader's examination. Be aware also that there is material here that may be disturbing to more sensitive readers.]

"Fear and Loathing" in Las Borreliosis

"T," Catawba County, North Carolina

[T's story was told in the September 2007 issue of Psychology Today *magazine by journalist Pam Weintraub.]*

Having Lyme disease has its up side. It allows you to experience firsthand, all the major themes of literature, from ancient Greek tragedies and comedies, to the themes of Shakespeare, and other great writers. Also mixed in are some of the seven "deadly sins," which I find rampant with this disease.

Love: of good doctors and good friends, the kind that stick around. Love also of family who helps out when the going is very tough, and of the times when you feel well.

Hate: of the disease and its process, and the ritualistic hunt for a good LLMD, the money to get there, to stay there; dealing with insurance companies, broken PICC lines, nurses who don't wash their hands, hospital doctors who refuse you your first mandated hospital delivery of a new IV drug, then write a letter to your primary caregiver telling them you don't need it, you don't have "*LYME'S*" and that you are considered drug-seeking (for antibiotics!)

Envy: of those who are cured right away, or who find a good doctor, or have tons of money and life is a bit easier for them, if that exists. Or envy of those who manage to stay healthy.

Gluttony: Those ticks really engorge themselves, don't they?

Abandonment: That's easy, no need to elaborate there.

Humor: If you are lucky enough to survive the first year of treatment, you find a sense of humor that tends to run to the low end of the spectrum (movies you never thought you would laugh at) and the sick-o end – the jokes that really make you laugh, as you have been there.

Tragedy: Seeing a child suffer, or worse; your own child, and watching those you know who have this disease, but choose not to pursue it, despite your efforts to help, go downhill.

Victory: In knowing someone who has beaten this disease, who is well, or "well-er," able to continue with their life, or having a courageous, optimistic doctor who pushes and cajoles you into taking your medicine and getting better. That happens, and it happened to me.

Betrayal: It happens all too often, by many in and out of the medical system. It's painful, yet part of life. Just because we are sick doesn't mean we get any respect or sympathy from anyone.

Despair: The luxury of complaining about treatment isn't ours. We are too busy trying to find it, fund it, and keep it to complain much. Despair usually takes place among us in private. The dark deep hole of depression that comes with disease is so bad, and so black, that I rarely meet anyone who can fess up to the depths of their despair. Just be assured, if you have been there and thought things, so has everyone else.

Hope: A wonderful, renewable gift that we can receive from others, our LLMDs, our advocates, our God, and our families.

Fortitude: This disease either gives it to you if you don't have it, or takes it away if you do. This comes and goes and is a daily process sometimes. We learn to borrow from others when we are low, and give to others when we are strong, or fake it when we don't have anything left, simply because we know strength is a commodity not measured, but is a mystery to give and receive. It is the best gift.

Character: Our character is enhanced when we get sick. It's a process of seeing what is there, building on it, losing it, realizing we have lost it, and working to gain it again. It's a work in progress.

Lust: This happens when I remember the times before I was sick, how I could do things without paying a huge price. I could teach art, I could dance all night. I could ride my horse into the wind, bareback, not caring about a thing. And not hurting afterward. I lust after those times.

✢ ✢

Three weeks ago on a Tuesday afternoon, I got hit by lightning. It was by far the best thing that had happened to me all day. I had been to a therapist, one that I had to see in order to see a new Psychiatrist. The one I had for the past three years was moving away. I had completed the intake a month prior, and on this day was seeing him for the first time. During the session I had laid out the bullet points of the previous year.

He told me that many of those things were just unbelievable and that I was either "delusional or had one helluva story to tell." I told him that part of my story had already been told in the September 2007 issue of *Psychology Today* in an article about Munchausen by Proxy mothers. He responded by telling me that **in order to see the Psychiatrist there, I would have to prove that I had "Lyme's" disease**.

(We really should give in and just change the name of the disease to the possessive noun form. Any time I hear someone say "Lyme's," I know I am talking to someone who doesn't know anything about Lyme.)

"Here we go again," I thought. I am here for an unrelated (sort of) health or medical issue and I am being questioned about the presence of Bb in my body. Good GOD woman, don't mention Bartonella, nor the fact that it took three years, four antibiotics, a great doctor and much intestinal fortitude to rid oneself of Babesia (no sir I have not traveled to any exotic lands) and both Ehrlicheas...that just confuses them more.

Though I had heard similar things many times, I still was too taken aback to respond right away, other than to request that our next meeting *not* include a Lyme discussion. I have privately sworn *not* to educate any more ignorant, closed-minded medical practitioners. They certainly must own computers and more than likely know how to do a "search."

About an hour later I was sitting in my car beneath two electric poles, waiting for my daughter to come out of the feed store, when it began to rain in a downpour. I stuck my hand out the window and touched the top of the car to wet my fingers which were covered with oil from some terribly good southern fried chicken, a treat not usually partaken of by me, having taken on the shape of an engorged tick from being sick and in treatment for many years. BOOM!! "Someone" hit my hand with a large wooden stick which sent an interesting jolt up my arm, past my elbow and then up into my neck and head. Was there someone behind a grassy knoll? No, I think that was lightning...uh oh. That was on my "bad side," too.

I have *Neuroborreliosis* and it likes to mess around with the right side of my body. That night I felt the stroke-like symptoms come and go. I felt the electrical "burn," felt the pain and tried to talk on the phone to a friend, who indeed thought I was having a stroke. My daughter gave me a B complex shot, and I took my medication that is just for this very thing, and waited it out. So really, the best thing that had happened to me all day, besides the illegal fried chicken, was the blast from the sky. A wake up call came from Donner, Thor, or God as I understand Him. "Get the hell out of that office..." (I hear you loud and clear, madam or sir, thank you.)

The next day I could talk well enough to leave the therapist a voice mail. I said that I felt I did not need to prove to him or anyone that I have Lyme, and that it was perhaps a bit discriminatory of him. If I had said HIV/AIDS, or MS, or Parkinson's, would he demand the same of me? I think not. My other Psychiatrists or any of my therapists have not asked for proof. In fact, three of them had Lyme. I told him I had ordered a lab kit from a good lab in California and needed to be tested again anyway, as I had been exposed to five tick bites this spring while staying somewhere else. I could bring the lab slip in for him to sign, and we could see for ourselves what was frolicking around in my body. That got a quick response from him, negative to the tenth degree: **"Oh no, we don't do that kind of thing here."**

I thought, well, gee, you have told me that from what you have read, a month of treatment cures "Lyme's," and my last test was three years ago, so why not, let's do this test. All you have to do is sign the lab slip, you don't have to treat me. I already have a doctor for that but I do need a Psychiatrist now, so I'll bring that lab slip in. That didn't work. He said the three-year-old test would be fine. I called back two days later and said I have found another Psychiatrist (though I will have to travel 60 miles, she is highly recommended) and I do not wish to continue therapy, thank you very much. I got a "cover-my-ass" letter from him a few days later.

We have all been-there-done-that-got-the-tee-shirt. Just change the names, locations, but not the disease. For you I will revisit this mucky nasty past that Lyme has left, and bring dear readers to the future. The author of this book assured me I could tell the truth and nothing less, and it would not be edited except for obvious names. The truth as I see it has gotten me kicked off the most famous of Lyme cyberspace networks that really doesn't want you to tell the truth, unless it suits them and the association behind it.

I joined an elite crowd fairly early in the game when I wrote an in-depth article about a doctor and his renowned neurotoxin web site, where for only $8.95 he could tell you, if indeed you have Lyme or not (having "borrowed" a visual contrast test from a reputable and accomplished vision scientist). He really ticked me off. That doctor no longer claims to be able to cure Lyme, at least not on his web site, which is good, as many of the people who went to see him got dropped by their insurance, and when his treatment didn't work, they got sicker and returned to their old LLMD's and low and behold had a heck of a time getting coverage again.

The advocates that helped them were really not happy about all of that. We all got kicked off the Lyme board then, so I was in good company. We have badges of honor and secret meetings once in a while where we swear to uphold the truth and tell our experiences no matter what. The article was to be published in a Lyme magazine, but when a very famous and beloved doctor included a nod in his new guidelines to this doctor, I asked the editor to pull the article. I did not want a good doctor being hurt at that time in particular, as he had just gone through the wringer, having spoken to a Congressional Hearing about the Lyme epidemic and was promptly punished in a cruel and long, drawn out way. I owe my life to Dr. B – a good man to the core.

The article did find its way to a few internet sites before I was banished from those too. I had learned a tremendous amount during the 4 months I feverishly toiled away at researching, interviewing, fact-finding, and driving everyone in my life *nuts* with the things I found out. I was crushed and astounded at first, but then got used to the fact that some "doctors, lawyers, and Indian chiefs" can lie, and the patient be damned. "Show me the money" seemed to be their motto, and if not money, then some type of fame might do.

To begin at the beginning, using 20/20 hindsight and my now informed brain to the likings of this disease, it seems I first showed symptoms probably in high school. Having graduated in 1970 in North Carolina, I then proceeded to college in the same state, and earned three degrees in art: a Bachelor's, Master's and a teaching certification. I topped out my testing into graduate school by making the highest score on one test that the secretary of the Art School at East Carolina University had ever seen. It was the Miller's Analogy Test. It had been fun and I had been finished in about 20 minutes.

I knew in high school that something was amiss, as the guidance counselor, (in her only meeting with me), told me my IQ was around 145, give or take some points. All I knew is that I was terribly bored, and wanted out of that small town. My horse had been fatally injured my junior year, and with all the stuff going on at my home, I was ready to get out of town. I remembered having to pick a lot of ticks off my horse and myself. They got as big as grapes and would burst before I could totally remove them. Who knew not to let the blood get on me? Who knew Babesia came not only from an exotic land, but also from the blood of horses (and also their urine, for those who don't know).

In college, I continued to spend as much time outside as possible, camping, riding, rolling around in the grass, hiking, and gardening. I continued to suffer from bouts of depression which would roll over me almost in a tangible way, like a curtain coming down. That can still happen, but it's only when I am much too stressed out emotionally, and I take a break when I see it coming. It took almost 30 years for me to say "uncle" to that feeling. I always worked so hard in school, not wanting to accept anything less than an "A" in my art classes. I also "partied" hard then, which probably didn't help my immune system.

In 1983 I had moved to a house in the country, and realized one day there were ticks crawling all around the head of my bed and on the window sill. I moved out as fast as possible, but not before some strange things started happening which pushed me into my first ever medical work up, at the wonderfully comprehensive medical school at ECU. The only test I flunked was called a visual contrast test. The very kind Neurologist said that this was just a diagnostic tool which told him something was wrong with my neurological system. At the time, it was the definitive test for MS. Thank goodness I did not know that, or I would have caved in and not lived to become the horrid pain in the backside of so many MD's that I am now.

I went on with my life, as well as I could. I taught for the defense department schools in Germany for four years, and met and married a German National. I got very sick somewhere along the way, and into my fourth year had already had several miscarriages, including twins. Fatigue was a way of life, and my panic attacks had returned. I quit drinking, went to AA, went to a therapist, did everything. I had constant upper respiratory infections and pneumonia several times. It got so bad that I had to resign my job, and in shame, hanging my head, (especially after a near-successful suicide attempt), I went back to the states.

My daughter was born nine months later in Pensacola, Florida. After 8 miscarriages, I was almost in disbelief that she was here. Miranda *(a pseudonym)* had a spinal tap before she was two hours old. Seven doctors stood around my bed, with me exhausted after 32 hours of labor, and they had me sign off on a spinal tap, which was negative for menigitis. They treated her aggressively for an infection of unkown origin and put the fear of God in me, that if she ran a fever during her first two years, to skip the doctor and go straight to the ER.

When she was two, we moved up to Cape Cod. We stayed there for most of her formative years. I got sicker and sicker, and after many misdiagnoses, was sent to Dr. D who tested me though BBI labs. I was found to have about 17 markers for Lyme. He started me on a combination of antibiotics, warned me of the herxheimer, and somewhere into my second bedridden week of pain, I remember him mumbling the words "will feel like shingles" and he was right, I guess. I only remember elderly women that I sewed for asking me to bring their clothes to them, as they had shingles and couldn't get out of the house. Gee, what the heck was that? *Pain*. That's what it is, nerve pain. I lived with it and still do on occasion.

Well, one day about three weeks into it, the herx stopped. I got out of bed, and on with life, sort of. I got better until I was switched to tetracycline, which did nothing for me. I got worse and worse and I knew I was going to die. Sometime along the road Miranda started verbalizing about her symptoms, and so I had her tested. She was also positive for Lyme. Who knew it was congenital?

Her treatment started, but the tetracycline did nothing for her. Finally, one day I got up enough guts to take her to Dr. J, the renowned Lyme pediatrician. I felt like I was sneaking around, knowing the other doctor seemed very possessive of his patients, and indeed, he did scream at me when he found out that Miranda was in the care of Dr. J, who brought her along to remission in about 3 years. She did well. I started seeing Dr. B, and was finally tested for co-infections (I had them all). We got the party started with IV, IM and orals. Three years of mepron topped off with bicillin, rifampin, rocephin, two pick lines, and one groshung. Somewhere in there came the birth of "Ticktoons" *[T.R. draws humorous tick cartoons.]* He got me free of Babesia and the Ehrlicheas, but I didn't start feeling really human until he started treating me for Bartonella. That did the trick. I remain on a "cocktail" of IV, IM and oral antibiotics, and I do well unless my treatment is interrupted. It has been, on a few occasions, and each time I have gone downhill fast. I would be the poster gal for Parkinson's if my treatment for Lyme was discontinued.

About a year after remission, Miranda was in a car accident in which she suffered a concussion. Slowly but surely her symptoms returned. It took a year, but we finally got another Lyme test done. Dr. J was beginning to feel some heat from the powers that be (i.e. those who would deny us our lives and right to treatment) and required several positive tests before he would retreat her. We obtained those, but it took a second mortgage on my condo, and treatment was limited.

A contact from high school in North Carolina told me about another doctor. I read about his treatment protocol on his website, posted on a Lyme board, asked a lot of questions, and got no negative feedback. Dr. B merely said in his kind and diplomatic way, that I could still continue to be his patient if I moved to North Carolina. We made a preliminary trip, met with the doctor and his team, looked at real estate, and my tiny condo on Cape Cod got me a five-acre farm in NC. We had horses, land, pasture, trails, open air, and treatment within 30 miles, for both of us! How wonderful...until...

Due to financial concerns (not ours) we were denied IV treatment. I had been a home IV patient for years, and with the regimen I was on, was doing very well. I was nearly symptom-free. Miranda on the other hand, was intolerant at that point of any oral antibiotics. She knew at the young age of 13 that she needed IV treatment if she was going to get better. She had been taking bicillin shots, but a wrongly placed needle set off tremendous nerve pain in her that to this day prohibits the delivery of bicillin, which requires a large gauge needle, and a long one. I myself was so afraid of them that I put it off for nearly six months. Once on them I wish I had started right away. They returned my mind to me, and my intelligence, and my depression began to lift. Again, those things have become controllable *unless* I lose treatment or am under too much stress. Then I can have problems, and it's a daily regimen, watch out for stress...it's real and it will get you.

And there is the "Catch-22." How can a single mother on disability raise a daughter who is also chronically ill and avoid stress? Answer: she can't. Stress took its toll on me and my daughter so many times. To even think of all the problems, denials of treatment, and doors slammed in our faces, is stressful.

The second doctor soon passed my calls and our appointments onto his panel of co-workers, and each sang a different song but all to the same denial tune. No IV, no this, no that. Finally I was told that he would provide back-up treatment if we found an out-of-state doctor. Well, that ride home contained all the cuss words in the universe. It took me five weeks to secure an appointment for my daughter with a doctor in another state. Then when it came time for the appointment, I called to make sure I had the date and time right, and I was told by her secretary that I had called the day before and cancelled it due to money concerns. I said no, you must have me confused with someone else. This appointment is for my daughter, and I would sell my blood (ha ha) to get her there. The time was still open, so we went.

Miranda was ordered on IV and also on oral vancomycin, which is the only oral antibiotic that she can tolerate. She got much better, but had problems with her port due to improper access by a home health nurse. She eventually had to have it taken out, but she got in nearly a year of IV treatments and got much better. She also got a lump in her breast, and of course the denial machine was in full force there too. No one would take it seriously. It took two years for anyone to really take it seriously, and by then so much more had happened that made that little lump seem like nothing.

In the meantime, I had also secured my first appointment with the new doctor, and she continued my regimen of medication. (I had previously begged my primary care from Cape Cod to write my IV orders for a bit, and she granted me six months, bless her.) She knew me well, and saw me get better, and also saw a practitioner in her own office go from a productive intelligent provider of health care, to a bundle of pain who couldn't leave her couch due to a tick bite. So many doctors find out about Lyme in this manner. But she was wonderful and got me back on treatment. I had gone terribly down hill in the five months I was off of treatment.

After Miranda had her port out, she remained on just the orals, and seemed to do all right until she was the victim of an attempted assault on her life from a young man in her church group. After that, she developed some pretty serious symptoms of PTSD. I got her into counseling and into a Psychiatrist's office. I kept a close eye on her, but though she told me things were all right, I didn't think they were. She took an overdose of medications in July of our second year here on the farm. I took her for help and they put her in a psych ward for four days, which did her absolutely no good at all. In fact she was assaulted there by a "doctor" or someone who was playing doctor; and the Psychiatrist on board was emotionally battering. He refused to move past the diagnosis of Lyme.

Miranda was discharged against medical advice when she told me she was given a breast exam in a strange room, lingered over by a big, tall, bald man who had an "MD" badge. No one of that description works on that unit, nor was the room used for anything but storage. Nevertheless, I believed her and still do. She continued with therapy, but the following October after many weeks of running a fever and a recent visit to our LLMD (who wrote a long note about the breast lump, would someone please take it seriously) she underwent diagnostic tests for endometriosis, such big things for such a young girl.

After my daughter's initial visit and my last orders for IV had run out, I was "kicked out" of the doctor's practice. This had never happened to me before. I had since been to see the doctor myself, and had continuing orders for my therapy, but not without the same problem as before. My appointment had again been cancelled a few days before we were to return. I had been in the habit for some years of keeping a book-size calender with me, and wrote all appointments down in the book. I also would tape (and keep) cards, contact numbers, fax info, all of that, in the back of my books. I have kept them all, so I can trace the history of appointments, changes in medications, onset of symptoms, or visits to the ER, things like that. So, I was in the habit of calling to make sure my appointments with the LLMD were set, and we would show up on time. I often had used *Angel Flight* to travel, and those pilots need not make a trip for a fouled up appointment time, so I always double-checked important issues.

For the second time, our appointment had been cancelled. I set up a password with the secretary, and called the clinic. I asked that all records be sent to me, and that no one contact our current LLMD. The only people on the planet who knew the "who, when," and "where," were employees at the clinic. Even my family didn't know the name and exact whereabouts of our current LLMD.

I was sent our records, and along with them, some pages with names and phone numbers of other patients; their test results and diagnoses (there goes HIPAA). I did contact those patients to let them know, and I returned their records to them. I wondered how many of *my* records went somewhere else. When I did get my records, they read like fiction. There were so many mistakes I couldn't count them all. I had briefly worked as a medical transcriptionist on Cape Cod, and never would I have passed the course if I had completed tests in that way. I wondered how many other mistakes were made from that clinic.

It wasn't long after that, big news hit. One of my nurses, and a friend, called me to say my doctor was on TV. It was the beginning of a long and probably (for him), painful profile in the media. He had a patient arrested. It was a dentist from Statesville. I called the TV station and got his name from the reporter, and called the dentist. He was very forthcoming, and told me the horrid story of what happened to him and his family at the hands of this doctor. His entire family had Lyme, and they too had moved from up north to see a doctor who would care for his entire family. It turned sour quickly. He told me of another practitioner in Statesville who had also suffered maltreatment, so I knew I was not the only one.

At the same time, a friend was planning on moving from Illinois to North Carolina to obtain treatment for herself and her children, who were about the same age as mine. I advised her not to. She, like myself, had heard nothing negative about the doctor until I told her what I knew, and that her hopes for obtaining IV treatment with a medicine that in the past had worked wonders for her, would probably be dashed. Desperation kicked in for her, and she moved, only to have her family nearly fall apart under the stress of it all. She has since moved back and is seeing a very kind, thorough LLMD in Missouri. As of a few months ago, she was starting to improve. It had been a long, slow slide from near-death for her.

Our current LLMD asked me, when I went to the first visit, if that same doctor was a good doctor, in my experience, and why was I there? I had the best insurance to cover treatment that one can have. I was asked what pushed me another 8 hours from home, when a man held in such esteem was so close to where I lived. I answered, "I really do not know if he is a good practitioner or not. He is brilliant, but he never really took care of us, was not forthcoming, and there remains that unanswered mystery of why he would not treat us with IV. I don't wish to talk more about him, but I would like to continue to see you. My daughter is much improved already, and it is worth the drive to come here."

Turns out my former clinic had its own IV pharmacy and IV treatment clinic. I didn't know that, as Medicare restricted me from being treated on-site. I could however, have continued IV therapy at home, which I had done for many years, and continue to do presently. The only conclusion my nurses and current IV pharmacist could come to about why I was refused IV treatment, was perhaps there wasn't any money in it for the doctor. I called Medicare and NC Medicaid numerous times, and would get the same answer. All the doctor would have needed to do was call in the orders, and I could have continued.

In my opinion, regardless of what he did at his clinic, on his property, he could still have this done for me. I did meet, through e-mail, two patients for whom this was done; one a doctor from South Carolina, and one woman from Colorado. The other patients lived within a day's driving distance at the most, and I know of several patients who would drive to pick up IV medications to last them two weeks or so. They would have to pay enormous sums, and had to learn "gravity drips." No pumps were issued. **That is the drawback that Medicare told me held back my orders. Medicare will not allow patients to use the "gravity drip" method; as with most medications, it is not safe.**

Imagine this: a sleepy, forgetful, sick Lyme patient hooking up an IV pole and starting the drip. When the drip is finished, the patient is asleep. No beep goes off, there is no warning bell for an air bubble, and no safety measures. When the IV has run its course, it then begins to suck back, and will start to fill the bag with the patient's blood. I spoke with several patients who had this happen, and it terrified them. They would have to have a family member sit with them during their IV, which some days can take hours.

They also were trained at the clinic to change their own dressings, a *huge* no-no in my opinion if you have a PICC line. It is nearly impossible to do this yourself without dislodging the line. Infection rate goes way up. The only advantage to this is that a doctor would be protected, or would maybe stand to earn the money that a home IV nursing company would receive. So, for stating the facts as told to me by Medicare, Medicaid and professional agencies, I was kicked off of a Lyme board. (I had joined again just to post about this doctor). This Lyme board is supposedly "the place to go" to get all your questions answered. But, what if in my opinion, it is run by an organization with its own agenda? Suppose the agenda is not really to help us poor old sick Lymies, but to prevent legislation from passing, or amending legislation that has been painstakingly written to include phrases like "the insurance company will determine the length of course of treatment."

What if I feel someone from the organization has meetings with the CDC and won't disclose what is discussed. What if I know that someone hired a private investigator to check on the claims of the leader of the organization and the PI finds no record of the children upon whom the association was founded in their honor, or whom were said to both have Lyme and life was made hard because it was so difficult to find treatment? What if, after all these years, we have, in my opinion, been backing a group which isn't actually helping patients, but may be holding us back in some way? And, what if I feel I have nothing left to lose by saying this?

Meanwhile, back at the ranch, my daughter was suffering terribly. It was summer, and she was getting sicker and sicker. She had fevers every day, no energy, and insomnia. Her Psychiatrist, who was so helpful, had moved on. She had changed church youth groups to get away from the young man who had tried to harm her, and had poured her heart, soul and precious energy into serving that church. She dragged herself out of bed every Sunday morning to go, would volunteer for everything she could, and made it to the Wednesday night youth group meetings.

Too bad that one of the richest people in the area had a daughter who set my child up to be the recipient of slander. Her photograph was posted on a *My space* internet page of another young man we had never heard of. Along with that photo were pornographic pictures. We knew nothing for months. The following November, Miranda received some very purient requests for more images to be sent to a cell phone. She brought me her cell phone, dumbfounded at what she was hearing. I listened to the two calls, and wrote down the numbers, and did a 4-1-1 reverse phone number look up. It turned out to be the same girl in her youth group who had befriended her, whose family has more money than anyone, who set her up.

We took appropriate steps to end it all, yet in January, during a ski trip, it came to light it had not ended. Once again the law was called, I ended up in the hospital with what appeared to be a stroke (it was a worsening of Lyme seizures which have now become a bigger problem). But for Miranda, it was the beginning of a slow, downward spiral. Nearly all adults in her life, in some fashion, had abandonded her. Neither minister at either church would own up to what had happened.

Despite her constant pain and lack of energy, she put everything into that church, her home school program, and her horses, which she intends to pursue as a career. She has a natural talent for training horses. Much to be jealous of, and a lot there that others her age might want to have. Perhaps envy or hatred was in the hearts of those who went about systematically to destroy her reputation.

Sexual abuse is soul-eating abuse; it is the gift that keeps on "giving," and takes chunks out of your self esteem. Pornography is no exeption. What is the problem is the law concerning minors in this state. If the offenders are within 4 years of age of the victim, no "crime" is committed. Let me state that again, *no "crime" has been committed.* So, unless we wanted to pursue the matter in civil court, nothing really would happen to the perpetrators, who admitted that this was done as a "joke."

Miranda stood up for herself at a meeting that she called at the church, and one of the youth group leaders quit, in disgust. She walked out of the meeting before it was over. My daughter was left in that room with no one to defend her, but herself. What a strong person. Over time, pressure got to her. Pressure to continue going to that church. Pressure to forgive, although no one had asked for forgiveness, and pressure from the minister to deny it all. There was so much pressure and so much sadness, I was so afraid of what she might do to herself.

Knowing about this illness, and knowing the depression and the deep dark bottomless hole we all read about really exists with this, and having been there and come out with treatment, and having recovered, made it all the more difficult to watch helplessly as my daughter went further and further downward. She refused to change therapists to one who might help her a bit more, and in October of that year, she took a tremendous overdose which could have killed her many times over. I happened to come into the house to ask her where she might have left a tool, and found her, non-responsive in her bed.

I immediately called 9-1-1 while I tested her gag response. There was none. She was rushed to the hospital, and immediately intubated, her stomach was pumped, and treated successfully. I took a short break from her bedside, after she had regained consciousness the next morning. Her hands and feet were tied to the bed. She was still intubated. I reassured her that I would be right back, as a family member was calling. Not five minutes went by when I returned to the CCU and there I saw the minister from that church, Pastor "Denial," leaving her curtained room. I was infuriated. I asked him what he was doing there. He said he had free-roaming privileges at the hospital. (I found out later they don't know who he is, and he is not on the visiting pastoral list.) Regardless, I had informed him previously he was never to speak to my daughter again. Yet there he was, in her room, while she was tied and intubated. When I got in there, she motioned for something to write on. Miranda wrote: "Keep him the hell away from me!"

I calmed her down, and told her he would not be back. The nurses came in and began to extubate her. They then took away her blankets, as she had a fever, and they could not transport her until she had no fever. They gave her Tylenol and left her cold in her bed. I lost it. I started screaming to get her a blanket and warm her up. Little did I know it was just for their convienence to ship her out. She had chest pain and a fever and I was concerned since she had vomited and aspirated over the tube several times, that she might have fluid in her lungs. They refused an X-ray. They shipped her out in handcuffs to another county, and put her in the psych ward.

She continued to have a fever and chest pain, and upon lab results they realized she had a urinary tract infection. So an antibiotic was ordered, which was one that in the past had given her leaky gut and terrible stomach pains. She refused to take it by mouth. Miranda was the one who asked for an IV, and I agreed that would probably be a good idea. What a mistake. Who knew that asking for an IV in a hospital would prove difficult. Miranda was afraid in two ways. She was afraid that the medication would cause her the stomach and gut problems, and she was afraid that those problems would be seen as "failure to cooperate" and that she would once again be tied up.

When Miranda would have this problem at home, with food or as a result of some medication, she would not want to go to the ER. I have had the problem too and I know the pain. Labor is not as painful as the overwhelming nausea, cramping, and projectile diarrhea. There were times when I asked her just to stay outside the bathroom door. I wouldn't be able to move, much less try to go to the hospital. I would hang on to the towel rack, or push against the wall, riding out the pain. So I knew what she was afraid of.

No one cared. I would not budge from that hospital. They sent the head of nursing up. The on-call pediatrician was in the ER and would not order an IV. I found out later it would mean discharging her from the psych unit, and admitting her to the hospital. In other words, it was too much paperwork. So they let her suffer, but finally ordered up the liquid form of Cipro, which Miranda said would still have to go through her stomach. They made me leave, but at midnight the head nurse called, and told me the medication had arrived and she was taking it down to Miranda. She also said she would tell her that if she didn't take it, they could hold her there for up to six months.

Then the crying started for me. It didn't stop for nearly a year. Things got very bad after that night. They wouldn't let me speak to my daughter, to tell her she had the right to refuse any treatment, period. (Later I found out she already knew that.) I had encouraged her before I left, to try to sip the medication and spoke to the nursing staff to please take any sign of a gut problem seriously. They threw me out. I was a thorn in their side, a pain in the ass, a mother who cares. Take me out and put me in front of the firing squad. God forbid that my daughter should be treated with kindness. God forbid she get the help she needs.

The next day I got a ride over to the hospital with a nurse friend. I was told I was not allowed to see my daughter for the remainder of the stay. My friend went in to visit her, and since she was a nurse, was able to check her out fairly well. She had taken one fourth of the medicine, and it had caused stomach problems. I urged my friend to tell her to keep trying, even the tiniest sip. That was on a Saturday. The following Monday morning she was released. The discharge papers said "no depression," but "stress" and "anxiety."

Tuesday afternoon, we returned home from running errands to find a card from DSS on our back door. I called, and they wanted to send someone to the house. "Standard proceedure in a suicide attempt," they told me. I had never heard of that.

Miranda had said in the hospital that she was "sick of being sick," and that she was "sick of having Lyme." Certainly understandable, and on top of that, with the sexual victimization and subsequent abandonment by the church, its leaders, and her friends there, she was certainly lined up for feeling badly. Her therapist was less than helpful. Little did I know that the therapist was also a direct pipeline to DSS.

I had never dealt with DSS except as a teacher, being a mandated reporter of abuse, I sometimes had to call them. Other than that, I knew nothing of them or what they are really all about. I do know now. I was always puzzled at some of the questions on forms at LLMD offices, in particular, "have you ever had legal problems from having Lyme disease." Well, I was about to enter the biggest fight of my life, not because of Lyme, but because of the denial of it.

The following day, I suggested to the social worker that we meet at the library. I didn't know much, but intuition told me not to meet at our home. We did talk, and she interviewed Miranda alone. She asked her about "Lyme's" (here we go again) and told Miranda that *she* had it in the past. She said her dentist had treated her with antibiotics for two years straight for gum disease, and did Miranda think that could have helped her with her "Lyme's" disease? Miranda, smart girl that she is, was friendly but guarded. She said it *may* have helped. She asked many more questions, but I limited the time as I was concerned what might be going on and what wording might also be misconstrued.

I asked the social worker what exactly were her concerns. The case worker then uttered words which sent a dagger of fear deep into my heart, followed closely by the knowledge that we would not win this, and that if I fought in court too long, that it would probably kill me. She said that **DSS was concerned that I was treating my daughter for a disease she didn't have, and that I was not having her treated for depression. I knew that meant "Munchausen's By Proxy," and no way out.**

First, both statements are untrue on several levels. *I don't treat my daughter for any illness and never have, the doctors do.* And she had been seen for depression and followed along with that, for years. But just to cover their tracks, they tacked on a myraid of other accusations, like medical neglect. How can I take her to the doctor too much, and then not take her enough…oh never mind. I used to work for the federal government and anything can be said or done without it making a lick of sense.

They insisted on coming to our house. I was frantic, as I knew enough by virtue of having been an advocate for many years, and knowing other Lyme mothers who had "Munchausen By Proxy" charges leveled upon them. **No one ever wins, ever. Their kids are taken, the mothers go to jail, and their Lyme gets worse.** That much I knew. I didn't however, know my rights. I did think that I had the right *not* to let anyone in my house unless I wanted to, unless they had a court order.

I checked with the county sheriff's office, and the officer said I was correct, and furthermore, if it were him he wouldn't let those people into *his* house. He would make them get a search warrant, and bring a law officer. He said basically that most law enforcement cannot stand DSS and hate to work with them.

Well, all of them except who is usually termed the "kid snatcher" – he's the one who grabs your kids...he kidnaps them in the name of the law. The one who was dispatched to my home **entered forceably with no warrant, and hit me.** The social worker who gave him the call to come here knew my daughter had already run away, yet she sent him anyway. He was exonerated in an internal affairs investigation. No harm, no foul play, no warrant, who cares. **I am just an overweight loudmouth mother bear who dares to suggest that someone follow the law.**

When I suggested to the social worker that she come with a search warrant, she was aghast (or at least gave a good perfomance). Perhaps no one had ever reminded her of the first amendment rights given to us by our Constitution, but they do exist. I asked her to please see the magistrate, get a search warrant, and come on to the house with a law officer.

I was thinking, what would go on the search warrant? Are they looking for *antibiotics?* How ridiculous of course, as surely that would never be granted. I know to this day, had I stuck to my inclinations, that it would have been dropped right then and there. DSS refused, and I refused. I said I would be happy to let them in with the warrant and an officer. I hired a lawyer (big mistake). Better to find out your rights through one of the internet groups, but be careful there too. MAMA, CPS watch, and AFRA all have excellent web sites and you can gather information and find out your rights.

I eventually caved in. The social workers were so nice, the lawyer accused me of being paranoid. I told him that it didn't matter if he thought I was paranoid, there still might be something to be afraid of. I fired him when he wanted yet more money, but by that time my daughter had run away. We had let DSS into the house three times and they told me each time that they "just wanted to see this or that," and would then drop the case. But each time they lied, and things got worse. HIPAA laws were broken so many times. Family lawyers can work very well, but only in family court, not for the client. (Mine actually returned most of the money I had paid him...maybe he does have a conscience.)

The next few months, (nearly a year), is a blurr and a nightmare. I cannot talk about much of it. I cried myself to dehydration a few times. My daughter hid out at different places for many months. The court tried each month to put me in jail for contempt. Contempt didn't begin to touch what I felt about family court. Go sit in court for a day and see what does go on there. See for yourself. It is horrible. **Families are torn apart, kids are ripped out of mother's arms.** Babies are taken from delivery rooms into custody. The death rate is sky-high in foster care homes.

Not one part of our lives has gone untouched. We will probably lose our farm. DSS got my daughter's SSI allotment and it has never been returned. In fact, yesterday I got a notice that I have been overpaid. Our broodmare lost her foal and my horse was attacked when I had to leave her quickly, and place the horses where I thought they would be safe during this process. They were not. In two weeks, years of conditioning were undone. Many things were taken from my property – just stolen while we were away. Gates, tools, our saddles and tack, lawn mowers, and flower pots. The total damage done is too lengthy and painful to list.

Worst of all is the damage done to Miranda. My daughter, at the time of this writing, has left home. She dodged DSS and their stormtroopers by getting married at the age of 16. Unfortunately, she married #6 on the list, not the first choice by any means. He is 11 years her senior, and a master manipulator.

He managed to seperate us, and had her in another part of the state for 3 weeks before they married in South Carolina. Her head is twisted and turned and yet if DSS had gotten her, she would be locked up in a psychiatric ward, deemed crazy (their words, not mine) because (now read closely), ***thinks she has "Lyme's" disease.***

Test results, and letters from her LLMD, none of that matters. What does matter is that the mother of one of her friends, works at the hospital that she was transferred to, and heard that there was a girl in for attempted suicide that "thinks she has Lyme's disease." This woman made it her business to try to see her, but wasn't allowed. She did make it her business to talk to the other nurses on staff, and did make the initial report to DSS. She also got herself signed up as a foster caregiver (read: money) and tried to have Miranda turned over to *her*. She wanted me to convince Miranda to live with her. I said no thanks. If she goes into the foster care system she can be removed from a foster care home for no reason at any time, and they probably won't tell me where she is.

DSS had all the paperwork ready for *me* to pay someone else child support. That's the way the system works. I never signed anything, and I believe the original case worker, who was supposed to have me sign a safety plan, got into big trouble over that.

Now, after a year of hiding out and full of stress from every angle... Miranda has heart problems, worsened anxiety and PTSD. She is also in the hands of a controlling, abusive man who has a criminal record three inches thick.

I have had many fingers pointed at me, and have been called a lot of names...and as a mother that goes to the core of my being. As a human, I am getting past that. It's easy to label people, and believe the worst of them. It is harder to dig for the truth, and the friends I have now, new and old, know the real deal about Lyme, the denial system, and the government agencies that just make things worse.

I pray my daughter will be able to make a healthy choice for herself, and return home. To be emancipated at age 16 by marriage got her away from DSS but also gives her the legal backing to do as she wants. There are reasons why the legal age to do certain things is 21. At 16, we are still learning, and our brains are still growing. Had her first choice worked out, it would have been fine. As it was, we were backed into a corner, and after so many months, (years really), of abuse and denial and disrepect by a medical system and government agencies, and frantically we made the best choices we could at the time.

Now, I hope and pray that we have a chance to start to repair some things; to recover, to move once again toward the future, and to work toward recovering Miranda's health, her self-esteem, and her life. I pray that she makes it out of the hands of this man who brags about his assualt-on-a-female charges. He is someone who can charm a snake out of its venom, and then spit it back at the serpent and laugh. **Oh, he also doesn't think Miranda has 'Lyme's.'"**

It will come full circle for the fear and loathing that manifests itself in the bite of a tick, in faulty research that determines our unreliable tests, and doctors fed lies by peer-reviewed articles; those who take advantage of our desperation, and clinicians who are lazy and in the wrong business. Also for our government who propogated and dispersed this disease, and the denial machine that is well-oiled by our leaders, and the insurance industry who passes around millions to keep it hushed up; the medical journals who publish, every spring, during the height of tick season, their lies. Our "leadership" who is not to be trusted, pretends to help us, yet is not able to fool and con all of us.

We mimic AIDS in our problems with leadership, Agent Orange in our goverment denials, the Tuskeegee and the Nazi medical experiments in the cruelty extended to us, their little lab rats. We sit at the bottom, clawing our way out, slipping down and accepting the blinders handed us because we are too tired. I want to scream from the top of the highest mountain, with the biggest megaphone in existance...***wake up!***

I have removed myself from the Lyme information lists that I haven't yet been thrown off, and ask people please not to send me news until there is a cure. I no longer will advocate except through my "tick-toons," with a percentage going to a foundation I think is filled with good people, and with whom my doctor, Dr. B has aligned. In that lies hope, he is a good man, a rare find, and a gem.

I am never going to shut up, and I won't always say things diplomatically, but what I do say, and how I say it, maybe perhaps won't be easily forgotten. This is dedicated to Jodi Swift, whose voice whispers in my ear from the clouds above, "keep going, keep going. I am keeping watch." May she rest in peace.

❖ ❖ ❖

Multiple Therapies, Long-Term Antibiotics and Persistence Pays Off

Laura Zeller, Adirondacks, New York

[Laura's story was featured in a 2007 Discovery Health Channel Mystery ER *television episode]*

Before I got Lyme disease I was a mountain climber, and an athlete full of energy! I had an exiting career path set out for me, full of endless opportunities in freshwater ecology and environmental science. Helping nature and animals was always my dream. My dreams motivated my life, and I had an intense passion for the outdoors. I had plenty of experience climbing mountains, but never in my wildest dreams did I imagine the mountain I would have to climb in my life. This mountain climb would be the most challenging journey I could ever imagine. The mountain climb began in my back yard.

The house I grew up in had a nature preserve behind it which was home to a large deer herd. As a child I lived for the woods, building tree forts, camping outside, and wandering for hours in the woods. I was also the only kid in my class to get the award for perfect attendance. I camped out under the stars more nights than I slept in a bed, and loved every minute of it. I bushwhacked up mountain trails, always seeking the pass less taken. I worked for the Conservation Corps in the summer, blazing trails while working in thick, dense wooded areas. Ticks were always crawling all over me, and I did not think it was anything to worry about. At lunchtime, I would take off my work gloves, and flick ticks off my arms and scratch them out of my hair. When I got home at night, I would get in the shower and use tweezers to pull the ticks out by the dozens. Back then, what was Lyme disease?

Lyme disease is a horrifying and potentially deadly disease lurking in our backyards. When I was growing up in the 1980's, Lyme disease was thought to be easily treated with a couple weeks of antibiotics. I had no reason to fear ticks, so I continued doing what I loved – being outdoors. I used bug spray of course, and found out I was allergic to that. Doctors used the *wait and see if you get sick* approach, before prescribing antibiotics. Many doctors now agree that if a tick bites you, treatment should begin as soon as possible. The *wait and see if you get sick* approach is no longer a logical option. Everyone is different and treatment must be tailored to meet the individual's needs. Many times a person may not remember being bitten by a tick. Since it is a relatively new disease discovery, scientists and doctors still have no idea what other insects carry these diseases, scientific research is lacking, and anything is possible.

Even if I had known about the dangers of ticks, what was I supposed to do? Should I have avoided the woods and spent my summers indoors? The outdoors was my life! Can you see how this was the prelude for disaster? Mix a healthy human with dozens of ticks. Expose your skin and let the tick bite you daily. Go to school and work while the spirochetes replicate out of control. Add in steroids to wreck the immune system, mask your symptoms, and bite again. Another year, another tick bite, this time add-in co-infections like Babesia, Bartonella and Ehrlichiosis. Add a camping trip, another summer of trail work, a few dozen more tick bites, and bring to a rolling boil for 8 years. Follow this recipe and try to survive as a host organism. People ask me all the time, "How did you get Lyme disease?" They often sit there with a puzzled look on their face when I tell them I have been bitten over a hundred times. I think to myself "Don't you people ever go outside and enjoy nature?"

I began to experience fatigue in my early teens, and questioned the possibility that I might have Lyme disease. My Mom took me to a doctor who tested my blood; and the test came back negative. Eventually we went back to the doctor and he prescribed 10 days worth of doxycycline, *just in case*. The medication made me feel worse, and the doctor told me to stop taking it after only 3 days. I was nauseated and exhausted, my joints hurt, and I had pain in my eyes. All I wanted to do was sleep. I was so weak I had to drop out of my high school basketball, volleyball and softball teams. My heart was broken because I could no longer play on the teams with my friends. My identity was slowly being taken away, piece by piece. Instead of riding my mountain bike and rock climbing on weekends, I was sleeping all day. I missed out on so many activities, dances, sports, parties and fun with friends. Eventually the doctor diagnosed me with mononucleosis and told me to go home and sleep some more.

After another couple of doctors, I was told that I had Chronic Fatigue Syndrome (CFS), and that there was no cure. Months turned into years, and the overwhelming fatigue continued. I struggled my way through college with a limited course load, and many incompletes. The fatigue never went away, and all I ever did was sleep. If I had only known what the true cause was, I could have begun treatment. Once infection becomes established, symptoms of Lyme disease may include pain in muscles and joints, fatigue, swollen glands, fever, upset stomach, headache, forgetfulness, sleep disorders, depression, and sensitivity to light and sound. One of my re-infections manifested as a sinus infection. I had no idea it was Lyme, and when I took Zithromax, I got a herxheimer reaction, but I did not know what was happening.

The medical community is often perplexed by the complex nature of Lyme disease. Some people experience Lyme disease as a minor illness that appears to be easily treated with antibiotic therapy without any long-lasting complications, but others are not as fortunate. My Lyme disease went on for at least 8 years undetected, undiagnosed and untreated. The bacteria spread deeply into my brain and all over my central nervous system, my heart and other organs, tendons and joints. This late-stage infection resulted in a wide variety of physical, emotional, and mental/cognitive symptoms. I often thought to myself that I would rather take my chances with cancer than have this disease, just as I would gladly have an arm or leg amputated if I could be cured.

As in my case, one tick bite can give you multiple infections. If you are still feeling sick after a good strong dose of antibiotics, you either did not kill the bug completely; you have one or more co-infections, or both. I cannot stress enough the importance of being tested for co-infections, and working with a doctor who treats Lyme disease as his/her main practice. Based on my personal experience, I estimate that 90% of primary care physicians and family doctors have no idea what they are doing concerning diagnosis and treatment of tick-borne diseases. They will probably look at you like you are crazy, misdiagnose and undertreat you, not treat you at all, or try to send you to a shrink. Lyme disease is everywhere. It is very serious and is spreading all over the world. It is really difficult to find a good Lyme disease treating doctor if you are located out in the middle of nowhere, or off the east coast of the United States. There are a few LLMDs out there, but it's not easy to find one. If you have a difficult case, and you are far away from NY, CT, and PA, consider flying in to see one of the best doctors, nothing is more important than your health.

If you go untreated for weeks, months or years, the late-stage list of symptoms is long and confusing. My symptoms included low energy, poor stamina, sore throat, unexplained menstrual irregularity, upset stomach, abdominal pain, chest pain, rib soreness, shortness of breath, cough, heart palpitations, pulse skips, heart murmur, joint pain, joint swelling, stiffness of the joints all over my body, muscle pain and cramping, twitching of the face or other muscles, neck pinches and cracks, neck stiffness, neck pain, tingling, numbness, burning or stabbing sensations, shooting pains, skin hypersensitivity, facial paralysis, (Bell's palsy), double and blurred vision, increased floaters, light sensitivity, buzzing, ringing, ear pain, and sound sensitivity. I also had increased motion sickness, vertigo, major facial flushing and bizarre skin rashes, poor balance, lightheadedness, wooziness, panic attacks, anxiety, and tremors. Additionally, confusion, difficulty in thinking, difficulty with concentration, forgetfulness, poor short-term memory, poor attention, disorientation, getting lost, going to wrong places, difficulty with speech or writing, mood swings, irritability, depression, disturbed sleep, (too much, too little, overwhelming need to sleep 4 hours every afternoon), and a complete intolerance to alcohol. In my case, I dragged myself though 4 years of college missing many classes and taking it slowly. It was up and down for a long time and I was never quite "right."

Many Lyme patients fail to receive a conclusive diagnosis long after they first become sick. Although depression is common in any chronic illness, it is more prevalent with Lyme patients than in most other chronic illnesses. There are many causes, including a number of psychological factors. From a psychological point of view, Lyme patients are psychologically overwhelmed by the large multitude of symptoms associated with this disease. Most medical conditions primarily affect only one part of the body, or only one organ system. As a result, patients with only a few symptoms can still work, and do activities, which allow them to take a vacation from their disease. With chronic Lyme disease, there is no escape for periodic recovery.

This has been the case with me for going on 15 years now. In many cases, this results in a vicious cycle of disappointment, grief, chronic stress, and demoralization. I used to get so frustrated that I wanted to swallow an entire bottle of bleach to kill the Lyme. *[Of course this is poison – do not do!]* The annoying depression is not only caused by psychological factors, but physical dysfunction can directly cause depression. Endocrine disorders such as hypothyroidism, which cause depression, are sometimes associated with Lyme disease and further strengthen the link between Lyme disease and depression. In my case, the swelling of the lining of my brain (Lyme encephalitis) was the cause, in addition to poor adrenal function; brain lesions and vasovagal syncope, also known as neurally-mediated hypotension (NMH). My Lyme disease did frightening damage to my central nervous system. Lyme encephalopathy results in the dysfunction of a number of different essential mental functions. As a result, I experienced cognitive, emotional, and neurological symptoms on a daily basis.

One day in 1997, I was driving my car while running an errand for my boss at work. I was driving along looking at the mountains when I felt a shooting pain across my chest, right below my bra line. I thought, it must be the bra, is it pinching me? It was the beginning of paralysis, and in the following weeks, I began slurring my speech, stumbling, getting lost, and going out in my car and having no idea where I intended to go. I started to wonder if I had some kind of mental illness, since I was so confused in the head. I started to become increasingly forgetful. I could not remember what errands I was supposed to run. I wandered, lost track of time, got lost in my own town, and spent 4 hours in the supermarket for no reason.

My eyes hurt, they ached from the inside out, my vision went blurry, I could no longer sleep with the blinds down, or the window open. The slightest spot of light in my bedroom sent a violent shock wave through my entire body. It was very painful, the only way I can explain it to a healthy person would be to compare it to not having slept in 48 hours, being punched in both eyes, while having the flu, then drinking a six-pack of beer, getting smashed, finally going to sleep, after puking, sleeping for 4 hours (while having nightmares of dying) and then someone opens the window, the sun hits your face, and you scream, "no!" I went to the Emergency room unable to feel my own skin and with tingling and numbness all over my body. They sent me home telling me I had an anxiety attack.

It took too much energy to scream. I needed to sleep with a blindfold on, and wear sunglasses at night. I also did really dumb things without realizing it, like putting my clothes in the refrigerator and a box of cereal in the dishwasher. "Lyme brain" is what that is called. A few days after the shooting pains started going down my legs and across my face, and my face sagged, I had the first of many tearing episodes while driving my car. While on my way to work one morning, my eyes suddenly went haywire and I could not see. They were super-sensitive and could not take the light. I swerved and pulled over on the highway, and tried to recover. I must have allergies I thought. It was so scary, and it would not stop. Tears were streaming down my face, and I could not see.

I also felt dizzy, and had cold sweats and exhaustion. I needed 12 hours of sleep per night, and still woke up tired. Something is really wrong with me, I thought to myself. What am I allergic to now? All I eat are organic foods. The steroids that have made me gain 30 pounds are supposed to block allergic reactions, so what the heck is going on here? I closed my eyes until I could see again, and then drove on to work, still screwed up. I ended up passing out in a dark closet at work, so exhausted I could not stand up.

Now looking back, I know that the light sensitivity was a major sign of neurological damage. My ears were next to go, and I became a very light sleeper. When I tried to sleep, I needed to run a fan right next to my ears. The sound of the phone ringing, car horns, music, and especially car alarms and motorcycles were so loud. When you have Lyme, everything gets amplified, and it's like you can feel every little sound vibrate through your whole body. Damage to your nervous system makes you ultra-sensitive, and puts your startle reflexes on overdrive. People around you will be scared, and not understand. It takes a lot of time and patience to understand the complex nature of this disease. If you are a family member or friend of a loved one going through anything like this, you have to be strong for them. It is not their fault that they are sick. Be as loving, giving and sweet as you can. Let them sleep, be quiet, and take care of them. Although this is not easy to watch, you cannot give up on people you love. My loved ones had to deal with me sleeping in a walk-in closet with no windows – my cave, my little womb, and the safe haven where I could get what my body craved…sleep!

As my symptoms increased, I sought the help of over 40 doctors. I was misdiagnosed with CFS, Fibromyalgia, MS, immune dysfunction, Hypoglycemia, Rheumatoid Arthritis, Lupus, chronic Mononucleosis, and Addison's disease. Most of the doctors I saw referred me to specialists because they had no idea what was wrong with me. I have had some horrifying encounters with doctors. The worst of them all are Infectious Disease Specialists. Since the testing for Lyme disease is so poor, many of my blood tests were normal. As a result, **two-thirds of the doctors I saw though told me I was perfectly healthy on paper, and that I should see a shrink.**

Ironically, when I finally did see a shrink, it was he who thought I was really sick, and so it went in circles for years. I was the victim of verbal abuse by 3 doctors back-to-back. The Infectious Disease doctor, Rheumatologist, and Neurologist were all probably getting kickbacks from my insurance company to *not* order tests, or diagnose Lyme. Insurance companies do not want to have to pay for the extremely expensive long-term treatment of Lyme disease, so they pay these doctors to make sure they never diagnose Lyme.

An Immunologist told me I had Epstein-Barr virus and that I had less than 2 years to live. A Gastroenterologist in NY told me I was suffering from hypochondria. An Infectious Disease doctor in NY told me that all cases of Lyme disease were easily cured in 3 weeks. Because I took 3 weeks of treatment, they told me I was "cured" and to try some Prozac. A really heartless and stupid Infectious Disease doctor in Colorado told me I had all the symptoms of active AIDS. Infectious Disease "ducks" also told me that Babesia did not exist, and that if I had Ehrlichia, my organs would be failing by now. Infectious Disease doctors I have found to be among the most heartless, cruel, and stupid of all doctors. I have had so many nights full of panic and worry that I was dying from some mysterious deadly infection, that it is a wonder that I am still here.

Doctors who know nothing about Lyme disease are referred to by the majority of the Lyme community as "ducks." To say I went through a lot is not telling the whole story. I went through hell, and enough of it for a lifetime. I was so sick and desperate, I would sit there in the ER waiting room dripping with sweat, with a 102° fever, my left side numb, my face drooping, my feet purple, having slept 16 hours and woken up tired, with no appetite, massive anxiety, nausea and facial flushing that made me look like a homeless drunk, and I would be dismissed as perfectly healthy by the doctors. They would go on about me finding a Chronic Fatigue support group and that I needed a shrink.

What everyone needs to realize is that Chronic Fatigue, Fibromyalgia, and Arthritis are not diseases by themselves. Of course, they are real, but they are *symptoms*, not diseases. If you go to the doctor, and complain of being tired all the time, for 6 months or more, you are probably going to be diagnosed with Chronic Fatigue. You have to use common sense here. You have a symptom, and you are being diagnosed with a symptom. It makes no sense. You need to find out the cause! Lyme disease and the bacteria *B. burgdorferi* are often the cause of Chronic Fatigue. People join Chronic Fatigue support groups, they go on disability, they tell their family "I know what's wrong with me now, and I have Chronic Fatigue." I still find it amazing just how many people get sucked into this giant conspiracy and line of thought. None of it makes any sense, yet we are so happy to have a diagnosis, we accept it. Meanwhile a cause is not found, and the person is left with an undiagnosed and untreated infection.

Many thousands of people believe they have Fibromyalgia, Chronic Fatigue Syndrome, Depression, Multiple Sclerosis and more, and still they have no idea what the cause is. Normal, healthy people do not just suddenly come down with MS, or are exhausted all the time for no reason, there is always a cause. Do not buy into the word syndrome either; it is just a word for a collection of symptoms for which the doctors label a syndrome because they have no idea what is wrong with you. The same thing is true for treatment of diseases. People seek out a cure, and what they get is not a cure, but medication to treat the symptoms. An example of this in Lyme disease is anti-inflammatory drugs, NSAIDS, or steroids prescribed to treat painful joints. The medications will work on the symptom, the pain, but the cause of the pain goes untreated. The smart treatment would be antibiotics, which directly kill the cause, plus supportive prescriptions to treat the symptoms and make the patient more comfortable. Therefore, in the previous example, the patient benefits from treatment aimed at the cure, plus they get symptom relief. **Seek the cause people, always seek the cause.**

In my story, I set out for a diagnosis and treatment for my cause. I was mis-diagnosed as a crazy person with Chronic Fatigue. I heard the previous responses from so many different doctors and medical staff that I have lost count of them all. I was told repeatedly that I was crazy, in perfect health, depressed, have Chronic Fatigue and that I could not possibly "still" have Lyme disease. It is all one huge Lyme conspiracy. Insurance companies do not want to pay for long-term IV antibiotics that can cost upwards of $3,400 per week, so they pay these dirty doctors to misdiagnose and undertreat possible Lyme patients, diagnosing them instead with Chronic Fatigue or similar made-up disorders so they do not have to pay anything. I had been severely wronged for 8 years and too sick and poor to do much about it.

As the months dragged into years, I kept getting sicker. A few doctors took blood, and some interesting things were found. I tested positive for Rheumatoid Arthritis, HHV-6 and Epstein-Barr virus. I was told I had a stealth virus infection that I got from a contaminated childhood polio vaccine. I took ganciclovir and other anti-virals, all of which did nothing. The MRI of my brain showed white matter lesions on my frontal lobe, and I was told I had MS. My natural killer cell level and function were low. I had a result of 3, and a function of 88%. My adrenal glands were shot and not producing cortisol, and I was diagnosed with Addison's disease. My red blood cells were low, my platelets low, and my immune system was weak. I was put on prednisone for almost 3 years for my bad adrenals. Now I know that was a huge mistake, and is one of the worst things a person with Lyme disease can take. They make you gain water weight like a hippo and there is nothing you can do.

I tried many alternative treatments, diets, and supplements. I had all my mercury fillings replaced, and I did the chelation protocols. I even traveled to the Dominican Republic to a special chronic disease clinic seeking help. I tried treatments from Europe that were "new and amazing" immunology. I was treated with anti-viral drugs combined with a supposed "targeting agent" called hyaluronic acid (HA). I had to pay

$12,000 to receive the HA, since it was illegal to use in the United States. I later found out that some patients were getting it "sneaked" into their nutrient and antibiotic IV treatments without having been to the Dominican Republic. My treatment also included hydrogen peroxide IVs, ozone, UV-B photo ox therapy, IV vitamin C drips upwards of 75 grams, multi-mineral and vitamin IVs, detox therapy, Chinese herbs, homeopathy, and poly-MVA that was being used for cancer. I also did a German vaccine at the clinic. They took my blood and sent it to Germany, separated out all the bad stuff in my blood, and made a vaccine out of it that I would later inject to supposedly cure me. I know now that most of these clinics are just big money scams, preying on sick people with their wallets open. Be careful!

While I was seeking help in the Dominican, I came down with a life-threatening bacterial pneumonia. My throat closed up and I was rushed to the ER in the awful city of Santo Domingo (third-world medicine nightmare). Nobody spoke English, nor did they have any idea what was wrong with me or all the different chemicals and treatments that I was taking. I was on a breathing machine, and was out of it until I woke up in the clinic with IV's in both arms, a 105°F fever, shaking, sweating, and I could not talk. It was scary, and even though I was an adult, I wanted my Mommy! The doctors at the hospital gave me IV antibiotics for the pneumonia. I was very weak, and I had no idea what was happening to me when I got worse upon the addition of antibiotics. Now I know that was the first big herx of the previously untreated 8 years of suffering. The ducks in the Dominican waited until I could get on a plane, and I flew back to New York so my parents could take care of me. I was supposed to fly back to home cured, and have a happy life, but that did not happen.

Strangely, after a month in NY, I felt a little better. I know now it was because some of my Lyme was killed off by the pneumonia treatment, which was an IV antibiotic. At the time, I thought it was the IV vitamin C that was making me feel better. Unfortunately, I quickly crashed again, and became sicker each passing day. The time finally came when I could no longer work or take care of myself, and I was confined to bed. I truly began to believe that I was not going to make it.

My symptoms had progressed to the point of complete exhaustion, where I was too weak to brush my teeth, or even sit up to drink some water. If I did get up to go to another clueless doctor, I would be "dead" for days afterwards from the exertion. I spent weeks in the hospital, still untreated for Lyme. I was given painkillers, anti-inflammatory drugs, and diagnostic tests up the wazoo! Even while lying in a hospital bed, my Lyme tests which were usually false negative, were all positive, including the ELISA, and the Western Blot, even by the obnoxiously-flawed CDC criteria. I was released and sent home with antidepressants and Rheumatoid Arthritis drugs, and yet another diagnosis of CFS.

To make matters worse, I got bit by another tick in the summer of 1999. I found the little sucker right on the side of my armpit, it was so tiny. It was full of blood and had been there for 2-3 days. I checked myself all the time, and yet since it was so tiny, about as big as the period at the end of this sentence, I missed it. That night after I pulled off the tick and was sleeping, I woke up to a drenching sweat all over my body. My heart was pounding, and I was shaking. I thought I must have an allergy to something, or a stomach flu. But that miserable tick did this to me.

At daybreak, I had a friend drive me to the ER. They took blood, recorded that I had a 103°F fever, and gave me 2 weeks of Ceftin, another antibiotic. They sent me home with orders to rest, and said that I had Lyme...again. Oh my God! It kept getting worse. My heart went crazy, it was pounding at 150 beats per minute while I was lying down trying to sleep and it never calmed down. At the spot where the tick was attached I had a really annoying muscle twitching. The twitching spread to my entire body and never stopped. I had horrible sweating, a really weird, out-of-it feeling in my head, low blood sugar, nausea, and vomiting. I know now that is the exact day that my neurally mediated hypotension (NMH) started and Babesia blasted me into a whole new realm of infection. The spot of the bite twitched for weeks, calmed down, then started back up again. The hospital results showed a positive ELISA and Western Blot for Lyme. They told me to take all of my Ceftin and that I would be "fine." At least I received some treatment that time. Of course, they did not check for Babesia or Ehrlichia.

After 4 more mad dashes to the emergency room, now knowing I had Lyme disease, from a myriad of neurological symptoms, I finally found a piece of information that held hope. I bought the book, *Everything You Need to Know About Lyme Disease*[184] and found the name of a doctor who seemed to know a lot about Lyme. After reading the book, I had a breakthrough, and I had found out what was wrong with me. I did it all on my own, all these doctors could not figure it out, but I could read a book, and it all made sense.

After being verbally abused in the hospital for 2 weeks by Infectious disease ducks, Rheumatologists, and shrinks, I left the hospital once again, sicker then when I arrived, and half-paralyzed on my left side with my skin feeling like razor blades, because they took away my antibiotics. I was released and sent home with painkillers, Vioxx, and steroids for inflammation; sick with tingling pain sensations all over my body, and numbness; and was unable to feel most sensations on my skin. And still they refused to address my Lyme disease.

The same day I was released from the hospital, I went onto the Internet to research what I had learned in the book. I found an online forum for Lyme patients, a wonderful source of information. After posting a desperate plea for help, I got an answer, and along with it the address and phone number of a doctor. I dragged myself out of bed for an hour a day and went on the Internet having no idea how to use the thing, and I found help, answers, and treatment guidelines. I knew I could not give up now, I finally knew what was wrong with me since I was a young teenager!

The day my journey of mental and emotional pain and suffering, misunderstanding and abandonment came to a halt was the day I walked into the office of my LLMD. He read over my folder full of lab tests, and my 20 pages of typed personal history of the previous 10 years. He told me he knew what was wrong with me and said he could make me better. He said I had been grossly under treated and misdiagnosed. He said that although my health history was bad, that it was not unusual to him. He had seen thousands of patients just like me, who were sick and desperate. He examined me, discussed my diagnosis, and what treatment I would need. He said my case was severe, and that I may get over this all together but it will take a long time.

I cried tears of joy! Finally, someone had listened to me, and I found a doctor who understood this awful disease. He outlined my treatment protocol that would consist of IV antibiotics, hyperbaric oxygen therapy (HBOT), nutritional supplements and adequate rest. I had to have a minor operation to have a *Hickman* catheter, central line put into my heart so I could do my IV treatment at home. It is the same central line to the heart through the chest port that chemotherapy patients have to use. After my appointment, my Mom took me to the ocean and we cried tears of joy! The love and gratitude I felt for this new doctor was overwhelming. How do you thank someone who saves your life? I told him I would never give up, that I was a fighter, and that I would climb mountains again no matter what! He gave me a big hug, and sent me on my way to start the journey back to health.

My treatment began with IV antibiotics on New Years Eve, 2000. My co-infection testing proved positive for Babesia, Ehrlichia, and Bartonella. I had no idea just how much sicker I would get! When you start Lyme treatment, you get sicker before you get better. I had this herx sickness, which is a worsening of all symptoms, plus the addition of new ones for 8 months. I could not function at all, and lay bedridden with my IV's dripping day after day. My blood pressure dropped so low with the herxing that my LLMD prescribed IV fluid bags for me to do every day, just to keep my blood pressure up. I dripped the 4 hours of IV saline solution and magnesium sulfate into me, followed by the 2-hour drip of IV Zithromax. I also had to do IM Bicillin shots and swallow pills. I was concurrently being treated for the other tick infections I had, Babesia and Ehrlichia. The medication for Babesia (Mepron) is an anti-malaria drug, a yellow, nuclear-looking liquid I had to swallow. I did not leave my house for 9 months except to travel to see my LLMD, with a bed in the back of the car, and my IV bag hanging on a coat hanger. I was too weak to do anything except sleep. Reading was impossible, and talking to others made me have anxiety and panic attacks.

Hyperbaric oxygen, Flagyl and every single antibiotic I took for Lyme made me herx. The entire first year of my therapy was one big blur of "feeling worse before feeling better" herxing, and misery. As part of this reaction, many patients describe becoming suddenly aggressive without warning. When I would herx, I got foggy in the head, confused, slurred my speech, got totally exhausted, shaky, and weak and wanted to be left alone.

I flew into several Lyme rages where I had no idea what was happening, I started breaking windows and throwing things around and had the most painful herx, right in front of my family. A bad herx can last from several hours to several weeks. I herxed for almost all of 2000-2001, and on and off thru 2002. I never quit taking my antibiotics during a herx. Some people back off them. I kept going, it is the fighter in me, and I would not let the germs win. Flagyl was a real eye-opener for me. After I would take a pill, an hour later my muscles would twitch like crazy all over my body. My muscles would get stiff, and my whole body would be swollen and in pain. Flagyl made me so tired I could sleep for weeks and wake up acting like a drunken zombie. Once the disease has spread into the peripheral and central nervous system, hang on tight! It can begin as tingling sensations anywhere on the body, for me it felt like shooting and stabbing pains from head to toe.

I began hyperbaric oxygen treatment (HBOT) as an adjunctive therapy to my antibiotic protocol. My treatment plan began with a series of 60 treatments in a monoplace (single person) chamber. I did 2 treatments daily, Monday-Friday at 2.4 ATA *[atmospheres]*. The first dive took a little getting used to, but I did really well thanks to my "diver's ears." The chamber was nice and comfortable with a nice mattress to lie on, a pillow and a blanket if I needed it. The chamber was great. I could watch TV, movies, and listen to music in there. You have a hyperbaric technician, a nurse and a doctor all there for you while you do your treatment, so I was not afraid. It takes about 10 minutes to dive to pressure depth, during that time you have to equalize your ears. I found that very simple with the procedure the technicians taught me. Once at pressure, I could sleep the entire time.

The worst of my neurological symptoms came out during this therapy. I had panic attacks, hallucinations, nerve pains, muscle spasms, encephalitis, fevers, flushing, joint swelling, edema, and total exhaustion. I grew too tired to handle it and had to have my Mom come stay with me all the time, feed me and help me with my IVs. The flushing in my face was so bad it felt like I had a severe sunburn 24/7. It was not only disgusting to look at, but it hurt and I was so dizzy because all my blood was in my skin.

After the initial six weeks of HBO, I went home to lie in bed while the herx cleared (the worst it ever got, or so I thought). I had hallucinations and anxiety so badly I needed a Xanax pill just to go to the bathroom. I could not sit at the table to eat. I could not handle lights being on, cars driving by the house, any noises or sounds. Even people talking had me shrieking in pain from my brain. All I did besides sleep was stare at my lava lamp for hours. Those chambers made me herx so hard; I had visible shakes and muscle twitching, rashes and nerve pain during my dives.

Hyperbaric oxygen was a *huge* factor in my success. I continued with the treatments in the monoplace chamber for over a year. I started with 60 dives, and then did 10-15 treatments each month as maintenance. I infused my IV an hour before each treatment to maximize the effect. I also did hot bath treatments before and after each dive. Right in the middle of my treatment, I decided to try a different type of oxygen chamber, the multiplace (multi-person) chamber. It was less expensive than the monoplace, and closer to home, so I tried it. I wish I never tried it! My experience in the multiplace chamber was not pleasant. First of all, I was with other people, and it was very uncomfortable. You have to sit up and wear a mask over your head. The mask kept leaking air out of the neck gasket and deflating on my face. The other patients in the chamber were not instructed how to equalize their ears and my treatments were interrupted countless times. You cannot rest, and forget about sleeping, that is impossible in there. I got no help from those treatments; I got no herx, and felt no effect at all.

I found out later from my LLMD that in the multiplace chamber, I did not absorb the pressurized oxygen through my skin, which is where spirochetes like to hide. The hood had a design flaw, and it lost its potential effectiveness through air leaks. Every single one of my multiplace treatments were either delayed, or ruined by other patients who were claustrophobic, could not equalize their ears, or complained about the pressure depth and wanted to stay at 1.7 or 2.0 ATA. I needed 2.4. It was very frustrating, and wasted a lot of time and money.

Before I knew the facts, I tried another multiplace chamber. This one was a bit different. There was only one other patient with me who also had Lyme. We dove to 2.4 but it never felt like it. Again, no herxing, no nothing. The mask was better than the hood at the first place, but it still felt "wimpy." It is very frustrating to deal with the lack of individual attention in a multiplace chamber. Treatments are started and stopped so many times it can take hours just to do a single dive. Even though the multiplace chamber says you are at 2.4ATA, it is more like 2.0, and I could feel the difference. I got fed up with the lack of results, and went back to the monoplace chamber. As soon as I went back into the monoplace chamber, the herxing began. I experienced twitching, nerve pains, and even rashes coming back again on my skin from original tick bites...amazing things! It knocked me down hard, and my herx was so powerful I needed medical intervention to calm it down, and a break from the meds. After 2 days rest, I continued my dives, and did

90 more.

During my first few months of Lyme treatment, another medical discovery was made. I had a tilt table test (TTT) with Isuprel challenge done. This is an invasive test done by a Cardiologist. You are strapped onto a table with your arms spread out, and the rest of you tied up in Velcro like Hannibal Lector in the movie *Silence of the Lambs*. You are tilted upright, strapped in, and your heart and blood pressure are monitored closely. After that, you are given Isuprel and your heart beats at its maximum while you are lying still. When my heart rate reached 180, they tilted me up vertically and I passed out. My heart rate dropped from 180 to 65 in one beat, and my BP dropped from 140/70 to 50/0 and I fainted and was out cold until they stopped the test and administered the antidote to the Isuprel. It was an exhausting experience, however, this test turned out to be one of the most significant tests and discoveries of my health journey. I had a combined neurocardiogenic and vasopressor response, a double fail. This means that the Lyme infection had inflamed my vagus nerve, which is the major communicator between my heart and my brain. The inflammation caused the nerves to misfire sending the wrong messages to the brain, to stop the heart. The treatment for the symptoms is beta-blockers, Florinef, Zoloft, a high-salt diet, extra hydration and to avoid heat and stress. All these meds made me gain tons of weight, and it was no picnic. Still, at least I could walk around without fainting.

During this time, my blood pressure during this time was typically 80/50, very low and I fainted a few times. One time I fainted in the shower and passed out and smashed my head into the stone sink, and sliced my scalp open. I crawled to the phone and called 9-1-1 and the ambulance came, and said my blood pressure had fallen to 70/35, and my blood volume was dangerously low. I got 3 big bags of IVs, talked to some more clueless doctors and went on the steroids after that. Steroids are nasty! They make you huge and wreck your immune system. When I fell asleep for the night, I often wondered if I would ever wake up again. It was really scary.

Many times I felt my body ache with exhaustion so badly that it took too much energy just to breathe. As time passed, I did 120 more hyperbaric treatments, and 9 months of IV antibiotics. I gradually grew stronger, and watched happily as many of my symptoms began to disappear. I spent months without leaving my house and weeks without getting out of my bed. The IV's gave me herxheimer after herxheimer, and knocked me down hard for what seemed like forever. The IV Zithromax got rid of many of my most annoying and painful symptoms, but it took many months for them to clear. Treatment for Babesia took away my fevers, night sweats, chills, flushing, hallucinations, panic attacks, and anxiety.

I ended up switching from IV to oral antibiotics in September of 2000 due to 2 serious cases of blood infection from the IV line. It happened suddenly and without warning, but I got a 106°F fever with total delirium and went into septic shock (which kills most people) because a bad, gram-negative bacterium got into my IV line. When I started my infusion, I flushed it into my heart, and all hell broke loose in my body. I called 9-1-1, threw up all over my bed, turned white, shook uncontrollably and passed out. It is a miracle I lived. It is an even bigger miracle that I could even dial 9-1-1 because most people just die right then from the sepsis. The police kicked in my front door to get to me, unhooked my IV's and the ambulance came and got me. I had emergency surgery to remove the catheter. The doctors in the ER had no idea what was wrong with me when I first came through the doors. They thought I had contracted West Nile Virus since my temperature was so high, at 107°F.

I absolutely insisted through my babbling, valium-induced stupor that they call my LLMD. When they finally did, he saved my life over the radio dispatch from the ambulance and he told them to "pull that IV line right away, she has sepsis!" I have never been that sick. That call saved my life because the doctors in the ER were so stupid and Lyme illiterate, they were not even going to pull the line. You can't even imagine how sick I was, you don't want to, it was that bad. I woke up packed in ice and really scared. I remember then my Dad came in and I woke up traumatized from the ER.

After 2 days, I was home with the line out, a hole in my chest, and an appointment with the surgeon to get another Hickman catheter put in. To make a long story short, I had the operation to get the new IV line put in. This time the new IV line lasted 21 days before I got sepsis again. The second time it happened I called 9-1-1 again, and deteriorated over 3 minutes time to be a ghost white-faced, seizing, dying person. I was taken by ambulance to the hospital again, and this time they knew what to do, but yes, my LLMD called and told the ER docs what to do and he saved my life *again.*

I was due for another 6 months of IV, but after that my LLMD and I agreed to stop IV, and I went on long-term orals. The woman who pulled out my IV yanked the catheter out of my chest and dropped it on the floor. It hurt so much and she was supposed to use sterile procedures and culture the tip of the catheter. If you have a PICC line or a Hickman, please be very careful, and alert for any sign of sepsis. Ask your treating doctor what to do when, or if it happens.

In addition to the orals, I took a combination of Rocephin and Bicillin IM shots twice per week. Magnesium sulfate and methylcobalamin B-12 injections were added for support. I continued aggressive HBO until April of 2002, after which I was well enough to take a trip out to Colorado. I was so exited to be alive again, and feeling halfway decent too, I ended up overdoing it big time, and my friend and I put 3,000 miles on the rental car and we drove from Denver to the Grand Canyon. I was alive again, hooray!

I overdid it big time in Colorado, and felt totally wiped out upon returning to New York. I still say it was worth it to feel alive again in the mountains, and not be attached to my IV pole. Back into the monoplace chamber I went. I took high-dose combinations of oral antibiotics, and did hyperbaric oxygen during the week. On a break from my monoplace hyperbaric treatments, I tried out a portable, mild hyperbaric chamber that a friend of mine bought. What a joke. It did nothing for me, even after daily treatments. The inflatable plastic chambers can only go to 1.3 ATA. Some people even tried to convince me that these chambers would cure me, what a laugh and a huge waste of money. I also tried 2 types of Rife machine, but none of it did anything.

Many times throughout the years people would say, "You're *still* sick?" and it drove me crazy. People do not realize, or take the time to read about Lyme and understand it. **You are not going to get better in a few weeks to months if you have been ill for half your life.** Lyme patients are generally treated like dirt. We get little to no respect, and are not taken seriously because we "look" fine. This is not the common cold, people! We have no cure yet, so stop asking us why we are *still* sick! **Fighting this disease is harder than working a full-time job.** You have no idea just how precious life is until you lose your health.

The combination of aggressive IV and oral antibiotics, treatment for Babesia and Bartonella, and my hyperbaric oxygen therapy made an enormous difference in my life. I went from being bedridden to independent and functional again. I could do everything anybody else could; I just had to pace myself. Ketek was the last antibiotic I was on. It was powerful, and did a great deal of killing of spirochetes. After that, my Lyme symptoms lessened significantly. I gradually tapered off antibiotics using IM Bicillin in 2004.

As of the writing of this book, I have been off antibiotics for over 3 years and I am doing well again. I have had some gastrointestinal problems (*c. difficile* infection) one of the side effects of long-term antibiotic use. Despite the GI issues, I have yet to suffer any significant Lyme relapse, and life is so much more beautiful because of where I have been. Trust me when I say, if I can get better, so can you!

How did I survive this? My family raised me to be independent and determined. I was a mountain climber, and I was familiar with challenges. For the thrill of adventure in the outdoors, I used to risk my life on purpose before I got sick. Rock climbers, whitewater kayakers and mountain climbers know what I am talking about. It is our choice to risk our lives to make our lives fuller and richer by living wild, and on the edge. During my darkest days, I remembered the lessons I learned while mountain climbing. Mountains are beautiful, almighty and powerful. Reaching the summit requires physical strength and mental perseverance. You cannot give up if you want to conquer the mountain's majesty. My journey taught me patience and gratitude while strengthening my already fierce and determined spirit. Although I am still alive, not having my dreams come true has been a death of sorts. My identity and my freedom were lost. I learned that no matter how challenging a mountain is, the hardest mountains to climb in life are invisible. My love for life kept me alive, and fighting for survival. It has been a long and tortured climb, although beautiful at the same time. Sitting here writing about it makes me feel like it is a rare experience, and a true accomplishment.

As for the rest of my life, I am now a dedicated Lyme activist working hard to spread the word to others who are suffering from this life-sucking beast of an illness. I have made some truly wonderful and precious friends during this Lyme journey. When you are as sick as I have been, it takes one to know one. Most of my friends abandoned me when I got sick. Lyme turned out to be a blessing in that respect. A true friend is one who walks in when the rest of the world walks out.

At one point, when I thought I was going to die, I wrote letters to all of my family and loved ones. I put all my deep feelings down on paper and tucked them away so that if I died, they would get my letters. I have a great support system, and I love my life. No matter how I feel, I still go out and live each day. I work on my rehabilitation at the gym with my trainer every other day. Exercise is essential to getting better. You have to start slow, and rest in between, but it makes a huge difference in your stamina and immune function. I am into sea kayaking now and have been paddling around my lakes. Midway through my illness, I realized that I could be sick at home, or sick out having fun, either way, you have to go on! Going on with your life as planned is important people. Do not forget, you are still alive, and you still can do it if you try hard enough. Do not give in or give up, it just isn't part of the master plan. Climb the mountains! The beauty of the sunrise on the other side is well worth the journey.

As the dearly departed Christopher Reeve said, I am "*still me,*" only stronger! I am still the same person, I just have limitations. My outlook on life has changed very much, all for the better. I feel very lucky to have been saved. I am very grateful to be alive and feeling healthy again. I will always be eternally grateful to my brilliant Lyme doctor for saving my life. Never diminish your dreams, and try to enjoy your life no matter how badly you feel. Remember, if you have hope, you have everything. Healing thoughts!

❖ ❖ ❖

Lyme By Any Other Name Is Still Lyme

Karl Odden, Connecticut

[Karl's story is published on the web at www.cpnhelp.org. See *patient stories, top of the page, titled "Karl's treatment for MS"]*

I was diagnosed with "MS," May 4, 2006 with 23+ lesions on the brain and spinal cord. **I was found to have suspicious Lyme (otherwise negative),** Babesiosis and C. Pneumoniae (respiratory infection). To me this is what caused my MS and I am eliminating all of it and expect to never live with "MS" again. In 10 months I'm getting close to normal but have some symptoms that keep me from working and driving yet. And so, I wanted to notify you of my story.

I want everyone to know how much the CAP *[chlamydia pneumoniae treatment]* has helped me. I have always been a good picture of health. Never in a hospital, never flu-like, no broken bones, vision 20/20 and fantastic overall. I rarely missed a day of school or work. At most, I would have one cold each year, a fair amount of headaches as I deal with stress internally, and I just slowly became chronically fatigued. My aunt (father's side) and my father's cousin in Minnesota and Wisconsin both have "MS," diagnosed approximately in the 1960's. My aunt has had a few exacerbations over the years but my father's cousin has been in a nursing home since his mid-late thirties. We didn't really know anything about MS until after my diagnosis.

Six years ago, I moved into a great career of sales in the dental industry. I worked like a dog and bought my first real home. We knew nothing about MS and CPN. I was happy, healthy and took most of life for granted, I guess.

At that time, I had a tick bite marked only by the bull's-eye, no other rash or symptoms. The Lyme test, (ELISA), was negative. One month of antibiotics was given just in case, and I moved on. No other testing was done.

Since then, I've married my dear Alyson in April, 2005. In October of the same year we attended her brother's wedding in Jamaica. Many of the guests became ill after the wedding, returning home. My wife had a walking pneumonia for nearly two weeks. I had some respiratory symptoms, but I wasn't as sick as my wife (or so I thought). My wife got better and we forgot about it. We moved into a new home December 2005. Our daughter was born February, 2006. All through this time, I was fine, "healthy," except for headaches, and growing fatigue that I attributed to a large sales territory and to work stress. Who wouldn't be tired consistently driving an average of 4,000 miles a month and flying as much as the birds?

Mid-April 2006, the fatigue was epidemic and for 3 days my right foot was always "asleep" and numb. Two days later my left foot became numb like the right. I was sleeping extra and stumbling through work appointments. I had to pull over on the road and power nap so I would make it home alive. Numbness ascended my legs and then my entire body within days. My head was in a fog, (cognitively), and felt swollen. I started having trouble swallowing, speaking and the dexterity in my right hand lessened. I lost abdominal reflex on the right side. I became so weak and I knew this was serious – that I wasn't well. Due to extreme work stress at the end of that day, I experienced severe changes in mood. I was enraged, spitting and ready to break anything I could get my hands on. I literally and seriously noted increased saliva with my anger, no joke. That night, April 28, 2006, I became more alarmed and scared, and we went to the local hospital. The first ER doctor said, "Oh, numbness like that in your legs happened to me when I started running. It'll go away. This isn't anything like MS or such, don't worry." Blood tests were negative (ELISA and Western Blot) for Lyme. "I don't run," I told him. "Let's just watch it," he said.

The symptoms worsened. I had more fatigue, trouble swallowing, weakness, and numbness. No further testing was done. The next morning, I took a hot shower and realized I was extremely weak and shaky all over the body and more numb throughout immediately after. I couldn't feel the towel against my skin anywhere as I dried off. We went to a more prominent hospital ER that morning.

The second ER doctor did more of a work-up and blood tests, but the end result was the same as the first. "Let's watch it," he said, although it was not attributed to running, but rather to depression. Was this "all in my mind," or work stress? I was wondering what this was, maybe menengitis, mad cow disease, anthrax or even ricin poisoning? I started to research these and realized I was not suffering from any of them.

A few days later, I went to see a Psychiatrist (also an MD) who also thought this was "all in my mind." He felt depression, anxiety, work stress and negative thoughts regarding company management were causing this. He even tried to reason that I was depressed after the birth of our daughter in February and that I felt "left out" of the relationship between my wife and daughter! No such thing. I was highly involved with my wife and baby and laughed when he told me I wasn't. He prescribed Zoloft and Xanax. I tried them since we didn't know what we were dealing with. I took only one pill. It actually made me more depressed with what was going on and more mentally dull. The Psychiatrist said, "This isn't MS or such, let's work on anger management, self-esteem, and dealing with work stress and management negotiation."

My symptoms were growing and we still had no idea what the problem was. In late April, my wife set up an appointment with another GP as we were not happy with my current one. Doctor #4, a GP in

Connecticut, didn't have a clue. "This isn't MS or such, let's watch it. I don't know what this is." Overall, at this time, I was still functional, able to drive, and had good coordination and reflexes. I was just numb and hugely exhausted with brain fog and growing issues with swallowing, speaking and lessening dexterity. The doctor kept me on antidepressants. That messed me up further, making me more depressed at times and mentally out of it. No further testing was done.

A few days later, I went to see my primary GP, since she knew my history and had treated the tick bite before. Again, we still had no idea what this was, but Lyme was in the back of our minds as Lyme is very prevalent in New England. "I don't know what this is," she said. Now I was really having trouble writing and using utensils with my right hand. She tested my finger strength on both hands and found weakness in my right ring finger and said I should see a Neurologist for the weakness in my ring finger. Again, I was still quite functional, otherwise.

In hindsight, it is amazing that *each* doctor simply stated, "This isn't MS or such," yet no further testing was ever discussed or done. On May 4, 2006, I went to see a new Neurologist. He tested me, and was amazed at my functionality but noticed a loss of abdominal reflexes on the right. He ordered an MRI right away within the hour. The MRI showed 18+ lesions on the brain and spinal cord, all of which showed new enhancement with GAD (injected dye). There was no evidence of any old lesions. The doctor told me, "You have MS. You're lucky... these are not tumors. I'll hand you off to our MS specialist here in the clinic." Another Neurologist in the same office said, "you have MS, we'll start you on Solumedrol (steroids) to start getting the symptoms abated. We'll see how you do. You also have your choice of 3 standard MS medications that are injectable interferons to keep the MS in check and it's something you'll learn to live with. You're not dying." "Is there anything I could or should do concerning diet or physical therapy?" I asked. "No, do as you normally do. You just may want to increase vitamin D." That was all he ever recommended even in the following appointments.

On May 5, 2006, I started the steroids. Over the next few days, my health declined further. I was bedridden, and slept most all day, which reminded my wife of her grandfather after he had a stroke. She and I both wondered whether I was dying. After 3 steroid IV's, I was much worse. I began having double vision, and the fatigue became even more extreme. Further, the swallowing was more difficult and the brain fog became heavier. I was even speaking slower and the numbness was worse. I lost taste and appetite and didn't want to be around anyone.

On May 16, we went back to see Neurologist #2. He prescribed 2 more doses of the steroids and also Elavil. It didn't work, but seemed to worsen the symptoms and gave me insomnia. I was having major insomnia, for which Melatonin was recommended. We read the label which states not to be used by those with autoimmune diseases. We questioned the Neurologist and he said it was "okay" to use, so I tried it. The Melatonin made all the symptoms worse. I only used one. After finishing the steroids, the symptoms again gradually worsened. On May 19, 2 days after the fifth steroid, I started the Betaseron Interferon. Still the symptoms continually worsened. I experienced some night sweats and headaches along with injection point irritation and bruising.

On May 25, we returned to the Neurologist even though we didn't have an appointment. We were so desperate that we sat in the office and refused to leave until we saw the doctor. He agreed to see me, and I asked him about the elevated saliva level. He said there was no connection to MS. I asked him about the trouble breathing and was told it was not connected to MS, either. **I asked him whether this could possibly be Lyme disease, and he said no.** My wife pressed him and asked him if he could guarantee I didn't have Lyme. Of course, he was unable to guarantee that since he didn't do any further testing. He agreed to put me on Minocycline, ostensibly because "it's good for MS as an anti-inflammatory." At this point in time, I judged myself to be 8.0-8.5 on the EDSS scale *[expanded disability status scale]*. I was never classified by any Neurologist other than to say this is MS.

Shortly after the appointment on May 25, my wife learned about CPN/Wheldon/Stratton antibiotic CAP treatment through her extensive research. She was not going to accept MS for me, for herself or for our 3-month old baby. She remembered the illness she had suffered from in October after the Jamaica wedding and wondered whether it was CPN. She decided we would try the antibiotics as my health was declining every day and the standard MS treatments were clearly not helping. They were only causing irritation and bruising. We asked our Neurologist to do the prescribing, which he agreed to do if we saw Dr. S personally and if I agreed to stay on one of the standard MS medications. He said he was interested in the treatment, but we knew he would never validate it. He wouldn't prescribe anything other than the Minocycline until I saw Dr. S. He ultimately said to me, "Well, good luck with it. It is at your own risk." We were ready to do anything we needed to, in order to get healthy.

We considered flying to the UK to meet with a Dr. W. We even considered stem-cell therapy in Holland for $20,000.00, but felt the need for much more research and also that this would simply be a last resort. We began making arrangements to see Dr. S, and at the same time posted on *cpnhelp.org* asking for referrals to a local doctor who would be willing to prescribe the CAP. We were given the names of two local Lyme doctors, one who is a Neurologist and one who is an Internist. We called for appointments, but were unable to see the Lyme Neurologist until June and the Internist until September. On May 22, 2006, we went to see another Neurologist for a second opinion, (Dr. #8, Neurologist #3).

At this time, my symptoms were worse. I had more fatigue, more trouble swallowing, a swollen head, trouble walking, and vision and balance issues. The balance problem was severe and prevented me from walking properly without aid. I was experiencing diplopia (double vision) and nystagmus (eyes shake left and right). The new doctor was amazed at my functionality, coordination and strength considering the number of lesions. He tested me for Devics disease, but the test was later negative. He confirmed the diagnosis of MS and recommended 5 more IV steroids. I continued to get worse. At the end, I had a total of 10K grams of steroid infused. I was ruined. My double vision was worse, and I was more exhausted. Numbness was still very heavy throughout my body. Steroids should have made me hyper, I thought, but instead I was growing more and more fatigued. The steroid withdrawal was mentally shattering. I wanted to break things as well as myself and be done. I didn't want to see or talk with anyone; not even family.

I consulted again with the third Neurologist, and he recommended a plasma exchange. We agreed, but found that insurance would not cover it. The Neurologist was to appeal it, but never did. The doctor's next recommendation was chemotherapy. We refused and asked him to prescribe the CAP while providing him research articles, etc. He refused to prescribe the CAP and we fired him.

On June 1, I started the CAP vitamin supplements and Alyson began to order antibiotics online in case we needed to start on our own. I couldn't wait for relief any longer. After starting the NAC (600 mg, then 1200 mg/day) alone, I began having major herxheimer reactions. I was lying in bed and felt as if my entire body was swollen. I felt like I was 400 pounds instead of my standard 165 pounds. I felt so large I couldn't move, and I felt as if I was actually floating. Also, my mind was racing with numerous old memories and dreams when I was sleeping, like my life flashing before me. Surprisingly, I actually thought it was fun and was laughing at times. This type of reaction validated the treatment.

The reactions then went away and I titrated up to the high dosage, 2400 mg/day and my body took it in stride, although I began to have major amounts of fluid draining mostly from my left ear, with some pain and tingling sensations working their way down my neck to the shoulder. There was also minor drainage from the right ear, but I did not experience the tingling or pain on that side.

After approximately 2 weeks on the Minocycline and the supplements, the fatigue felt slightly better and the numbness was beginning to slowly abate. On June 16, I went to see the Lyme Neurologist. He confirmed the MS diagnosis. We asked him to test my blood for Lyme and CPN and any other infectious diseases. He did the CPN test somewhat reluctantly. "Everyone has CPN," he said. The results of the tests were as follows: CPN/Chlamydia Pneumoniae IgG = 1:64H, IgA = 1:16H (Positive old respiratory infection, positive new respiratory infection). Lyme Serology: Non-Reactive ELISA, 0.10 C6 Peptide; Negative ELISA 0.59, Negative Western Blot IgM (Indeterminate-41 and other "CDC" non-specific bands-93); IgG (Indeterminate-41, 93 and other "CDC" non-specific bands-43); Babesiosis 16H Titer Real Time; PCR Negative (Positive old infection only from tick bite-malaria like.)

Neurologist #4 was amazed at my functionality/coordination considering the amount of damage to the brain and spine. He agreed to prescribe the CAP, but insisted I remain on the standard MS medications. However, he also insisted I get a lumbar puncture to determine whether I actually had Lyme disease or what was going on. At this time, I was already on Minocycline (200 mg/day) and Betaseron (1 ml/every other day). He instructed me to stop the Minocycline for 2 weeks so any infection in the CSF would not be masked by the presence of the antibiotics.

I was off the Minocycline for 1.5 days and the original symptoms returned with a vengeance. I became more fatigued as in the beginning and the numbness was much worse than it had ever been. We called the Neurologist and told him I'm going back on the Minocycline and to forget the lumbar puncture. I went back on the Mino and the next day noticed the fatigue was slightly better. I also noticed a resurgence of the herxheimer reaction. I had constant itching, major tingling all over and severe night sweats. Several days later, I had an MRI which revealed growth in the lesion on my spine. I wasn't surprised as the numbness was so much worse. On June 27, I went back to see the Neurologist He increased the dose of Minocycline from 200 to 400 mg/day. He also put me on Azithromycin 200 mg/day. The herxheimer reaction continued in the form of intense itching and night sweats.

July 2, I went back to see him and he added Mepron at 750mg, in a 6-week cycle to treat Babesiosis. This meant I was currently on Minocycline, Azithromycin and Mepron. The herxheimer reactions worsened. I experienced a thick pain in the back of my swollen head/neck. The ear canal (inner ear) on my left was still draining clear fluid, regularly. At this point, I felt like something was crawling under the skin horizontally away from the Adams Apple on both sides of my neck to the back of my head. Night sweats, intense itching and tingling continued. On July 12, I stopped taking the Betaseron as I did not feel it was helping and I hated injecting myself. Also, I wanted to ascertain whether the night sweats were herxheimer reactions or a reaction to the Betaseron. I stopped the Betaseron and the night sweats continued, so I figured the sweats truly to be a herxheimer.

[Note: sweats can also be a symptom of Babesiosis].

On July 14, we met with Dr. S at Vanderbilt University. We initially made this appointment because Neurologist #2 told us he would not prescribe the CAP if we did not see Dr. S personally. However, by the time the appointment rolled around, we were less concerned with getting Neurologist #2 to prescribe as we had already found Neurologist #4, whom was willing to prescribe. Nevertheless, we kept the appointment with Dr. S and we're very glad we did. The doctor answered all our questions about the CAP, but most importantly, he gave us hope that I would get better. He told us he believed I could be cured, in time, which no other doctor I had seen had been willing to say.

On July 17, I went to see my eleventh doctor, a Lyme specialist who is an Internist. He checked me out and also was amazed at my functionality/coordination. In review of MRI reports, the lesion total was more around 23+ on the brain, 3 of which are on the spine. He stated that the suspicious titers in my Lyme tests were low, but **he determined I had Lyme disease, particularly because my CD-57 test count for killer immune cells was low (21).** He was aware of the research on the connection between CPN and MS, and he stated that he believes that the combination of Lyme and CPN can lead to progressive MS, which is what he feels I have.

Due to the number of lesions, he felt I should immediately be put on IV antibiotics (Rocephin, 2g/day, 3-month standard treatment). He also said that my case was so severe that I would probably need to be on antibiotics for life. He prescribed the first month of Rocephin, but told me to follow up with an Infectious Disease doctor as the rule in Connecticut says that insurance companies do not have to pay for more than a month of IV Rocephin unless it is prescribed by a Neurologist or Infectious Disease doctor.

By this time, the fatigue was better, but my vision was worse. It was keeping me off balance and it felt as if my eyes were not working together and therefore I couldn't lock in on moving objects. (For this reason, I was unable to drive and walking was problematic where before I had trouble with the actual mechanics of walking.)

On July 21, I began to wonder whether I should have stopped the Betaseron. I decided to give it a try again, mainly because I was concerned that the last MRI had shown growth of the spinal lesion. Shortly thereafter, I went to see Neurologist #4 again. He suggested IVIG (infused garbage to boost the immune system, for lack of a better description.) I initially agreed, but later changed my mind after reading the fine print from paperwork he provided that IVIG is made from blood plasma and isn't properly tested for other diseases, (viruses, HIV). Neurologist #4 then recommended chemo, which I declined as I felt I was already getting better from the antibiotics. Specifically, the fatigue was better and the numbness was lessening again.

August 1, I stopped the Betaseron completely as I really felt it was not helping. On August 3, I went to see an Opthalmologist, as I was very concerned about my vision and balance. We discussed my MS diagnosis and vision problems. My eyes were dialated for full testing. Diagnosis: 20/20 vision with Nystagmus (eyes shake left and right when stressed) and Diplopia (double vision).

It was interesting that this doctor was aware that MS could be treated with antibiotics as **several of his patients were diagnosed with Lyme-induced MS, and had gotten much better from antibiotics.** "Why aren't you on IV Rocephin?" he asked. I was floored that any other doctor knew of this treatment connection to MS and glad I decided to start the Rocephin (which was scheduled to start 1 week after the eye appointment). I had been unsure whether to start the medication as the daily herxing was already so bad and the numbness was so extreme. This day was particularly bad as I could barely walk around without support and my dilated eyes made walking impossible. I was at a really low point, so it certainly helped to hear from the Opthalmologist that he had seen people get better on IV antibiotics.

Throughout the treatment, I was only using activated charcoal to detox my body and would only use Ibuprofen for pain issues. Later I used the Vitamin C flush with success. I also used Ambien and Lunesta for the insomnia. The Ambien made me feel worse the next day so my choice from there was always Lunesta.

On August 26, I started IV Rocephin. At the time I started, I was also on Azithromycin, 200 mg/day and Minocycline 400 mg/day and just finished the Mepron cycle. The herxheimer reactions continued. I had intense tingling, itching, out-of-body experiences, sweats, and chills. The Rocephin did not seem to make it much worse. I was monitored very carefully with weekly blood draws to check white count and liver function. My white count dropped to 2.5 and the liver count was elevated, but the doctor said this was a normal reaction to Rocephin so I did not discontinue anything and the numbers rebalanced. I also had monthly ultrasounds and blood tests to test for gallstones and/or clotting in the IV line. On September 7, I began taking Tindamax, at 1500 mg/day.

At this point, I was on Rocephin, Minocycline, Azithromycin and Tindamax. The herxheimer reaction got more intense and the out-of-body experiences seemed more dramatic. The Rocephin made me exhausted, immediately during and after each infusion. The herxing was awful. I spent the days in bed doing what I could to get away from the herxing – sleeping, listening to music, trying to read or watch

TV. I experienced sweats and chills at different times through the days and nights. Every nerve was on edge and I experienced heavy itching and tingling. I was also dealing with leg and body spasms (restless leg syndrome) along with the extreme fatigue. With the reactions, I really wasn't able to sleep, either. There would be short periods of deep sleep and then up again at all hours. Overall, each symptom (numbness, vision, swallowing, speech, etc.) became elevated and my head was achy and swollen. Nevertheless, I stuck with it and did not discontinue any of the antibiotics or supplements.

Roughly one week after starting the Tindamax, I felt my head beginning to clear. The brain fog began to lift and I would have days with short periods (a few minutes at a time) of feeling cognitively "normal." The first day I felt my head was clear for most of the day was September 18, which was the day I met with the infectious disease MD. This highly validated the antibiotic treatment for me. I met with the ID doctor and he agreed to continue prescribing the IV antibiotic. I continued to get better. The brain fog continued to clear, and my walking started to get better as did my balance. Also, the numbness started to descend. First my head was no longer numb, then my chest, then the numbness left my legs. The remaining numbness was left to my hands and only periodic episodes in my right toe.

On October 2, my Lyme doctor added Diflucan at 200 mg/day to the mix. At this point, I was on Minocycline, Azithromycin, Tindamax, Rocephin and Diflucan. (Rifampin soon was added.) The only numbness I was experiencing was in my hands. Roughly two weeks after starting the Diflucan, I had 2 distinct moments of validation/success; each one early in the morning. The first time was October 17; the second was two days later. Each time, I had taken one Diflucan, 100 mg, at 5:30 am because I felt so bad I wanted to keep hitting it by stretching doses out. Both times, about 2 hours after the Diflucan, I felt the numbness "washing" out of my hands, up my arms, around my chest/abdomen and "out" of my body. The first time, the numbness in my hands abated, roughly, 60%. The second time, the numbness abated, roughly, another 30%. After the second time, the numbness in my hands was approximately 10% of what it had been at its worst. Today, the numbness in my hands is about 3-5% of what it was at its worst.

On October 28, I was started on Rifampin at 600 mg/day. Immediate reactions were heavy pins and needles in the hands and balance/vision was way off. I also was dealing with a shakiness in the head and upper body along with soreness of muscles and wanting to be "out of my body." On November 28, I finished the three months of Rocephin. Although IV antibiotics can be dangerous, (they can cause allergic reactions, gallstones, blood clots), I never had these problems with it. There was one evening when I felt as if my throat was swollen closed with caused more difficulty swallowing and also caused me to lose my voice. I wasn't sure whether it was an allergic reaction, so I went to the local ER and was treated by a doctor who injected me with high-dose Benadryl (5,000 ml). All standard bloodwork, etc., was normal. I was immediately high, silly, then exhaused. I slept for 2-3 hours solid in the hospital, and the problem cleared up.

The next day I spoke with the Lyme MD whom told me I should not infuse myself with more Rocephin unless in the presence of a doctor. Therefore, the Lyme MD spoke with the local ER and arranged for me to get the next infusion in the hospital. Unfortunately, when I got to the ER, the doctor didn't want to monitor me while I infused myself, and he refused to do the infusion for me as he claimed the risk of allergic reaction was high.

"Wouldn't you rather not deal with that? People have died from simple peanut allergies. Rocephin is so much more caustic," he said. He told me his daughter has MS and that he would never treat her with antibiotics as the treatment "would not work." I was really upset by his comments and by the fact that I was unable to get the Rocephin infused that day. I called the Lyme MD and we discussed that I do the next dose at the Allergist's office where the line was put in my arm.

I went in to see the Allergist the next day and the infusion was done in 10 minutes. No reactions or issues came up. The Allergist informed me any allergic reaction would literally happen in the first 10 minutes of the infusion if not immediately, so it was unlikely the throat symptoms had been from an allergic reaction, and was probably a herxheimer. Therefore, I resumed infusing myself at home with the IV. I never needed to use any of the Epi-pens I already had just for that reason. The only real reaction I had to dealing with the Rocephin was simply from the tube in my arm causing irritation. When I finished the Rocephin on November 28, the ID and the Lyme MD both advised me to go off all antibiotics and see how I do. If I got worse they would put me back on the Rocephin; however, if I stayed well they would just keep me on maintenancc antibiotics (pulsed orals).

I posted on *cpnhelp.org*, spoke with Dr. S, and ultimately decided to stay on the antibiotics, mainly because I was still experiencing herxheimer reactions and therefore felt I was not yet cured. I wouldn't be able to withstand any relapses. I asked the Lyme MD to keep prescribing for me, which he agreed to do and continued to prescribe Rifampin, Tindamax, Minocycline and Diflucan. On December 15, the Lyme MD discontinued the Diflucan. On December 18, the doctor replaced Minocycline with Doxycycline at 200 mg/day in an effort to help counter the balance issues. The symptoms and reactions at this time (numbness, itches, tingles, etc.) all got more intense in the early evening which lasted through the night and early morning. As I got up and moved, they abated and balanced out. The numbness in the hands I could feel coming and going like it was "washing" out of my fingers through the hand and out my wrist. He also replaced the Tindamax with Factive (320 mg/day). At this point, I was on Doxy at 200 mg/day, Factive at 320 mg/day and Rifampin at 600 mg/day.

It took some time but I slowly experienced a resurgence of herxheimer reactions, with deeper extreme tingling and itching (mostly in my head/face and neck/upper chest). The Factive was ended shortly thereafter because I began to experience tendonitis in my legs and wrists. Accordingly, the Lyme MD put me back on the Tindamax.

Today, I am on Tindamax 1500 mg/day, Rifampin 600 mg/day and Doxycycline 200 mg/day. My head is completely clear, my balance is much better. I'm regaining strength and energy, I am able to walk more properly and the numbness is gone save for 3-5% in my hands. My vision is slightly better but I still can't drive. The fatigue is better but still periodically there. I still have some trouble swallowing. I still have the daily/nightly herxheimer reactions, but it's not nearly so severe. For example, I no longer experience sweats, chills or body spasms. The itching and tingling are not as severe. I'm slowly beginning to be able to sleep better and through the night. My doctor's next step is to discontinue the Tindamax, Rifampin and Doxycycline with one week off to allow my body to balance. We'll see how I do and then he will put me on high-dose Tetracycline at 2000 mg/day with Biaxin at 1000 mg/day, and Doxy at 200 mg/day and Mepron for another 6-week cycle.

On January 26, 2007, I met with a Neuro-Opthalmologist to again look at my vision issue. After 90 minutes of testing, he concluded I do not have Nystagmus. I currently have prescription glasses that work to counter the balance issue and to allow me to read without skewing lines or becoming tired too quickly since my upper vision is over-compensating for the lower. Time will tell whether it is successful. If not, I may be looking at vision therapy on a much higher level.

My thoughts on the treatment path I chose are as follows: I am amazed by how much better I am in a fairly quick timeframe. It's shocking to be so ill; mainly bedridden due to exhaustion and muscle weakness, numbness; and to be so much better 9 months later. As I said earlier, I still have 3-5% hand numbness, vision imbalance, some fatigue, minor balance issues, deep and wicked itches/tingles mostly in the head/neck but it is lessening and I have slight trouble swallowing at times. I also have shakiness in my head, which I attribute really to atrophy of muscles. I've lost roughly 25 pounds throughout this ordeal. I was 165 lbs before this hit me, I'm only 140 lbs now. We feel I am 90% better today. My biggest hurdle is the vision issue. Balance, I am mostly able to control as long as I take it slowly so my vision works with my body. Numbness, I can deal with if necessary but I expect it to go away completely at some point.

Despite how much better I am, I know I have a long way to go yet. I wish others could feel my symptoms just for a moment because they look at me and think I'm fine and normal. They don't know what I am experiencing mentally or physically each day. I plan to stay on the oral antibiotics for a minimum of another 6 months. This will give me a full year of treatment, which is discussed as minimum standard for the CAP treatment. I don't want to stop in the middle and get a relapse. After six months, I will further evaluate the situation, but I do think that I will need to take pulsed boosters for the rest of my life in some form, most likely in the form of pulsed orals every few months. I'll always do what I need to do to stay on top.

I am actually glad this hit me so severely in the beginning only in respect to push us to find what was really happening. As we found it early, I'm also happy I had the chance to take so many antibiotics so quickly and that my body has dealt with it. Find it early, treat it fast and hard, equals less damage overall. Every case is different, but in my case, I truly felt the disease process was so progressive that I risked being irrevocably damaged if I didn't hit the bacteria hard and fast. I am not a doctor, so this is just my personal opinion.

I expect the lesions to heal in their own time. The last two MRI's I had showed that the disease process stopped in its tracks. All the lesions were still there but no longer enhanced with GAD. There are no new lesions. My Lyme doc says the healing of lesions will take 1+ years. To me, the MRI results are the biggest validation of the antibiotic treatment.

Mentally and physically, this treatment is extremely rough, but the diseases it treats, ruins lives. It's not easy day to day, either herxing or living with symptoms. But in the larger picture this treatment can be rather quick and less problematic than the approved MS treatments such as chemotherapy, which help very little and can be very difficult to take. In my opinion, the CAP cures "MS." My validation of the CAP came in stages. With each herxheimer episode, my symptoms abated a little each time and I felt better. Every/any herxheimer is not easy physically or mentally, but literally each one made me feel better or more functional in the following days. Simply, if you have symptoms like I've written about, you might ask to take a trial of strong antibiotics and the vitamin supplements. If you have herxheimer reactions, you would know there is infection within to ruin before it ruins you.

[Author's note: December 15, 2006, 8 months out of treatment, Karl and his wife were interviewed by ABC News for a prime-time medical mystery spot intended to air in 2007. The spot is titled, "Chronic Lyme Disease as it Pertains to ALS and MS." The slot is expanding into 60 minutes at this time; but has not yet aired.]

❖ ❖ ❖

Tackling Loss, Life, and Lyme Disease

Glenroy Wolfsen, New Jersey

[Note: a brief summary of the following story was published in the Hunterdon County Democrat, Flemington, New Jersey; and a short story appeared in the book "Confronting Lyme Disease," by Karen P. Yerges and Rita L. Stanley]

This is the story of my life with Lyme disease. What must be emphasized is just how very different every individual is. While Lyme has some characteristics which are common among patients, it is also a disease that manifests in each person in different ways. Because it is a systemic disease, it also tends to find weak spots or previous illness and attacks those areas more than others. It is important to remember that what was effective for me as a patient may not be as effective for another. Each of us with Lyme must walk our road essentially alone, and it is a very lonely road. We must become our best friend and advocate.

Because Lyme can be so isolating, it is very important that those who know Lyme patients help them stay in contact with others and have some sort of support group. Many times the difficulties of Lyme symptoms may cause a spouse, lover, friend, or relative to abandon the patient. Lyme can be a tragic disease and cause great financial hardships and a loss of other resources. It is my hope that this story will help all who have Lyme and those who know people with Lyme to learn more about the disease and become better teachers, supporters, and fellow advocates for those who suffer. Though it is almost impossible for those who have never had Lyme to understand what a patient is going through, perhaps this story will bring many closer to that understanding, so compassion and companionship might replace ignorance and abandonment.

It is my faith and conviction that everything that comes to us in this life has a meaning that needs to be found and understood and acted upon. This story is my expression of that faith. I have learned from my disease some very valuable lessons. Though Lyme disease has attacked me, it has not defeated me. Though it has changed my life, it has also deepened it. Though Lyme disease has asked me questions, it has also given me answers. Though Lyme has shown me my weakness, it has made me face more clearly than ever my dependence on the Love, Mercy and Strength of God. I offer to you my own journey then, in the faith that it may touch you to a deeper appreciation of the uniqueness of this illness and the great need for more education and support for all who face their own journey.

My wife Patricia and I had lived in New Jersey for over 30 years. We had 4 children, three girls and a boy. We both were professional people. She had been a public school music teacher for many years and a gifted soprano who sang in churches, arenas, schools, and numerous functions both sacred and secular. She grew up near Wilkes-Barre, Pennsylvania. When it came time for college, she studied voice at

Westminster Choir College in Princeton, New Jersey.

Like my wife, I was also a person born with musical gifts. My life on the farm in New Hampshire was the usual farm boy's life. My wife and I married in 1964. We both graduated from Westminster and moved to Massachusetts where I was organist-choir director for a large church and she began teaching music in the public schools.

We next moved to High Bridge in Hunterdon County, New Jersey. It was there where we were to raise our children. While she continued to work in public schools, I entered the same profession, but continued postgraduate work at Trenton State College with a major in Musicology. Later I received a Master of Divinity Degree from New Brunswick Theological Seminary in New Brunswick. She continued to teach school and I taught while serving as organist and choir director in churches throughout the area. Eventually I entered full time Ministry in Protestant Churches in Pennsylvania and New Jersey.

Then events began to take a turn that would affect our entire family in ways we could not yet imagine. From early childhood, our daughter Julie was always having hospital visits because we could not understand the petechiae *[broken capillary blood vessels]* that were showing just under the skin. Many tests were done including a bone marrow test. Eventually tests revealed she was suffering from a blood condition knows as idiopathic thrombo-cytopenic purpura (ITP). This is characterized by blood having few platelets, but those she did have, were extra large. With this condition, there was always danger of excessive bleeding from minor cuts and bruises. In her teenage years, great care had to be taken even during the menses, and we were always on guard to monitor her condition.

One day in her late teens, she and her boyfriend were driving on one of the back roads in our area, and came to a hill with a stop sign at the bottom. They were going too fast and as the roads were wet, they slid through the stop sign and into the fence of a farm at the other side of a cross street. This was just a minor accident with no injuries, but a precautionary hospital visit was in order just to be sure. Maybe this accident was a blessing because they found protein in her kidney. She was taken for tests which revealed a kidney condition. The doctors told us that she did not need any special treatment, nor did they expect any problems with the kidneys for perhaps many years, if at all. At this point there wasn't even a discussion of dialysis. She was simply to report for occasional monitoring.

Our other children were coming along very well, and my wife and I continued in our professional work. Suddenly one day while at school, my wife had a fall while going up the stairs to teach a class. After that, she noticed difficulty negotiating stairs on a regular basis. She had never been sick before, not even during childhood. Then she felt a tightening or a "banding" sensation around the waist, followed by a frightening bout of optic neuritis. We decided to see a Neurologist for a check up. With her symptoms and the rapid changes, they decided to do a test for Multiple Sclerosis. It was quickly determined that she was having symptoms consistent with the onset of MS. They wanted to do more testing, so she was hospitalized for a week. The results confirmed she was suffering from MS. After the initial shock and attempts to adjust, she returned to teaching. This helped get her mind off the diagnosis and gave her a sense of purpose and accomplishment.

As time went on it became more and more difficult for her to get from one class to the other. After a lot of discussion she came up with a plan of what to do. United Cerebral Palsy was an agency out of which aides for handicapped persons were employed. We submitted a proposal that I be hired as her aide, and this would give her the possibility of making her 25 years in teaching before retirement. But the catch was that a spouse was not normally hired as an aide. We came back with the idea that I was the best possible choice because I was also trained in music and could assist her at the technical level that another aide could not possible fulfill. They accepted our idea. I left my work and dedicated myself to taking care of her during her school day. A full day's work at school was more than enough for her.

Meanwhile, our daughter Julie was doing well. No bleeding, kidney problems or treatable dysfunctions. When her boyfriend decided to go to college, Julie decided to go to school with him at Florida State University in Tallahassee so they could continue to be together. We arranged 2 teams of doctors in Florida for the continued necessary monitoring of her blood and kidney conditions, one team for each. Once this was in place, we wished them well and waited to hear how they were doing. We were excited to get tape recordings and letters from them. Not long into the school year Julie wrote and taped that she was having fatigue walking around campus, and seemed a bit puffy and would sometimes get nose bleeds. We weren't overly concerned at first, but soon the nosebleeds had us quite worried.

Her doctors saw her in hospital and couldn't find anything wrong. They would do things to stop the bleeding, and send her back to the dorm. One night she was discovered on a stretcher outside the emergency room by one of her doctors. The doctor was horrified at her condition and rushed her in. Within less than an hour, she was in a coma. We were called and were in shock. My wife made emergency arrangements to get down as quickly as possible, leaving me with the other kids and the house. She called as soon as she got there to tell me that I should rush down right away.

We learned that the two teams of doctors had not consulted as they were supposed to do, and the blood doctors had given her a drug to help with bleeding problems that was contraindicated for a person with her kidney condition. It was the drug that had begun to shut down her kidneys and eventually shut them down completely putting her into a coma. Because of the size of her platelets, the dialysis machine was not filtering the kidneys properly and she was near death. When doctors got all this straight they took a measure to get her out of the coma and stabilized with constant blood transfusions and special dialysis equipment. After that, it was a matter of many more blood transfusions to try to get blood with normal palettes to stay in her system so dialysis could continue. But the blood always reverted to its former type. It was determined to get her stable enough to fly her home to New Jersey and have her hospitalized here. There the decision was made that the only type of dialysis that would work was peritoneal or "hemo" dialysis, done at home with a special machine.

The hospital and our family decided that I would be the best one to administer this dialysis and to maintain the equipment. Once home, I got used to this nightly routine. It was a constant struggle with clotting factors and the peritoneum tube.

But Julie had an extraordinary spirit – one that was to become for me, years later, a living example. I know she would not mind me sharing with you a secret that she had told me when she was very young. I promised not to "laugh" as she told me she had been visited by an angel every night who told her calmly that "everything was going to be all right" and not to be afraid. We accepted this during those young years without realizing the significance of those nightly visitations. It was just during the days and nights of complications from dialysis that

Julie reminded us that her angel was still with her – a secure presence in an invisible certainty which made Julie radiate confidence when the rest of us were sometimes in a panic.

During the few years of dialysis it become more and more apparent that there was going to have to be a transplant if Julie was to live. Dialysis became less efficient and more problems added to the stress on her body and heart, though, as usual, her spirit was not flagged. Her doctors were becoming concerned and thought it was a good idea to make preparations for a transplant. So eventually I went in for match and test. I did fine. Then our oldest daughter went in for the same tests. She was a match as well. The hospital and doctors thought our daughter might be the best donor, but they had to have a talk with Julie first. They told her that the staff was divided on the idea of a transplant. Some thought it too risky and did not want to he held responsible for the operation, and others would be willing to perform the procedure, feeling that it was the only chance she had – but Julie was told that ultimately she needed to make the decision. This she did in short order, deciding that life was to be lived with quality and a new kidney, or it was not to be lived at all. This was her stand and her faith. So she went to hospital in Philadelphia with her hopes, her angel, and a few stuffed animals. We prayed and cried and trusted. She was an inspiration.

While she was being prepared for the operation, all of us gave a lot of blood. Julie's friends came to give blood, too. Knowing her bleeding problems, we anticipated more than the usual need. The day of the operation came and the two sisters became one in a mystery that was out of our hands. After the operation it was a real joy to see both daughters recovering together, the giver and the given, both happy to be alive. Soon Julie began to have expected problems with the blood – again this was a crucial factor. This time they had trouble getting a balance between clotting and bleeding. It eventually became a battle that took them into many more blood transfusions and into the operating room to tie up bleeds and to make sure some clots were out of her legs.

Julie and her sister laughed together the first day Julie went to the bathroom as a normal person in a long, long time. Then her sister finally went home confident Julie would soon follow. Still, blood problems persisted. Then one morning Julie wanted to tell me another me another secret. This time it was a vision of the Buddha and her favorite pastor appearing on a door opposite her hospital bed watching over her all night. That day a sudden need for water overcame her. The doctors were not pleased and told us that this usually means a massive internal bleed. They gave her water, but then said they better take her to the operating room quickly, and so she was put in the stretcher for the trip down stairs. As she was about to go out of sight down the hall, I saw her turn her head to me and wave her hand as she said quietly, *"I won't be back this time."* I will never forget her angelic face and the calm words she said that afternoon. The doctors were soon back without her – they tried to tell us in the best way they knew how – but I already knew. She was gone. They had worked valiantly to bring her back, but her angel had other plans and our Julie went with her angel to learn to fly.

I must say that I was never so proud of any of my children than I was of my oldest daughter. She was just recovering from having given her kidney to Julie. She worked as a funeral director near by, and arranged her sister's entire funeral. Not only that, but she also delivered her own personal eulogy to the sister she loved so much. Her courage and love is something none of us will ever forget. They truly loved each other with a love that lives on in eternity.

With our daughter's death my wife's condition began to worsen more rapidly, no doubt the shock and sorrow of losing our daughter was very hard on her system. She continued to teach, but had more and more difficulty even though I helped each day. I could also begin to see how the school administration might be looking to find ways to get her out. It was something I didn't really want to tell her and make her feel bad about (I knew she already did), but I was afraid they might eventually succeed. Finally I convinced her to retire so she would have the well-deserved benefits from years of teaching. It was well she did, because at one of her physical therapy sessions, the therapist discovered a well-developed subcutaneous ulcer near the bottom of her spine. It took almost a year to clear this up. Being in bed so much for the wound healing left her limbs much less flexible and far less functional.

Now her mother's birthday party came up, to venture out of the house and into the van was more of a struggle than ever. She tired easily and could not enjoy events of any length. It was a warm, humid day in the Poconos in June of 1998 when we finally reached the Hotel Center for the birthday celebration. It was a hot drive and hotter when we arrived. My body seemed very tired from the trip and I didn't look forward to the physical work of getting my wife out of the vehicle and into the party. After I did and she was settled and the other kids were with her to keep watch and help, I stayed in the van. I had (as was my habit for years) brought books to read and paper to write on, so I stayed and read and wrote and tried to relax and enjoy the magnificent view from up high in the mountains of Pennsylvania. My kids from time to time would bring me a drink and a little food. They asked me if I wanted to come in, but I didn't really feel like it and declined. I put my head back and rested every so often. I waited and hoped they would be done soon. Stretching my legs with little walks in the humid air wasn't really as enjoyable for me as I thought it would be. It was a long trip back to Hunterdon, NJ and I was anxious to leave.

By the time everyone came out of the hotel, it was mid-afternoon. As soon as we hit the pavement of the main road, something happened. I had a sudden sensation that the outside world was being seen through a "glass darkly." It seemed strangely unreal and distant. I also felt more tired, but not the ordinary fatigue I was used to; something more pervasive, and sinister. Of course I had to drive home, but it required a very concentrated kind of attention and sense of purpose and focus to maintain the usual automatic driving skills and to remember the way home – a way I had traveled many times before.

This strange new feeling stayed with me all the way home as I struggled to stay alert and finish the trip safely. Once we arrived outside of our house, it was time to get my wife into her wheelchair and inside. Evidently the long party and the heat of the day had taxed her stamina. Usually I set the chair outside her van seat, secured the wheels, then I'd take hold of the "gate belt" around her waste, then with her legs as a pivot, lift and gently set her into the chair seat. But this time, her legs had no support, and she folded like a rag-doll; half in, half out of the van. I yelled for the children to help. My wife was heavy and it took all of us to get her in a position where I could try the swing movement again – and this time it worked, but we were all soaked with sweat from the effort and the heat. Once I got her in the house and in bed I felt such fatigue I could vomit. I never felt this tired in my life.

Because this was so unusual, I went to the doctor the next day and he told me I must have nearly suffered heat stroke. He made sure I drank the appropriate electrolyte liquids for recovery. But even with that it took about a week for me to feel "normal" again. By September, I was feeling a strange tiredness not at all characteristic. It was a more systemic and pervasive kind of tiredness I had not known before.

Care taking was difficult and time-consuming. As my wife's condition became more progressive, I had more to bear. My body, mind and emotions were all under stress. Day and night I had to be alert to breathing and swallowing problems. I had to watch for bedsores, lung fluid buildup and infections. I had to watch her and try to understand what she wanted or didn't want, as her ability to communicate became more and more restricted. It was no wonder, I thought, that I often felt tired, and sometimes more than tired – what I would call weary.

One afternoon after feeding her lunch, I went into the living room and leaned in at the doorway, taking a break to appreciate the leaves just beginning to turn. I felt in my chest that my heart was not beating right. It felt like it was going very fast – and I was sweating. It took me by surprise, but I didn't make much of it. I was just tired, I supposed. The next afternoon something like it happened around the same time, but this time my heartbeat was not rapid like the day before, it did a "flip-flop." It would beat a few times, then stop, then beat a couple of times real fast, then stop again. I got one of the blood pressure cuffs I had used for Julie and checked myself out. I was a little on the high end, but nothing serious. This continued to happen every few days, and I made an appointment with my doctor.

He did the usual kind of check-up plus took a good look at my heart. He found nothing wrong and came to the conclusion that caregiving was taking its toll. He suggested getting some relief in the schedule and taking a little more time away, have a little wine in the evening to relax, and take the pressure off. I took his advice. I thought the wine would help, but to my surprise, I found it made me feel more "unreal" than ever. **It was as if I had no tolerance for alcohol.** I had always been a beer drinker and was surprised as I tolerated alcohol before, but now it seemed different.

Now Halloween was coming up. My son Michael and I got into the van and headed out. On the way out of town I felt like I was shivering, but it wasn't particularly cold. I stopped at a light. When it turned green, some other cars started pulling out before I did, and just as they did I had the distinct perception that I was traveling backward at a high rate of speed. It was bizarre and scary. I went on, and we arrived. I parked and let Mike out and wished him a great time. As soon as he closed the door, I noticed the surroundings were unfamiliar. I thought, "Where am I? What road is this? How do I get out of here?" I sat in a blank stare as if in a sudden amnesia. I don't know how long this lasted before I snapped out of it, but even after I got my bearing again, nothing was quite as "real" and sharp is I was used to. Yes, I knew where to go now, but it was all shaded with unfamiliarity. What an eerie feeling. I was thankful that Mike called me later to say his friends were going to bring him home.

From the very beginning these seemed like isolated incidents, (trip from Poconos, heart rhythm, disorientation, strange tiredness). Almost imperceptibly it began to feel like these odd symptoms were happening closer and closer together; a little more elevated and intense each time. Slowly days became harder to get through. My heart would bother me, by mind was not sharp, my beloved reading periods made my eyes hurt, my moods where more changeable, and I even began to have an overall low-level anxiety creep over me. Taking care of my wife was more difficult. I knew something was wrong, but had no idea what. Even the doctor's suggestion that I was worn down by caregiving didn't seem to explain everything happening.

It was convenient for me that a pharmacy was close by, where I could get the necessary supplies my wife needed. The pharmacist was always helpful and supportive. He seemed to appreciate the weight of taking care of a chronically ill relative. One day I mentioned to him some of the strange things I had experienced. When I got to the part about anxiety and feeling panic from time to time, he said something to me that would make all the difference in my life from that time forward.

He said he had suffered anxiety and panic attacks. He said that he would sometimes have to stop everything and lay down on the floor with his legs up to alleviate the attacks, and on other occasions had to stop his car in mid-trip because of them. **The reason, he said, was because he had Lyme disease and some of the co-infections that often occur along with it.** I was to learn later that not only was he affected by Lyme, but many of his family members were also sick and being treated. He said that from what I told him, it was very likely that I had Lyme disease. He asked me a few more questions for his own confirmation and said that it was his strong opinion that I should get some money together and head for his doctor as soon as possible. He gave me the doctor's name and assured me it would be much better to find out as quickly as possible, because early treatment was crucial. He had a sense of urgency in his voice. He didn't want me to hesitate, because, as he explained, the longer Lyme is in one's system, the harder it is to treat and the more damage it can do.

I took his advice and called his doctor in Pennsylvania, about an hour and a few minutes from my house. He thought I should come in right away and made an appointment for me. I got help for my wife and had one of my daughters drive me down. I didn't feel confident enough to drive myself. Little did I know that on the day I went in for my wife's supplies, my pharmacist friend would be the right man, at the right time. Nor did I know that he had already helped and would be helping innumerable people take timely steps to diagnose Lyme, and that he was keeping literature about the dangers, a symptoms list, prevention and other resources of help for others with Lyme disease. He was not just a pharmacist; but a man of compassion and healing. I am sure he does not know how much suffering he has helped to prevent and will continue to prevent in the future.

When I arrived at the doctor's office, blood was drawn. During this process it was pointed out to me that my blood was "very thick." I noticed it was taking quite some time for it to flow into the tubes. When the doctor saw me and interviewed me, I told him about my circumstances and all my symptoms. On the basis of listening to me and observing me during the visit, he said that he was quite sure I had Lyme, and therefore as a precaution he started me on an antibiotic right away. This was to prove a very important decision, because my blood tests and urine tests were all to come back positive for not only Lyme disease, but for two of the co-infections that can accompany Lyme. In my case they were *Basesia*, and *Human Granulocytic Ehrlichiosis* (HGE). Not only did my test results confirm these parasites, but they also came back with photographs of my blood showing the presence of the spirochetes. How scary they looked when I saw them!

From the combination of tests, observations of my condition and my history, my doctor was of the opinion that I had been infected with Lyme for some time. He described my psychological symptoms, characteristic of late-stage Lyme. He said that treatment would continue for an extended period. This was important information. All that I had experienced from the first strange episode in the Poconos to the latest anxiety and heart symptoms must have all been signs of Lyme disease, but I never knew it. I had never heard of Lyme disease, nor did I know that some Lyme-infected people develop a "bull's-eye" rash soon after being invaded by the bacteria. **I never recalled having such a rash.** If I had, then I might have been saved from the infection I had, and from the long struggle that I had no idea that lay ahead. As all Lyme patients learn eventually, prompt treatment is essential, but without the rash or proper diagnosis, that never happened for me. **I also learned the majority of people infected do NOT demonstrate a rash.**

How long had I been infected? No one knows. It could have been a short time before my Pocono event, or it could have been long before that. I could have been infected years earlier and it did not manifest or become active until stress triggered the bacteria to begin its active course. Stress, sudden life changes, prolonged periods of physical or psychological events can be triggers to long-standing, but latent infections. I will never know, but the doctor gave me clues. He suggested that caregiving had compromised my resistance and lowered the effectiveness of my immune system, allowing the infections to get a stronger hold on me than usual. He thought I must have had Lyme for quite some time as my symptoms were more typical for what he called "late-stage" or "chronic" Lyme.

On the next visit, my diagnosis was confirmed. I had additional tests to monitor the status of the bacterial and parasitic infections as well as to check my liver and other internal functions. My doctor had sent the blood to IGeneX labs in California for analysis. This was the very best laboratory at the time and was using the ELISA and Western Blot tests. These tests were accurate to some degree, depending on the condition of the bacteria, which changes shape and cell form, and on the condition of the body and immune response to the infections. This is one part of the diagnostic problems many Lyme patients suffer, and is sometimes why diagnosis is delayed or missed.

For treatment, I was prescribed 3 antibiotics. They were Doxycycline, Ceftin for the Ehrlichiosis, and Mepron for the Babesiosis. All of these were powerful antibiotics and are very effective against the bacteria and parasites, but they also kill all the important "good" bacteria in the intestines, allowing the build-up of candida or yeast, with potentially devastating results. This killing of the good bacteria and resultant yeast growth seriously reduces the power of the immune system. It also leads to "leaky gut" syndrome allowing improperly digested foods to pass into the blood, which the immune system identifies as "the enemy," resulting in serious, multiple food allergies, and reducing the assimilation of food nutrients. To prevent these problems, I had to take "probiotics" which replace the good bacteria in the intestine. Yeast is tenacious and aggressive, and I had to take Diflucan to reduce the yeast. In addition to the antibiotics and probiotic, I was given a host of vitamin and mineral supplements along with heart enhancing products that included CO-Q10.

I knew I had been getting worse, but it was at least good to have a name for what was wrong with me and to have medication that would "make me better." I was trying to figure out how I ever got bit in the first place. I knew I mowed the lawn behind the pool areas were two trees had very low branches which forced me to go underneath, and I was always getting them in my face. The area also had tall grass and was at the bottom of a downhill slope where lots of moisture flowed. I also had three dogs. When I let them out during the day, I would stay out with them to keep an eye on one of them. I often brought a book with me, as I was an avid reader. I remembered that before I was aware of Lyme symptoms, I had been out with the dogs, reading. I wondered if I got a tick on me from the high grass and brush in the dog area, or perhaps one got on a dog and then on me.

While I was pondering these things, I continued to take care of my wife and do things around the house. Our son also had to be cared for and given attention. I was always aware of how much attention I should be giving him, because I was always so occupied with my wife' care. I hoped I would begin to feel better soon; I had so much to do and was looking forward to getting my energy back. But, instead of feeling better, I noticed I began to feel worse – not a little worse, but much worse. I started to have my symptoms mushroom and I was scared.

When I went into the pharmacy, I told my pharmacist friend about what was happening. He told me that I had to expect to "feel worse before I got better." He explained it was a part of the healing process. He told me all about a "herxheimer reaction." This is something that all Lyme patients should know about and they should make a little calendar and keep track of when this happens, because it was cyclic so you could watch for it and know that when it happened, that you weren't regressing.

My own experiences of the herxheimer reaction began right away. I was glad I learned about it right from the beginning, because otherwise

I would have been caught between two very negative choices. I would have felt very discouraged thinking that I was getting worse in spite of treatment, or I would have thought the antibiotics were making me sick. I was not always faithful in keeping records of these reactions and I am sorry I wasn't. This made my phone calls to the doctor's office more frequent than they really needed to be. I could have saved both of us time and trouble. But I did keep enough records to get a general sense that my cycle was between 3 to 4 weeks. What varied with me was the length of the herxheimer, because it was unpredictable, and it always made me worry.

Depite treatment, I had 2 sets of symptoms which were both increasing. The physical body was involved in the heart irregularities and fatigue, and my mind and emotions were involved in increasing neuropsychological manifestations. The latter were the ones that were beginning to have the most impact on me. Caring for my wife and son involved physical work. I had no choice but to do it, and I could not rest when I wanted. I would find myself calling the doctor in the morning telling him that I was afraid to get out of bed because I felt badly.

His advice to me was specific and pointed. I needed to get out of bed and begin moving and doing what had to be done whether I "felt like it" or not. He assured me that this was best for 2 reasons; the first was that lying in bed too long actually would make be feel worse because I was not allowing the toxins that build up in the system that needed to be emptied, circulate. They accumulate in the lymph system and become poison and that causes great discomfort. The only way to "empty" this accumulation is through muscular motion, or some sort of movement and exercise.

Once I got moving and over the initial struggle, I would actually feel better. The second reason was to give me a psychological motivation and a sense of accomplishment. I was not to allow myself to feel totally dominated by this disease. I was to maintain some control over my life. The doctor's advice made it easier for me to do what had to be done. If I had not *had* to move, I probably would not have. If there were no *necessary choices*, I would have made the wrong ones.

Motion and action were good, both physically and psychologically – but that doesn't mean they were "easy" – anything but! And as far as the heart problems were concerned, that was the issue that scared me the most. Here again, my doctor pointed me in the direction of doing more, rather than less. He had told me early on that I must establish a habit of doing some walking every day. He didn't care how short or long; the important point was to be consistent. "If you get out there and walk," he said, "you will find the heart will begin to regulate itself." Now my problem was to believe and to act on this advice.

My other growing problems were neuropsychological. All my early symptoms seemed to be escalating. Mild anxiety was increasing. I began to have panic attacks. Seeing or meeting other people frightened me. Tasks that had to be done became exaggerated out of proportion. Every molehill became a mountain. I had constant, loud ringing in my ears. One ear didn't hear as well as the other. I became sensitive to loud noise, and sound in the higher frequency ranges was intolerable. I could no longer listen to my classical music, because I was not able to endure the emotional intensity. My eyes were inconsistent in clarity of vision. Bright light hurt. I became tired when I tried to read, and I had to stop after short periods of time. Sometimes the print on the page of my book looked as if it were slanting to the right. The first time this happened, I called my doctor in a panic, I was so frightened.

I began to have the sensation that my head was filled with cotton, or that I was living in an internal "fog." Everything was slowed down and my actions and reactions were slower. I had to concentrate to do simple tasks, and they took too much mental and physical energy. I remember sitting beside my wife's bed to write checks and pay bills. I had to concentrate and I struggled to write and make sure I was doing it correctly. It seemed like things once "automatic" now were done with conscious effort and directed will.

Talking to people was a real challenge. I knew what I wanted to say, but the wrong words came out of my mouth, or they came out "twisted up." My writing and typing was a mess. The word order was scrambled, and my short-term memory wasn't working. Mental and physical exhaustion set in after simple tasks. I was caught in a trap. I couldn't get out of this tired, aching physical body, and to me what was even worse, I couldn't get outside of my own head. My head seemed like a cage through which I would see and hear, but as if from a distance; as if I were somehow buried under cotton and fog, lost in a maze of confusion and anxiety, oppressed by fear and paranoia. Indeed, I felt like I was drowning in self-doubt and terror. Then there were the chemical sensitivities; every odor seemed intolerable. What I once hardly noticed, now made me sick. I just could not stand chemicals of all kind.

Another impossible activity was driving. I could drive no more than a mile or so without beginning to get "car sick. Vertigo and terrible disorientation accompanied stomach tightening and panic with my heart racing after trying to drive more than a short distance. Thankfully I could manage my wife's supplies and groceries as they were all close enough. But my doctor's office was more than an hour away, and that was impossible, so one of my daughters and her boyfriend came to my rescue. On these trips I had to bring a pillow or two and lay back and keep my eyes closed so as not to see the motion of things moving past the car. I had to make believe I was in my house and not a car. I was still very sick – each motion, sharp turn in the road, each bump felt like a tidal wave at sea. By the time I got to the doctor's office, I didn't feel like sitting in the waiting room, but preferred to stay in the car lying as still as possible until it was my turn.

Sometimes I went in, but I would become anxious around other people, especially if they tried to evoke a response from me. My anxiety was so high that when I was in the office I was talking all the time, and when I was about to leave, I would ask the doctor questions about what he had just told me over and over again. I felt like everything he said was leaking out of my brain, or that it never really got in there in the first place. Of course, my doctor was well aware of my anxiety and panic. He added Buspar to my medications to help control anxiety. He gave me a bottle of homeopathic pills to put under my tongue to dissolve. This product was called *Hyland's Insomnia*. When I would come into his office panicked and anxiety-ridden with a rapid heartbeat, he would reach in his pocket and stick some in my mouth. He would say, "Why are you torturing yourself like this? Why don't you take these – this is what they are for!" The product almost immediately brought calming but it had another interesting and helpful effect as well. The active ingredients stimulated the vagus nerve to regulate the heart rhythm, so not only was I able to retain some control of my emotion, but my rapid/irregular heartbeat would return to normal.

I continued on my same 3 antibiotics and Buspar. I found that with Mepron I began to have problems. I took the prescribed dosage but could not tolerate the sensation. My head felt like it became detached from my body and rose to the ceiling, while the rest of me was in my "normal" place watching it, and my "self" was somewhere in between. I felt like a ghost. It was all too bizarre and frightening and I had to call the doctor when this continued to happen. He understood this was a terrible sensation and symptom and allowed me to cut back on the dosage, but said that we had to maintain a certain level in my system at all times in order to eradicate the Babesia.

Meanwhile I had continued my walking exercises even while at the doctor's office. Instead of waiting in the car or the office, I walked around the building, or went for short trips down the road. I also noticed patients in wheel chairs there. I wondered if Lyme would cause me to have to come to that. I asked the doctor one day about those people. **He said they were all "MS" patients who had been misdiagnosed. They had Lyme and/or co-infections instead of MS, and were now responding to antibiotic treatments.** He said some of them found him just in time – their previous treatments had made their Lyme much worse, among which he mentioned, steroids. I told him my wife was often on steroids after an exacerbation, (prednisone). He had asked me about my wife before, but this time he suggested that perhaps she may also have Lyme and that he wanted to see her. By this time her condition had deteriorated to the point where getting her out of the house was nearly impossible. We had even stopped taking her to the Neurologist.

Taking special care of my wife was a commitment I was dedicated to. Comfort, love and encouragement were nourishment for her spirit. And yet there were times when this seemed all too much for me. I kept a little vase in the bathroom just off her bed area with one pink artificial rose. For me it was a haven pointing to a better time. Why this symbol became my safe place I do not know, but it always lifted me out of my pain and feelings of entrapment. How I wanted her to get well, but how I sympathized with her when she would say to me, "Don't you think this should be over?" What was I to answer, and how to respond to that cry? Could anyone blame her for not wanting to live without moving from her bed day after day? Could I judge her for wanting to find that place where there was no more suffering, and no more tears? But meanwhile, it was my duty to make her days as safe and comfortable as I could.

It was suggested that I get more help by the visiting nurse service. I applied and was granted assistance. Caregivers would come in a couple times a week, and when it was time for me to take a break, I found myself reluctant to leave, and many times did not. Some of those who came to help just could not manage the bed changing by themselves. My wife was too heavy and too helpless. I knew all the tricks, and did it myself. I could tell the aides were glad I helped, but they were also compassionate and sad that the two of us were living in a land of devastating illness. Some days they left feeling down, but other days they left being inspired.

Out of these depths I cried to God. Morning meant facing the struggle to get up and begin to move. Bedtime meant a barrage of terrible feelings. At night when I lay down and tried to rest, my body seemed to feel the entire weight of the day in every cell. All the pain and inflammation was pulsing in my joints and muscles. My body would get "electric shocks" all through it. My legs would suddenly jump. Sometimes from the very center of my brain a sudden loud noise radiated, accompanied by bright lights behind my eyes, and then pain would spread down my neck and into my back.

Once asleep I would be awakened by vivid, bizarre dreams that caused me panic and a rapid, pounding heartbeat. One such night I was awake and dreading falling into fitful sleep. Then, from my Bible the sound of the twenty-third Psalm came into my mind. It came gently and softly; and I saw each word before me as a gift. I began to repeat them in a silent interior voice. "The Lord *is* my Shepherd, I shall not want." Then, eventually an unimaginable calm slowly descended upon me and I fell asleep. I was to repeat this Psalm many nights when I experienced the dreaded symptoms that made falling asleep so difficult. It always had the same calming effect. I wrote the Psalm out, analyzed it, and meditated on it. I brought it with me to the doctor's office and studied it while waiting for blood to be drawn. I went to the wonderful Lyme-Aid and Lyme groups and sent it to people with whom I sometimes corresponded. These mailing lists were to become a wonderful resource of understanding, support and information.

Before I was aware of Lyme disease, I had been reading the writings of, and about George I. Gurdjieff, a Russian spiritual/psychological teacher. To me his words and work were as a rope coming down from above, and I was reaching up and holding on. During brief rest periods I would read as much as my tired eyes would allow and as much as my confused brain would absorb. The writings taught me something

I needed to know just at the time I needed to know it most. He taught that we are responsible for our own states of mind and heart. I was to find that my "self" was *not* Lyme disease, and "I" was *not* my symptoms. "I" was *not* my moods and fears; or my self-pity and darkness. I learned of the terrible loss of precious physical and psychological energy which leaks away when we entertain negative thoughts. Fear, anger, resentment, sadness, loss of hope, self-pity, black moods, lack of motivation toward the future, but most of all, an inability to know the present where life is. I lived in the "disease" of yesterday and tomorrow as well as a present of "Lyme" disease. I didn't know how to be or how to "do." Essentially I was letting Lyme disease run my life. This was a key step, which opened the door for help from above.

There was new self-acceptance. I worked for myself and soon for others, to the best of my ability. Lyme disease was an "alarm clock" which forced me to become aware that my ability to work and separate from my symptoms was the essential goal. No previous training had allowed me to know how close the Divine is to each person when they are ready to open the doors. I now know that Lyme disease was an important key to the door within.

Everything continued getting worse as I struggled to get rid of the Lyme bacteria and the parasites. While the antibiotics were working, I had a lot of toxins from the die-off in my system. I had to walk, but I was very frightened. I used to fill out a piece of paper with the names and phone numbers of all relatives and close neighbors to keep in my pocket, just in case I became unconscious or died on my walk. I really felt that it might happen that way and I wanted whoever "found" me to know whom to call.

A neighbor at the top of a nearby street used to talk to me in the mornings before he went to work and that was a big help. I would go to his house in the morning and walk inside and wait when he wasn't quite ready. How wonderful it was to be able to get my mind off myself by talking to this man while walking, and to not be so afraid. We walked together every morning when he was home. But whenever he went away I was in a panic again. I would walk to his house anyway and look around his yard as comfort and remember that I had been able to walk with him, so why couldn't I do it without him. That was rational, but my mind was not feeling rational, it was chemically and hormonally imbalanced and my thinking was abnormal.

Other changes came along during this time. My body had increased cramping and my muscles went into spasms often. Encounters with people became harder to handle. I could not express myself the way I wanted and do not think I was understood. I felt that no one could identify with me, or really understand what was happening inside me. This was difficult because I didn't *look as sick on the outside* as I was on the inside. This was a major problem for me with relatives and friends. **Either I wasn't taken seriously, or I was made to feel like I was just overplaying my sickness for attention or sympathy.**

Soon the body cramps and spasms became unbearable. The doctor said that they were due to magnesium depletion, and that it is essential for a proper heart beat. From then on I received large magnesium injections. I also took calcium/magnesium supplements and *Dale Alexander's* cod liver oil for the omega fatty acids. Nevertheless I continued having the same symptoms.

I had my daughter's boyfriend drive me to the doctor in an emergency one afternoon because I could hardly move from muscle cramping and spasms. The doctor decided I needed to have shots twice a week. He called in supplies to my pharmacy but could not find a doctor willing to give me the shots (my doctor was quite a distance from my home). Finally the doctor taught my son how to administer the shots. My son faithfully shot me twice a week with a big dose of magnesium. I was so thankful for these shots and to be relieved from the terrible muscle problems. Eventually, I found a doctor's office that could give me my shots and which also accepted insurance. I was as thankful as my son was because although he was faithful administering them to me, I can't say that my son ever enjoyed the process.

While I was looking for a doctor, I noticed my son having problems. It was very hard on him to be around the house watching his mother deteriorate, and to see his father struggling with an illness which had changed him in so many ways from the father he had always known. I wasn't able to be the kind of father I wanted to be. I didn't have the kind of time I used to, and when I did have time, I usually had to rest. What little attention I gave him was my best under these circumstances, but it wasn't enough. He was slipping at school, and there were friends of his that were not what I considered the kind of kids which were a good influence.

Finally, we hired a family counselor and things were difficult due to my wife's greatly diminished ability to communicate. Sometimes she could be understood, but other times I had to interpret what she was saying. Other times I knew she was saying things that she wished or imagined, rather than what was true. I did not wish to contradict her in front of our helper or show that she was not always living with the reality of what was going on around her. This made my son and I very uncomfortable during these sessions. I always had to take anxiety medicine before the visit, and often more than once before each session was over. My son tried his best to admit to himself how he was feeling and to express it to the counselor. Some of the exercises we were given to work on were overlooked or left incomplete. I found myself in the position of trying to hold everything together without any help for myself.

Now there were changes in the wind I could feel, but could not see with clarity. There was a pervasive sense which overshadowed the days. My wife's condition was getting worse. The visiting nurses and the equipment dropped hints that her "MS" was affecting vital functions. Her swallowing and breathing were of concern, along with her frailty.

A home with 2 sick family members continued to take a toll on our son. His schoolwork and attendance were slipping and I had concerns about his friends. All of this was too much for a young man to handle. My oldest daughter voiced the opinion that it would be better if she obtained temporary custody and kept him until he was 18. At the time I thought having him live with her was a good idea, but I did not feel obtaining custody was necessary.

I felt bad enough as a parent struggling with our collective illnesses. Now we were having our son taken away from us, but I did not fight her decision. I knew she was doing what she thought was the very best for her brother. It also helped to get him out of some trouble that might have led to worse consequences down the road. But still, how lonely it was without him and his boy-like cheer and the help he always offered so willingly.

One day the nurses made it clear to me that it was time to look for a home for my wife's care. How sad I was. I was so used to caring for every need and soothing every pain. Now I had to tell her what was going to happen and why. My symptoms became much worse as I filled with sadness and felt the coming emptiness. The day finally came and I tried to be brave for her as they transferred her to the ambulance. I was crying inside and smiling meekly on the outside. My daughter went with her in the ambulance and I went back into the house. Oh, how terribly empty our home now was. In the morning my body was a mass of inflammation and my head was throbbing. My eyes were swollen and my heart was breaking. It was time to get used to being alone.

The next week I went to the pharmacy to get probiotics so I did not get candida, or a yeast infection. I had taken my supplements before heading for the pharmacy. By the time I got there I felt strangely warm and sweaty. When I walked in, the pharmacist looked at me with a horrified expression and asked what was wrong, "Only a little hot," I said. He told me I better get home and take Benedryl because it appeared I was having an allergic reaction. I rushed home and took Benedryl and within 45 minutes, the reaction began to subside. That evening I felt very panic-stricken and "wiped out." I was so scared, weak and shaky that I didn't want to be alone. I called friends whom lived nearby, and they let me stay with them. They made warm soup and kept me company.

The next day I tried to determine what caused the allergic reaction. I ate nothing unusual and took the usual supplements. The only thing I was taking in large amounts was magnesium. I decided to check with the pharmacist. I remembered that when I came to the pharmacy I had just taken my supplements. Among them was a large calcium/magnesium pill that I took a couple times a day. I stopped taking that pill for a few days and I was fine, so I decided to try it again. When I did, I began to get the same reaction. My friend the pharmacist and I wondered if it was more magnesium than I could handle, or if there might have been a filler in that particular pill. The latter idea didn't seem plausible, but I stopped that supplement altogether.

From this bad experience I had a setback and my anxiety and paranoia increased. Everything I ate and swallowed seemed threatening to me. It made me ever more watchful for reactions. I was prone to imagining and therefore, creating symptoms. I felt I was creating some of my own anxiety, but at the same time, I was powerless over the "Lyme-brain." My own mental chemistry seemed to stand between me and reality. This was my Lyme brain working overtime. My life became a maze of fears. I could barely stand to take any of my pills. Every time I took one, I waited in anticipation for a reaction to follow. I finally felt the need for magnesium, but refused to allow myself any more shots or even supplements in pill form.

I learned from a neighbor who also had Lyme, of a different form of magnesium called *Natural Calm*. I found that I could take this without any reaction at all. But I still had the battle with paranoia and anxiety every time I took it. I waited to feel that warm sensation beginning in my feet and moving up through my legs and into the rest of my body. Now, it just so happens that getting a warm sensation in the feet can at times be a natural result of the Lyme itself. In my state of mind, I could not distinguish between the two.

I was always on the phone with my doctor acting out my paranoia over every little thing. One day he told me that calling his office all the time was making it hard to work as they had many patients and phone calls. He suggested that I call only when I had an emergency, but, didn't they realize that I felt that *everything* was an emergency?

My wife had more frequent hospitalizations. The very things I feared were now happening. Finally, the day came when the doctors told us an infection had penetrated her bones and that she had pneumonia. There was nothing they could do. We had to make a decision. As a family it was decided that prolonging her suffering in the face of the inevitable was not humane. She was to be given pain relief and allowed to die. My oldest daughter brought my wife home with her, and arranged for hospice care. As my wife was slipping away, I too was dying inside. I felt numb and alone.

The day came when I needed to say a tender goodbye. The family knew I could not take trips as far as my daughter's home. I could call there though, and let her know I was with her in heart and spirit. So the day came to say my last goodbye and we had our last embrace. I was able to call my daughter to try to talk to my wife. As time went on it was more difficult to understand the few words she could say, but I spoke to her as if she understood, believing at some level that she knew I was there.

My struggle with Lyme and co-infections had made progress by then, but I was still very sick and the combination of life circumstances and stressful situations contributed to my symptoms. This was also obvious to those around me. What little talking I did with neighbors on my walks showed them a man whose mind was imprisoned within him no matter how he tried to bring his thoughts outside. My confusing and repetitive sentence structures were something that I was aware of, but couldn't get under control. I would walk away thinking to myself, "they must think I am crazy."

My daughter finally said to me, "Dad I am not happy with your progress, you seem to be standing still." She told me that in New Jersey (where she lived), that she had met several people with Lyme who had done very well with another doctor. She wanted to see if I could get an appointment with him. I wasn't willing to give up my doctor, but I knew I was not gaining much and still considered myself very involved with Lyme and co-infections. The next time she saw me she wanted me to speak to an older lady who had been extremely disabled with Lyme and was making remarkable progress. I talked with her on the phone and was impressed, and finally I was ready to listen.

Dr. B's office was in Warminster, Pennsylvania. Those I spoke to who had been under his care, consider him a genius. My daughter said it was very hard to get an appointment with him and come under his care, but she thought that because so many of her friends were patients there, I stood a chance of at least an initial appointment. When I saw the doctor, it was an emotional experience for me. He acted as a friend as well as a doctor. I found myself in tears as I related my story and symptoms. He could tell how emotionally fragile I was and understood the damage the disease had done. He explained his philosophy and showed me many charts and graphs to help me understand his approach to Lyme and co-infections. He was very thorough and patient. I tried to absorb everything, but some of it I didn't retain due to my memory problems. He was knowledgeable of traditional antibiotic treatments for Lyme and knew doctors who had previously treated some of his patients.

His approach to Lyme disease does not involve antibiotics because of the effects of these antibiotics on the bacteria. The doctor is a Naturopath and Nutritionist, who also uses wide modalities of alternative treatments. He immediately made it clear to me the role of nutrition and the need to balance the body chemically and electrically. His approach in diagnostics and treatment was to do more than treat symptoms of Lyme disease; it was to repair and optimize the body to allow natural healing. After showing me his approach, testing criteria and treatment modalities, I decided to continue with him. He began his analysis with Vega Equipment. I was "off the charts" for Lyme, Babesiosis and Ehrlichiosis. He considered my condition dangerous and wanted to begin treatment as soon as possible.

One of the very first objectives was to begin to rid the body of massive toxin buildup with a *Bio-Cleanse Unit*. This was done in a room where rods with positive and negative ions were placed in water with my feet placed there to draw toxins out of the body through the bottom of the feet. I was amazing how dark, if not black the water became in a short time. This process was done while using the Rife Machine at the same time with the electrodes held in my hands. This was continued for quite a few sessions because of the high toxic buildup in my system. He also told me what kind of diet was essential. This diet had two purposes. The first was to stop taxing the body in processing foods which were inappropriate, and the second was to ingest foods for optimum nutrition and chemical balance.

At the same time I began homeopathic and herbal formulations for Lyme and co-infections. I began these gradually. He told me a gradual process was necessary as the body has to adjust to new protocols, and that the transition could be difficult. I would feel much worse at first, and this would last quite a while, but should be expected and must be gone through. He warned me the transition from an antibiotic protocol to his would be most difficult. He said there was much toxicity and so many bacteria and parasites to kill. There was a whole shift in body chemistry that had to take place over time. There would be a realignment of nutrition and metabolism and a revival of the immune system. I was soon to learn just how right the doctor was. But he kept encouraging me as well as always telling me what to expect. He also insisted that I exercise, especially walking, as much as I could without overdoing it. I had to learn to "listen to my body."

During this transitional time I suffered far more than I had before. All my symptoms mushroomed. This meant both the physical and psychological. One of my real problems during this early period in my new treatment was paranoia. Ever since the episode of the allergic reactions, my paranoia over what I put into my mouth intensified. I had no trouble with liquid medications, (the majority from the doctor), but anything in pill or capsule form was easy for me to convince myself not to take. Thus I ended up not taking many of the important supplements and medications I should have, early on. The doctor later told me that if I had been able to follow his protocol as he gave it, I would have improved much more quickly. But this was a hazard of my mental condition.

All my physical symptoms magnified and made it very hard for me to function. My walks made me feel like I was going to die. My legs were so heavy and my body felt so weak that just a block was all I could take before I had to rest. I divided my short walks in half, with a rest period in between.

My son's visits were always a time of light. We missed each other and he almost always came with me on my walks. While he was with me I had the courage to drive the short distance to Clinton, nearby. One day my son listened to me describe how hard it was for me to think and walk and how the head fog made me feel like a prisoner. He said, "You know, Dad, why don't you try to write some poetry again like you used to years ago." "How could I possibly do that," I said to him, "because my brain isn't functioning." He told me that he thought it would be good for me and said I should just try it and see what happens.

I decided to start the next day. I sat at a table and got out my pen and a note pad. I hadn't written any poetry for many years. What was I to write about, and how was I to "think" when my brain was in a fog? Nevertheless I put my pen to the paper. I did this twice a day almost every day. To my great surprise, this became a literal oasis in my life. I found that while I was writing, I was not as conscious of my symptoms. I was focused on something else for those brief moments – almost as if I were in another place. And when I read what I had written, it was as if I was reading them as a stranger – they sounded to me as if someone else had written them. It got to be the time of day that I looked forward to the most, something just for me.

I knew then that I wanted to share what it was like to live with Lyme and let poems tell it to others. It was for anyone and everyone who might find a resonance there, or find some hope or some wings to lift them above the hopelessness that Lyme brings into life. Now I had a purpose and a reason to live. *[A few of Glenroy's poems appear later in this book]*

In time, it became clear that my wife was nearing death. One day I got the call that she had passed away. Now my time to face her death had come. I felt so devastated. Needless to say, this sorrow and stress made what was already a very sick person, sicker. My mind was unable to respond to the reality around me normally. I could not face the public funeral with all the people and the length of the service. We made arrangements so I could be with my son and oldest daughter for my own private time with my wife. I can just imagine how the rest of my family felt. They probably thought I didn't care about her or was so self-absorbed in my symptoms that I neglected my obligations. No one ever said anything, but I would feel that way if I were them. The greatest insult to the family was that I felt too sick to travel out of state for the grave-side service with the rest of my family and her other relatives. I am sure I will never be forgiven for that. This is an example of the misunderstandings this illness can generate.

Lyme makes the patient's behavior seem bizarre that those around them feel that the patient is either indifferent, uncaring, or rude. It makes others interpret your behavior as intentional when it is not. They do not realize that your life is not totally under your control, nor do they understand how stressful circumstances exacerbate symptoms and how long it takes to recover from every kind of upset or emotional turmoil.

If there was a private hell, I was in it. I knew I had confidence in my doctor and I was being treated, but now I was at my lowest. My wife had died in February and my father would die in March. Now I was again facing an escalation of symptoms and fear of what lay ahead. How could I go all the way to New Hampshire for his funeral when I couldn't even travel nearby for my wife's? My family talked to me on the phone and told me they would disown me if I did not attend the funeral. How could I insult them all and dishonor my father, they asked. And yet I knew that this trip would be terrifying. I also knew that if I did go, my own family would never forgive me for not going to my wife's burial.

> *[This kind of dilemma faces many Lyme patients, where they often have to choose between their own health, their very real fears, and responsibilities. The pressures often leave patients with little choice but to select obligation over their own health. Even simple choices are difficult for someone suffering with a Lyme-afflicted brain.]*

I signed up for Social Security, and was awarded a widower's benefit. This was not enough to maintain my family home and I had to move. I had many bills to pay off many expenses from my wife's care. My wife had taken all of her pension benefits so there were none left. Her will was re-negotiated close to her death so I got the minimum allowed by New Jersey law. The executor of the will paid outstanding care expenses using that portion. The end result was I got nothing from the sale of our home, a place we had lived in for 30 years.

I was beginning to feel the effects of Dr. B's treatments during this time. Some of the worst symptoms in my head were getting less intense. I had a little more energy and needed to rest a little less. My moods didn't have such wide swings, and my ability to focus was improving. At the same time I was coming to terms with the losses recently suffered. I was able to drive as much as a half-hour each way. The head problems were lifting and the "head fog" would leave me sometimes for a few hours at a time. There were changes in my condition that I could really feel for the first time.

I also began to seek help from the social resources in our new town. I went to the employment center and got involved with a program of testing toward skill evaluation and proposals for therapy that might be helpful or available. One of the first things to be done was a psychological evaluation. I went to the therapist who used a number of standard tests. These were selected in part to see just what damage the Lyme had done in order for the social workers to be guided in helping me find employment. Here again, the testing showed neurological damage. My responses to certain types of tests showed impairment in pattern recognition and motor skills. This was no surprise to me. On the other hand, the therapist was impressed with the things that I could do well. He told me that my own motivation and involvement in reading, writing, thinking and sharing had kept much of my psychophysical integrity intact. I did not take advantage of their program because I soon found myself with a new job.

My new job was education. I was an instructional aide in a school that included levels K-8 in a small town nearby. It was within my ability to drive and was part-time, only 4 hours per day. My new job gave me a renewed feeling of worth through being productive socially. But it was not easy for my body and mind to adjust. Some days I had so much body pain that doing simple tasks was almost unbearable. Other days showed just how sluggish my brain still was. Simple elementary operations and concepts were not recognized at first without conscious effort. What was once so easy and automatic was now labor and for me, and an embarrassment. But the more I worked with the students, the more I was able to do.

A check-up with my doctor brought good news. He was happy to tell me that his measurements indicated that I had cleared both the Lyme and the co-infections. He put me on a "maintenance dose" of homeopathic and herbal formulations to keep from being re-infected. I was told to use them at the maintenance level and increase when I noticed symptoms. He said I was going to feel much better as I continued to become more active and retrain nerves, muscles, joints, ligaments, and my mind and heart.

On my way back from when I was taking care of my wife, e-mail has been an important outlet for me. The Lyme disease lists and web sites were my extended family. I am learning through writing and following my aim, a way to overcome my fear, hate, and my limitations. I am also learning to live each day one at a time, changing what I can change and not worrying about what I cannot change. But in addition to all of these things, I live life with the hope that the rose in winter lifts against a world of despair. There is beauty all around and gifts that abound, there is love to give and grace to take, there is mystery to unfold and history to make.

Up to this day, I still have periodic and cyclical times of symptom flare-ups. I continue to use colloidal silver every day along with my excellent diet. I walk at least three miles each no matter how I feel or what the weather. I have most recently added chlorella that is adding richly to my nutrition and hastening detoxification of heavy metals and neurotoxins from the Lyme damage. There is no complete consensus as to whether anyone who has chronic Lyme and/or parasites recovers completely. I do not choose to put myself into anyone else's box or prognosis. I will not entertain the idea or image that I cannot be completely well. Instead, I do entertain and hold before me the image of a completely well and vital person. This is the ultimate reality that bears my true image and this will never die.

I would add to this my own personal belief that sharing through writing and talking with other people in the Lyme community has added an acceptance of my illness that has its own healing power. For me, the profound spiritual lessons I have learned through suffering can never be replaced. I know that in my own weakness I have found the strength to trust in God.

Being brought to my limits by this illness, I no longer fear death. Accepting death has given me the ability to better accept life and its precious moment-to-moment miracles. I am learning to be here now, and not in the memory of yesterday or in the anticipation of tomorrow.

What I offer with this story is the invitation to be exceptional. I invite all who read to become involved in the life-long journey of learning and teaching. Life itself provides all the material that any of us need, but it is within each of us to decide to take the leap of faith. Everyone has someone to touch, someone to love, someone to share with, someone who needs you to make a difference. You could be that person. Burdens are there to be lifted and stories are there to be told.

Jesus said to all of us, *"You are the Light of the world. A city set on a hill cannot be hidden. Nor do they light a lamp and put it under a basket, but on a lamp-stand, and it gives light to all who are in the house. Let your light so shine before men, that they may see your good works, and glorify your Father in Heaven."* (Matthew 5:14-16)

I can tell you that I have not felt like a light with Lyme disease, rather, I have felt hidden, unknown, buried, and dim. But I have taken the leap of faith to set my light on the lamp-stand. I invite you to find your light, whatever it is, for be assured, you have one. The choice is always yours. When you do you will find that there is help and support, not only from this world, but also from above. Whether you write a book, talk to fellow Lyme patients, talk to their friends or relatives, join a support group, encourage another to come with you, share your suffering with one who suffers, offer compassion through understanding, and ways that only you might think of, all of these are a way to bring your light out from "under a bushel."

❖ ❖ ❖

Healing Arrives Through "Alternative" Treatments

"Amishdenny"* New Jersey

As a youth growing up in then rural NJ, I lived near some open woods and used to camp a lot. With ticks everywhere, I have to wonder if any of my other childhood friends ever developed Lyme. I have been symptomatic since 1954 when severe brain fogs developed. Slowly over the years, more and more symptoms developed, such as arthritic pain in my hands, chronic indigestion, chest and pelvic pain, and tremors.

By age 22 I was quite weak and easily fatigued. I had to stop long distance running which I loved so much. I had the exasperating quilt of symptoms that came and went, depending on the weather and my activities, but never lost the brain fog and muscle weakness, especially in my legs. I knew it was going to be a "bad" day if I woke up feeling a heaviness or slight tingling in my legs. During the years between the onset of symptoms and diagnosis, I had been to only a small number of doctors because I knew to expect the usual rhetoric of "you're not sick." Or, away at college I was told,"Oh, you miss your parents," or "it might be the weather," or "see a Psychiatrist."

Only one doctor in the early '80's took the time to run tests to look for something. I don't recall the exact year but it was around 1983. This doctor ran an ELISA test but not unexpectedly it came back negative. In 1993, I finally received a clinical diagnosis of Lyme, no lab validation, but a diagnosis anyway. Too bad the doctor refused to treat me! Infuriated, my advocate found another doctor 2 hours away in New Jersey, and before I left his office, I had a script for biaxin in hand and a soon-to-be-positive Western Blot ordered.

Four regimens of antibiotics later, including 3 months of IV clafarin, I was sicker than ever. With the cessation of each regimen of antibiotics, I inexplicably became sicker than before the regimen began, all four times. I could hardly stand, I missed a lot of work, and I was constantly sick with colds and other viruses. I was going downhill, starting in October 1997 and culminating in 1999 when I had to quit work. My (then) wife didn't believe I was sick, even with a diagnosis. She made so much trouble for me I had to leave to preserve my sanity; that was 1993.

Co-workers, up until my leaving work in early 1999, would harass me because I was always tired, made mistakes, and called off sick so much. 1999 was a pivotal year because that was the last time I went to a licensed allopathic physician for my Lyme care. That was also the year I had my fourth relapse after the cessation of an antibiotics session. I was so weak I could barely drive, go to the store, or even do volunteer telephone work. It was the year I switched to alternative therapies for good. I could not afford another relapse.

Allopathic medicine was killing me! I had tried a regimen of Hyperbaric Oxygenation therapy earlier in April of 1997. This glimmer of hope would affect my decision to treat myself in 1999. It did something because the herxheimer reaction lasted 3 months and I nearly went to the hospital, it was so intense. I was afraid to drive 3 blocks to the hyperbaric center on quiet small town roads. I could never walk that far. For 3 weeks, much of my day was spent on my bed with the radio on looking out at the clouds as they rolled by. It was horrible. Slowly I began to improve, and in 4 months I was back at work and feeling better than I had in 3 years. I wasn't a ball of fire, but I was fully ambulatory and able to work 8 hours with little trouble. But it was short-lived.

As so often happens, the first cool days of autumn brought a relapse in the form of debilitating viruses and 2 bouts of bronchitis in 2 months. This relapse was so severe I could barely stand and it never went away. I had to decline my usual shifts of holiday overtime. Also, had it not been for the good fortune of light work loads, I surely would have been fired sometime between then (October 1997) and my departure a little over a year later in January of 1999.

During this period, I cried nearly every day before work. Every day a fever would develop, reaching as much as 101°F. Every evening chills set in. I started my alternative regimen with acupuncture. The pain was too much to bear, so I had to quit it. I tried olive leaf, lomatium complex, calendula, LD complete, colloidal silver and European Mistletoe but nothing worked. I heard online, about Rife machines, the "EMEM3D" variety. My PCP, who later went on to include Chinese herbalism and acupuncture in her medical practice, said she'd heard good things about them and by all means to try one. Without disclosing brand or maker, I "rifed" for 2 years and made significant progress. I have cut way back on treatments because I am busy now and cannot afford time off due to herxes but I still improve. If you can afford one, it might be a valuable investment.

During the allopathic medicine days of 1994-1999 I developed a severe heart murmur. The muscle walls of my heart enlarged to the extent that the valves never fully open or close. Under the slightest activity, the valves flap around and don't move the blood, resulting in dangerous weakness and dizziness. This allowed me disability so at least my family and I could eat after I left work.

I continue to slowly improve, with no signs of relapse. I have added some alternative remedies to the machine usage as I mentioned earlier, but no other equipment. I recently started a neurotoxin binding protocol pioneered by Dr. S. of Pocomoke City, Maryland. By administering cholestyramine, any neurotoxins from dead lyme bacteria bind with the drug and leave the body. This, of course, is not without some level of hoopla in the form of a herxheimer reaction. I am entering my third week of herxing which may be unusual, but I've been sick with Lyme for over 50 years. Anyone who isn't getting better should look into this.

❖ ❖ ❖

Could Tick-Borne Illness be "All in the Family?"

The Author's Story: PJ Langhoff, Elkhorn* Wisconsin

*[*We now reside in a different city and county than the city of Elkhorn, (Walworth County, WI), where my family was "allegedly" infected with Lyme disease. Our story was also told in part, in the book "The Singing Forest, a Journey Through Lyme Disease," and in various articles.]*

I have included my story to let readers know that I too, suffer from the same illnesses as others in this book series. I also touch on my children's "alleged" Lyme and our family court history of discrimination due to Lyme Disease.

If you read the companion book to this one, "It's All In Your Head, Around the World in 80 Lyme Patient Stories" (Book II), you read stories collected from all over the world, and the common themes which run throughout – denial of a valid medical illness, the devastation it brings, and the ignorance which surrounds Lyme disease in general. Although we are many people from all backgrounds, and each story unique, we all have similar themes and experiences dealing with Lyme disease and other tick-borne illnesses.

I don't remember if I was ever bitten by a tick as a small child, but could have been when my family moved to Pennsylvania in the late 1960's, or possibly shortly after when we returned to Illinois. While in Pennsylvania, I spent a majority of my time outdoors playing in our yard, climbing trees, running in the fields by the railroad tracks, and wandering in the woods at a nearby school. It was highly probable that I would have come into contact with ticks and other creatures, as I thought nothing of these adventures – and I certainly knew nothing about ticks nor would have ever thought much about them back then.

In my younger childhood my mother seemed perpetually pregnant, and suffered several miscarriages, including one which had been substantially far along, and though young, I remember the "bump." Although she successfully carried four, she lost all good sense after, and suffered what our father deemed a "nervous breakdown." Poor mom was not herself after that and suffered from what I now recognize to be, depression. In retrospect, I wonder if she may have had more than loss going on, as her physical and psychological symptoms lingered and grew erratic over time. (My mother was born and raised in Pennsylvania by the way, an area that has long been endemic for Lyme disease.)

Her later symptoms mirrored those of Lyme disease – fatigue, depression, arthritis-like joint pains, headaches, agitation, extreme mood swings, unexplained fits of rage, hair loss, panic attacks, palpitations, and mitral valve issues. Later she received diagnoses of Chrohn's Disease, Ulcerative Colitis, Agoraphobia, panic attacks, Lupus and a few others which only partly fit her symptoms. Mom also sadly suffers from a complete lack of insight into her own behavior. Even as a child I never thought someone could walk around with so many concurrent diagnoses, but my mother never questioned the number, nor her doctors. She revered their opinions and wore her many diagnoses like so many badges of honor. In my observation, she actually seemed to revel in the attention and sympathy she could gain from others.

Further, over time one could see that our father had symptoms similar to those of Lyme. I wonder now that if mom indeed had Lyme, could dad have contracted it from her – if Lyme is sexually transmissible. Could it have been that his symptoms might have been Lyme all these years? He suffered from daytime sleepiness, fatigue, stiffness, easy agitation, fits of unexplained explosive rage, and eye "floaters." Dad also had episodes of extreme road rage and he was known to shout loudly, and occasionally throw objects across the room when angry. One time when he was very angry, he picked me up and bodily threw me across the living room in a rage. Because he died suddenly at age 56 of a stroke, which is fairly common in Lyme. I see clearly that Lyme or another illness like Bartonella which cause sudden rage-like behavior might have existed and caused these symptoms. In my mind, tick-borne illnesses can never be entirely ruled out.

For those who might be tempted to say that I am "obsessed" with

Lyme disease and that I suppose that everyone with a medical ill has Lyme, let me clarify those untrue thoughts for you. (I have been accused of this in family court believe it or not, despite my never even saying the words "Lyme disease" anywhere in the 10 years of trial transcripts that I have in my possession!)

There are perhaps thousands of medical ills in the world and any number of them might prove to be what affect(ed) my family. However, tick-borne illnesses cause many conditions within the body, because the organisms change the body and brain's biochemistry in order to survive within the host animal. And since Lyme is called "the great imitator," its symptoms mimic those which are routinely diagnosed as other illnesses, such as Alzheimer's, ALS, MS, Lupus, Chrohn's disease, Rheumatoid Arthritis, Fibromyalgia, Chronic Fatigue Syndrome, and even psychiatric diagnoses such as Autism, Depression, ADD and ADHD.

When one has been dealing with this illness for a long time, (in me, perhaps 16 years to 30 or more), you come to learn the hallmark symptoms of Lyme disease. Let me state clearly here, that Lyme disease is **not a rash and knee disease**, but something much more complex and destructive which affects every organ and system in the body, and each individual's disease course is unique.

Lyme disease has some very characteristic symptoms among the 80 or so that commonly manifest. Many of these are symptoms from which both of my parents suffered. In the case of my mother, are still suffering from, to this day. It is highly possible that like so many families in the world who are suffering from Lyme disease, that if my mother had contracted it before giving birth to myself and my siblings, that she might have passed it on in a congenital fashion. If she had contracted it after having her children, she could have passed it onto my father sexually or vice-versa.

I am not saying that it is *probable* that my family may have been touched entirely by Lyme disease, I am saying it's a highly *possible* hypothesis.

> *[There are some who will argue that there is no "scientific evidence" that Lyme is sexually transmitted. But in actuality, there are studies showing that spirochetes are detectible in breast milk, semen and urine, saliva and other bodily fluids, and that it is transmissible in utero. Without considering sexual transmis-*

sion, it is a challenge then to explain why entire families are suffering from the same illness, even members who do not spend time outdoors on a regular basis. Sexual and in utero transmission might therefore help explain a number of these cases.]

I remember a great number of fevers and unexplained throat and respiratory infections in myself and my three brothers when we were children. Someone was always sick with "flu" or an "ear infection" or a "fever." In fact, three of the four of us were all in the same hospital ward around 1967, getting our tonsils concurrently removed, in the belief that the joint operation would "cure" us of all of our medical woes. My bed was near the window, and I remember looking out at the street lamps and the new snow on the ground. I was the only one out of the three of us post-operation who got to keep the orange popsicle the day nurse gave us just before her shift ended, before the night nurse came in to confiscate the "illegal" treats. I cleverly hid mine under the sheet and swore I didn't have one, but my brothers lost theirs to the white hat. (My other brother got his tonsils removed later, as he was too sick to join the three of us at the time.)

Shortly after the surgeries, we began to be sick…again. One of my brothers came down with what my mother called "scarlet fever," but none of us were sick with it, which I find curious, as we lived in close proximity to one another, with two brothers sharing the same room, and my newborn brother and I sharing an adjacent one.

In the early years of school, I was an A student, a child who wanted to be a veterinarian, an archaeologist or a surgeon – I couldn't decide which. But suddenly in fourth grade (when we made the transition from PA to IL), things changed dramatically for me. My brothers were enrolled at a private Catholic school, but there was no room for me, so I was sent to the public school across town. The transition was easy for me, as I liked the independence the new school offered and I did well academically. After only a half a year however, there was a sudden vacancy in the Catholic school, and I was sent there to finish the last half of fourth grade. I remember getting a skin rash one day soon after the change of schools which my mother called "impetigo." At recess we spent time outdoors on the grassy schoolyard playground, often lying on the ground. I remember the rash was flat, and round, and it did not have blisters, like an impetigo rash might. In retrospect, the rash looked vaguely more like an *erythema migrans* rash. I remember it because it was so distinctive, and my classmates made fun of my "cooties."

Another time I had a similar rash on my leg which my mother called "ringworm," but interestingly enough, it went away over time, never to be seen again. My mother also later showed me a rash on her forearm that she called "ringworm." Perhaps she might have been infected with a tick-borne illness – who knows? It could explain her sudden onset rage episodes, emotional outbursts, obsessive-compulsive behaviors, verbal and physical abusiveness and other symptoms.

At the time, we were living in a suburb of Chicago, and I was spending all my waking hours outdoors. My brothers and I built forts out of the wood we took from nearby construction sights, (that was wrong but we were kids). We rode bicycles in the fields, we camped out at night, chopped fireword, we lay in the grass, and went fishing and canoeing on the river – all activities which certainly would have exposed us to ticks.

Soon after the rashes, I began to severely decline in school. I lost the ability to concentrate, and focus on daily activities. I sat blankly staring at the chalkboard and listened to my teachers drone on about things which didn't seem to make any sense to me any more. No matter how hard I tried, I couldn't seem to retain any new information. I also routinely fell asleep in class. Memorizing dates, times, places and math problems became virtually impossible for me, and I could never figure out why, nor was I able to fight the daytime sleepiness that plagued me in class.

My grades of course plummeted and I became severely depressed. Nobody seemed to know what to do with the girl who no longer could do her homework – a child who had her IQ tested before elementary school, with a very high score for my age from what I was told. Now I felt like a perpetual dunce. I was an excellent speller and absorbed things fairly quickly before that, but beginning in fourth grade, I lacked the interest, motivation, and ability to pay attention to anything going on around me. I was often "ill," sullen, and felt very sad, and I didn't understand why.

My mother took me to the doctor numerous times, but there were no answers of course. In seventh or eighth grade, I suddenly got what was called "mono," but I know it wasn't a true mono. I spent several days in bed with swollen glands, a fever and general malaise, and then returned to school. Nevertheless, my mother called it "mono." I had recurrent "flu's," joint pain, headaches, problems with my menses when they began, depression, weird "hallucinations" at night, sinisitis, and ringing in my ears. At night I would sleepwalk, and my mother would pass my room and I would sit up in bed and ramble on in a garbled, incoherent tongue while remaining asleep, which she admitted scared the heck out of her.

The sleepwalking, which some might consider "normal," went on for a few years, from about age six when we lived in Pennsylvania, until about my sophomore year of high school. It was a strange anomaly. I would awaken from sleeping and manage to get "stuck" in the hypnogogic state, somewhere between being asleep and being wide awake. In a semi-conscious state, I would sleepwalk around the house and do different things, completely aware of what I was doing and saying, but I was powerless to "snap out of it."

Sometimes I would awaken in the dark of night and hear what sounded like whispers of people talking who were not physically in my room. That was extremely frightening to me, but I told no one about it, because in my family, you would certainly have been ridiculed for something like that.

When I was about seven years old, I suffered a case of the "mumps" which was not really the mumps. I remember painful lymph nodes and a bit of swelling, but even the doctor said it wasn't "really" the mumps. As was a standard practice in my generation, I had also been vaccinated against them at the time, so whatever it was, it was an odd illness.

My brothers also had their share of problems. My younger brother suffered from what was diagnosed as "Osgood-Schlatter" disease of the knee. He had joint pain and swelling. My youngest brother suffered from smallness in stature – so much so that the doctor wanted to give him HGH (human growth hormone) and my parents entertained that idea for quite awhile before finally nixing it. He also suffered from hyperactivity. I suffered from somewhat of a delayed puberty, including underdeveloped breasts, joint pains, and "bone" pain in my legs, knees and shins. When my menses came, I had painful, copiously heavy cycles and other problems, including severe headaches and light sensitivity. I also had stabbing, shooting pains in my chest and ribs, accompanied by unexplained transient shortness of breath not brought on by physical exertion.

In fact I believe it was about this time that my mother began exhibiting bizarre behaviors. She was overtly verbally abusive, and became physically abusive toward me on an ongoing basis. She also began to perform unprovoked Bible-quoting rampages which were more bizarre than a television preacher on steroids. Being an ordained minister now myself, I understand scripture and dedication to God, but mother's interpretive ventures went way beyond even a preacher's comfort zone. I will say only that she was obsessed with things most people would regard as ordinary. I never quite understood where any of that came from, and I did everything I possibly could to avoid her wrath. But in retrospect, in a brain-infected Lyme or Bartonella patient, obsessive, single-minded fervor or erratically skewed, irrational, or aggressive behavior makes absolute sense.

You almost have to actually *be* a patient to fully appreciate and understand the process of brain infection and how it becomes a victim's puppetmaster. As intimately as tick-borne illnesses can manipulate the brain, once you have had the affliction, it allows you a unique "ability" to instantaneously recognize others who are probably also affected. It's like a weird club actually, one which I had never wanted to become part of. Ask other tick-borne illness patients and they will tell you, they can spot someone a mile away who probably also has a tick-borne illness. Go figure, because doctors certainly can't – and often won't.

In high school, things weren't much better for me. Although I could apply myself to the courses I liked (and hence got A's and B's), the rest of the time I was weirdly unable to apply myself, and I could hardly pay attention, because I was so depressed and had such difficulty focusing. I was also sick constantly with the "flu." Years of antibiotics were shoved down my throat by a well-meaning doctor, but of course, nothing ever seemed to lift the veil of fog that seemed to envelope my brain.

When I was twenty, I was accidentally bitten by a cat, adopted from a shelter. I was on my own and living with a friend in a suburb of Chicago. A short time after that, I developed swollen glands, a fever, profound fatigue, "migraine" headaches, sleep problems, easily provoked agitation, heart palpitations, panic attacks, and anorexia. I had no idea what was going on, and doctor after doctor performed tests, to no avail. I had no answers at all, but continued working full-time, attempting to deal with my health issues as best as I possibly could. At work I could be easily aggravated, and I often would fall asleep at the keyboard in the middle of my shift.

I believe now that I was probably infected with *Bartonella henselae* from the cat bite at that time, as Bartonella is easily transmitted by cat bites, licks, scratches, cat feces, fleas, ticks, and mites. Another time while living with a boyfriend, I remember a strange incident where I grew suddenly extremely angry and began smashing anything I could get my hands on, breaking glasses and other objects. I never did that before, and I can only put it down as a Bartonella or Lyme-rage type incident, because when the brain is infected, that is the kind of behavior that can quickly be revealed. Just as explosively as it appeared, it quickly disappeared.

One evening while driving home from work, I noticed that the green signs on the freeway were suddenly "blank." I had a moment of thought that was something like, "huh, that's really dumb, they put up a new sign but it doesn't have any letters on it." I did not realize that it was my brain beginning to show some of the signs of the "weirdness" that comes from tick-borne illness.

I had tremendous exhaustion and difficulty sleeping but put that down to my third-shift work schedule. But I also had a growing numbness to other people's painful issues. I sat on my bed January 28, 1986 after working a night shift, eating a "macho taco" and watching the space shuttle *Challenger* disintegrate live on morning national television. Not until later did the full weight of how numb I had become descend upon my shoulders when I told a co-worker (who had stopped by for a visit), my opinion of the disaster. "That's what they get for going up into space," I had instinctively said, most shamefully and coldly detached. My friend was so disgusted at my comment that he immediately got angry with me and went home. And yet I felt absolutely nothing at all at the time. I had obviously lost all insight into my own behavior. I can now put that down to the infections that were already raging in my body and brain. Now years later after treatment, I not only feel the tremendous loss of those brave pioneers, but I now cry during *Hallmark* commercials and other things which most people are perhaps far less sensitive to.

While in my twenties, I acted out sexually with multiple partners, took risks, and became inexplicably anorexic and depressed. My anorexia did not seem to be related to any "control" issues like you might hear about on television talk shows, nor did I have a body dysmorphic syndrome where I thought I was perpetually fat. In fact, I knew I was thin, I simply lost my appetite to eat, and had to force myself, because I would "forget" to eat! These are classic Bartonella-type symptoms. The loss of insight into my own behavior was profound during the most acute phase of the illness. For about a year and a half I felt no need to eat, and during this time my weight fell to under 100 pounds. I remember that my normal size 6 body could easily fit into a girl's size 14 pant (a typical size for an average 10- or 11-year old girl).

It was only following what I thought was a mild heart attack incident (paleness, chest pain, clammy, sweaty, palpitations, anxiety, weakness, etc.) that I finally recognized that I was going to have to force myself to eat food if I was going to survive. Doctors at the time performed all kinds of heart tests, but none of them ever ventured a guess as to why I was so thin, nor offered me any diagnosis or nutritional counseling. I spent days on the couch forcing myself to eat slowly. Soup, then soft foods, and when I could stomach more than one meal a day, my ability to eat, along with the size of my shrunken stomach, grew. I had no idea back then what might be the cause of the anorexia. But just as it slowly descended upon me, I worked hard to eat more normally again.

In 1984 I developed endometriosis, a painful condition where tissue grows on the outside of the uterus and other organs. My menstrual cycle was fairly regular, but it was still a horrible ordeal each month. I would get incredibly ill, nauseous, and have extreme pain and very heavy bleeding. I would miss at least 2 days a month at work due to heavy and painful cycles. I was eventually diagnosed with stage 3 endo, which necessitated immediate ablative surgery.

At the time, I shared a hospital room with an older woman who had just had her gallbladder removed. I remember making a comment once about that fact, and she said, "by the time you get to be my age, you'll probably have to have yours out too." Neither of us knew that her words would prove to be prophetic. My periods were somewhat better after that surgery, but the endo would return intermittently, and my ovaries became polycystic and painful. At one time it was thought I might have an ectopic pregnancy, but ultrasound showed cysts instead of an embryo, which was a good thing in comparison. That wouldn't be the end of my reproductive problems however.

I was married in 1987 to a man who grew up in the upper penninsula of Michigan. Suffice it to say that from his many years of erratic behavior and extreme rage issues, along with his recurrent health problems, I believe he could conceivably have harbored one or more tick-borne illnesses himself – it would certainly explain a lot of his behavior, but that is in another book I wrote, less I digress.

With each pregnancy, I had roller-coaster hormones, which to some degree could be expected. I was not diabetic but I had hypertension at the end of the pregnancies. I was a petite size 4, and my daughter was more than 8 lbs at birth. My son was more than 9 lbs – big babies for such a little person. Both necessitated C-sections due to malpresentation and being so large. After the pregnancies, my hair began falling out. We attributed that to hormonal changes. I lost about half of the hair on my head, so it was diffusely thin, but not balding. Doctors called it "female pattern baldness." I thought, gee, maybe I have bad hair genes, after all, my oldest brother suddenly lost all of his hair while in college. He also developed "lumps" of fatty cysts on his scalp; something my mother had, and I would develop myself, which I had removed some time later. At least I had *some* hair left I thought, oh well, the joys of motherhood, I guess. In time most of it grew back, which was good – until it fell out again, due to the Lyme and co-infections, most notably Bartonella which is known for this symptom.

I did breast-feed my children for some months after they were born, and my daughter was a most colicky baby. She would scream and cry and to no avail did I spend many nights rocking her dramatic, noisy little self until she would collapse from exhaustion. I looked like a walking zombie and believe me, I have the photographs. If I had Lyme or co-infections at that point in my life, I could certainly have passed them onto my children in utero or through breastfeeding.

After the two children came along, in December 1991, we relocated from a suburb of Chicago, to Elkhorn, Wisconsin (the southeast part of the state). It was my hope that our children could grow up in a safer environment, and I could stop working full-time nights and finally be a stay-at-home mom and attend college at night so I could finish my degree. I truly wanted a different way of life, as the area we had come from was turning into a high-crime area, and was no longer what we considered a safe place to raise children.

The year 1992 marked the beginning of a journey down a road filled with illness and uncertainty. I find this odyssey particularly frustrating since we had moved under the premise that we were "escaping" the bustle of the suburbs of Chicago for a "different" life – a new and supposedly, *better* life. The irony of that thought strikes me now as I did not realize that the "new and better life" I was seeking was going to be, in reality, one which would be forever life-altering for my family, and many people whose lives would be touched by an illness we would collectively share.

It was in our backyard in Elkhorn, in August, 1992 that my then two toddlers and I were bitten by black-legged, *Ixodes scapularis* ticks. I distinctly remember brushing one off of my shoulder. I would find them crawling on me from time to time, not really paying much attention to them, or knowing for sure what they were.

One afternoon I took the kids out into the yard to sweep up the early fall dump of leaves which came from the 200-year-old oak tree sitting "smack dab" in the middle of our back yard. The children played in the leaf piles as children often do, and I happily snapped pictures of their carefree, innocent fall frolics.

A day or so later I discovered, and removed a small black "scab" from my back left shoulder blade. The scab must have been an adult, partially-engorged tick, but I didn't think too much about it at the time, because I didn't recognize it as being an insect. I thought it curious that I bled a little after scraping off the scab. I could not recall injuring myself but shrugged it off at the time.

I do remember during bath time, attempting to dislodge the tiny poppy-seed-like "things" that were attached to my children's ankles. In reality, these were (I would come to learn later), nymph ticks which had attached themselves to their skin. I had to scrape them off with my fingernails to get them to come off of the kids' legs. "What the heck are these," I remember asking myself. I had no real knowledge of ticks or Lyme disease during that time. They resembled tiny black grains of sand, and were slightly larger than the period at the end of this sentence in size. My children were 3 years old and eighteen months at the time of these bites.

Within a day or two following the tick removal, I became acutely ill with a large bull's-eye rash. It appeared directly over the spot where I had removed the so-called "scab." I then suffered for weeks with 104°F fevers, "flu" symptoms, joint pains, nausea and vomiting, severe fatigue, migraine-like headaches, visual hallucinations upon waking, vertigo, and gastric symptoms, which landed me in the hospital, seeing several doctors. I began to spend all my free time in bed, as I felt truly horrible. I visited several doctor clinics, trying to find out what was making me so ill. (I had to make a few emergency room visits as well, for high fevers and dehydration, from some "viral syndrome" as it was called.)

The first General Practitioner wanted to focus on my digestive system, and even gave me a stool test which came back "negative" for parasites. I asked about the rash, and he told me not to worry about it. I hot-footed it to the library to see if an encyclopedia could shed light on my illness. I found "Lyme disease" at some point. And lo and behold, there was a picture of the exact same rash I had on my body. Returning to my doctor, I was told, "we don't have Lyme disease in Wisconsin." This doctor referred me to a Dermatologist instead. I was angry but wondered if it was possible I misinterpreted the pictures I had seen.

A couple weeks later the rash had disappeared but now I had new rashes developing. They looked like little red footballs and appeared first on my back. Then within days, I had developed about thirty of them, which were plastered on my back, waist, sides, chest, and neck. I looked horrible. The Dermatologist took one look at me and said "dermatitis." I asked him if I could possibly have Lyme disease, and I described the bull's-eye rash, my symptoms, and of course he saw the subsequent rashes. His reply was a flat, stern, "you don't have Lyme disease." He handed me some rebottled calamine lotion to put on my rashes that cost me more than what I would have paid for it in the store and told me to go back to my regular doctor. Of course the lotion did nothing and I felt at a loss to understand what was happening to me.

> *[Years later I would learn that this particular doctor might have been one and the same doctor directly involved in a Lyme disease study which was happening in our state at the very time he saw me. And yet he flatly refused to listen to my question of "Is it Lyme?" I would have to suggest that it might have been because it was a well-known fact at that time (via U.S. Army studies) that Wisconsin was already endemic for Lyme disease in the 1990's, but it was a closely-guarded secret. The number of billions of dollars annually that drive the tourism, real estate, boating, camping, skiing and hunting industries in this state are staggering. What would happen if people knew the truth about*

the state's endemicity? They would stop coming of course and we certainly can't lose revenue, can we...]

Still I traveled from one ineffective physician to the next in an attempt to try to discover what was making me so darned ill. Meanwhile my eyesight began to change. I noticed that I had "floaters" much in the same manner as my father had complained about. And I was suddenly sensitive to light, and sometimes saw halos around lights. I often wore sunglasses during the daytime – inside the house. When I drove, I noticed that at speeds above around 60 mph, that I had a tough time concentrating on driving. It was almost as if I could no longer process the motion and visual stimuli between my eyes and my brain.

I also suffered repeated bouts of "conjunctivitis," dryness and tearing, but only in my left eye, which I thought strange. I experienced weird visual migraines in my left eye which were akin to watching undulating shimmering lights dancing in my visual field, sometimes accompanied by pain and eye irritation. I went to the Opthalmologist and discovered that I suddenly needed prescription glasses to see objects up close, when I had perfect vision just days before. I was checked for glaucoma but that was not present. Some days I needed my glasses, and other days my vision was fine. It was very perplexing to me, and I wondered if this was "normal" for people to have vision that fluctuated that much from day-to-day, in their early thirties.

I also had new fatigue, and intense attacks of abdominal pain which were centered around my gallbladder. These would typically last between 9 and 12 hours, giving me no warning whatsoever. All I could do was to lie down with the heating pad and writhe in pain. Analgesics did nothing for me, and neither did my doctors. I would endure this pain for 10 long years. Repeated gallbladder scans would always indicate "no stones," so doctors accused me of fabricating my pain and other symptoms, or called it "gas." (It was far more painful than any gas I have ever had, even the painful gas trapped within the abdominal cavity following laparascopic surgery).

I heard more than once that I should seek counseling for my "obvious depression." I didn't have time to be depressed. I was working a full-time job as a self-employed person because my husband lost his job only a year after we relocated. So much for being a stay-at-home mom or attending night school. I worked two different jobs to support us, and when my employer closed their doors, I opened my own business and did fairly well for a year and a half – until I could no longer work due to my declining health. At that point I had to hire employees to come into my home and do my work for me. That was in 1994.

By then my husband had found new work and was gone 6 days a week. He had no clue what was happening to me or the children. When I'd complain of fatigue, he'd say "I work too." When I asked him to watch the children because I needed rest, I never heard the end of it. Needless to say he was extremely limited as a support person, and that only added to my stress. At this time I had seen probably 10 doctors; and all with different versions of diagnoses. None of these fit my symptom history to any large degree, and it was most disheartening. My husband started to believe that I was making up my symptoms to get attention. But no one invents the symptoms of Lyme disease, and no one can deliberately fabricate fevers of 104°F, either.

In time, I had 5 employees working in the half of the basement we had converted to office space, because I could no longer work even a part-time day. I hired a driver to take the job work back and forth the two hour round-trip to Milwaukee, where most of my clients were located. This was particularly difficult because I had built a successful home business making >$100K a year and now I was handing out all the profits to my employees and receiving practically nothing in return. I had no choice due to my increasing illness, but to scale down the business to a point which was manageable for one person on a part-time basis. I had to make the difficult decision to let the employees go after about a year of them working for me. This was very hard to do – to admit that my hard work had to be tossed into the trash can because I was now defeated by "something" physically wrong with me that no doctor was willing to diagnose. But by this time I had spent the past 10 months of my life virtually in bed when I wasn't directly dealing with two small children and the demands of running a household and business.

My children took slightly longer to develop obvious health problems. It was perhaps weeks after their rashes initially appeared that they first became ill. Then slowly and intermittently, they began to be ill, more often. When they did become repeatedly ill, I was very ill and tried hard to deal with their bouts of "flu" or "ear infections" while being ill myself.

My daughter suffered stomach aches, bronchitis and tonsilitis, fevers, strange rashes, a brief period of incontinence, and irritability.

My daughter supposedly had scarlet fever and roseola in addition to chicken pox and other "normal" childhood illnesses. My son, who was previously walking at nine months and beginning to talk at a year-and-a-half, found himself unable to do either very well. He constantly fell down, and his well-formed words became muffled slurs. He ran fevers of 104-106°F regularly with convulsions, and had episodes of unexplained rashes and upper respiratory problems. He was diagnosed with roseola like his sister, and curiously seemed to have chicken pox twice. He received 3 sets of ear tubes as doctors thought his eustachian tubes merely dysfunctional. This did nothing for his nightly fevers or extreme crying and agitation in a child otherwise reasonably healthy and happy-go-lucky.

Both children grew large, cryptic tonsils and my son developed a "geographic" tongue. They were constantly on Amoxicillin, Augmentin, Lorabid, Bactrim, Septra, and anything else the Pediatrician could throw their way. Practically every week I had one or both of the children at his office, and always with fevers, rashes, headaches, diarrhea, stomach or other problems. I was so well-known there that all I had to do was phone in the symptoms and the doctor would prescribe medications over the phone, without even seeing the children.

> *[This is an issue of competence and trust which in my opinion, can, and should be allowed between medical caregiver and patient. Parents after all are the primary caregivers of their children, and they know better than anyone when their child is ill. Physicians who are caring, compassionate and intelligent, are aware that "Mother knows best" and are generally willing to trust a Mother's basic intuition and judgment. They should be allowed to work via phone when appropriate once the doctor/patient relationship is firmly established, and this is ROUTINELY done by most physicians, especially when on-call covering other physicians' patients.]*

My daughter had regular fevers of 103°F and both children had multiple, ring-like rashes on their legs, which their doctor deemed a reaction to medication they were taking. "Hives don't look like little circles with a blank spot in the middle, do they?" I remember quizzing a different Pediatrician on the phone, (mine was out on vacation at the time). He was condescendingly dismissive and assured this "nervous" mother that her babies would be fine from their "summer flus."

During my own struggles to obtain any reasonable diagnosis for myself and 2 children from 1992 to 2005, I visited nearly 100 doctors, clinics, hospitals, and a major Midwestern medical center (Mayo clinic, Rochester, MN). I received many different "diagnoses." "Stress," and "hypochondria," and even "agoraphobia," and "premenstrual syndrome" were dictated into my medical chart, even though the diagnoses were inaccurate. Many other "diagnoses" followed, but more often than not, they described the physical symptoms rather than what could be termed a real illness. CFS, Multiple Chemical Sensitivities, allergies, Irritable Bowel Syndrome, Endometriosis, AV Node arrythmia, polycystic ovaries, fibrocystic breasts, bloating, Gastritis, Dermatitis, swollen glands, Agoraphobia, "possible" MS, slipped disks, Degenerative Disk Disease, Fibromyalgia and much more dotted my medical files. But nowhere did any of the doctors I contacted, ever mention the word "Lyme disease." Not even when I implored them to test me for it and upon my insistence that I had every symptom of it that I would come across in my later research (except for testicular pain, as I am female).

Yes, I had done a fair amount of research when I first became ill, at our local library because there was no such thing as the internet as we know it today at the time, and my doctors were incredibly dismissive of my sudden illness. But I did the research only *after my symptoms had occurred,* and *not before*. That photo I found in the encyclopedia convinced me I had found the cause. Any reasonable adult would do research when answers seem abundant but none seem to fit the model of personal experience and daily symptoms. Unfortunately I would later learn that not only *is* there Lyme disease in Wisconsin, (and that it is endemic here), but that at the state and federal level, that information was known in the 1990's, but not readily shared with the public.

It still isn't to this day, but not for lack of trying on patient advocate's part. Indeed, my LLMD was on a public television station recently, attempting to give an interview to discuss Lyme disease. His discussion was conveniently edited down to minimize the symptoms and to appear less "controversial" or "hazardous" to hunters, as it was nearly hunting season. In addition, attempts by myself to have the major Milwaukee television stations pick up the Proclamation that Wisconsin Governor Jim Doyle issued at my request that May 2007 be declared

"Lyme Disease Awareness Month" for the state of Wisconsin, went completely ignored. I couldn't get any air time even for a Governor's Proclamation in an endemic state, and it wasn't for lack of trying!

As I have explained, the first tell-tale clue to my illness besides my other physical symptoms, was indeed the large bull's-eye rash that many Lyme patients are not "fortunate" enough to experience. Thanks to a library reference book, as uneducated patient, even I knew that the rash meant possible Lyme disease; and yet I was unable to convince any doctors to investigate my hypothesis. Instead, doctors told me they didn't "believe in" my disease and handed me referrals to Psychiatrists. I received antibiotics for some symptoms when acutely ill, or IVs in the emergency room when dehydrated, but no intensive treatment or diagnosis until 12-1/2 years later. And despite the intermittent symptomatic treatments, my symptoms never fully abated, but slowly and steadily increased.

During those dozen or so odd years, I had experienced a myriad of unrelenting symptoms, all hallmarks of neurological Lyme disease. I had all the characteristic rashes, severe headaches, light and sound sensitivities, joint aches and pain, chronic partial paralysis on my left side, painful radiculitis, head and neck creaking, cracking and feeling stiff and frozen, facial paralysis and *borrelial lymphocytoma.* I suffered coordination and balance problems, and I would walk into things or miss putting an item on a countertop because I had no true idea of where my body was in relation to space and time. I suffered profound visual disturbances, such as floaters, the feeling of tunnel vision, feeling like something was in my eyes, flashes of light, eye pain, repeated attacks of conjunctivitis, and alternating blurry/normal vision. When I went to bed at night, I would "see" things – sometimes before falling asleep, sometimes upon waking, and always frightening because I knew those "things" weren't really there, and which, on occasion, included "people;" none of whom I recognized, and some of them had been deceased for years.

One night after going to bed early, I was awakened by "something." In my semi-conscious state, I thought I saw three menacing black blobs standing at the side of my bed. I had no idea what these moving entities were, but they scared me out of my wits. Without realizing where I was, I stood up on the bed, and stepped off, trying to get away from them. As the bed was some three feet off the floor, I landed on my left ankle and a loud crunching sound could be heard. Undaunted, I flew down the hallway in a blind panic and descended the staircase and made it all the way into the living room before I realized I had badly sprained my ankle. It was only at that point that the pain caught up with me and I became fully awake.

I suffered massive panic attacks, sometimes while driving my car. I would have to pull over to the side of the road until they would pass, which left me terribly frightened and confused. Sometimes in a panic I would stop at a store just so I could be near people in case I collapsed into unconsciousness. It is difficult to put into words the kind of insecurity that surrounds episodes of panic and anxiety of this magnitude. It is so pervasive that every moment you are worrying about when the next attack might occur. A sense of paranoia creeps into every thought, and each time a new episode occurs, it reinforces the worries. And yet this self-fulfilling process is beyond the Lyme victim's conscious control.

With each episode, I would feel like I was having a heart attack, with shortness of breath, chest pains, sweating, clammy skin and a feeling of doom or dread and it would come from out of nowhere. Sometimes it would be accompanied by the urgent necessity to have a bowel movement. It was the classic "fight or flight" response, as controlled by the sympathetic nervous system. These were debilitating to say the least. My children, who were young, wondered what the heck was wrong with Mommy and why she was no fun any more. I suffered incredible amounts of daily pain, blinding headaches, high fevers, auditory and olfactory hallucinations, nausea, dizziness, OCD, tremors, partial seizures in different parts of my body, and a whole host of other problems. Numbness and tingling, sleep problems, excessive daytime sleepiness, fatigue and irritability were all present and difficult to deal with. Needless to say this made raising children and working more than just a bit difficult, but somehow I still managed to function.

In 1994 after being unable to work full-time any longer out of my home, I went to a Rheumatologist and begged her to test me for Lyme disease. She flatly refused to test me, but she did consent to treat when I pleaded with her at length to *please* treat me with antibiotics *in the event that I had Lyme.* She gave me a combination of 2 antibiotics to be taken for 30 days, which I did, and which provided a small relief of some of my symptoms. One of those drugs was doxycycline and the other one I believe was erythromycin. At that point, my symptoms affected me daily. During treatment, some of the symptoms partly left. But after ceasing the prescriptions, the very same symptoms which never quite fully went away, returned with a vengeance. A new problem which had just begun to surface was a sudden inability to eat certain foods. I did not understand the intermittent food reactions at the time, however. I just thought it was yet another "weird" symptom to add to my perplexing repertoire.

Personal and family stressors in my life added to the severity of my symptoms, and little to no understanding was afforded to me by my mother or my husband at the time, which made raising 2 children by myself while extremely ill, next to impossible. And throughout the years, each time I was acutely ill with another host of symptoms, I was given more antibiotics for weeks at a time or sometimes months at a time. Always the end result was the elimination of some, but not all symptoms for a very brief period, a plateau of relative wellness, followed by their eventual return, in full force. And yet I managed to keep functioning, one way or another, until such time as a tumor and 3 major surgeries in 18 months and acute Lyme symptoms finally sidelined me for a period of several years until an accurate diagnosis and more aggressive treatments could be obtained.

In 1997 I divorced my first husband, and this additional stress and the necessity to find a job in a tight market caused an out-of-state daily commute of 176 miles round-trip to work. This while being a single parent who no longer had any savings, investments or anything of value, was not easy to endure. For several months I dropped my children off at school in WI, (they would walk to after-school daycare), as I commuted by car out-of-state to IL, to the only job I could land on such short notice. I reversed the procedure at the end of each day and worried every day that my children were at school "in another state" (of course I had several friends helping me with the aspect of ensuring my children were safe and cared for).

I cannot believe I endured that process for as long as I did, because I remember fighting with my brain and body during the long drive times, and having fatigue and horrible panic attacks while driving in heavy traffic. Many days I drove white-knuckled in the slow lanes – anything I could do to get from point A to point B safely. I was terrified and yet to others, I did not "look sick." This says nothing about the intense pain I had to endure from my left shoulder, neck and back acting up and the cognitive problems or the numbness in my hands and fingers. First I was sitting at a desk job all day, and then I was driving in a car for hours. The double-whammy was an insult to a very inflammed left upper body. I would cry to myself nearly every day through the anxiety and the traffic as I drove home to pick up my children. And the nights I could not sleep well made the travel much more difficult to bear. But persevere we do when we have children to support and no clear cut answers.

Fortunately I did find a new job, which was important because I could no longer afford to pay for the mortgage of the home I was living in, (which still belonged to my ex-husband and myself). After being forced to spend my entire 401K on the mortgage to keep it out of arrears for a year and a half, it was going into foreclosure. (I received barely any support from my ex). I found myself forced by my ex-husband and the courts to vacate it and find a new place to live, and quickly. Yes, the courts returned the house to my ex, who had previously moved to an apartment with his original statement that he "couldn't afford" to live in the house. But now just a year and a half later with no change in his employment or income, the court was suddenly *giving* the house to him, and he could magically afford to pay the back arrears, and live there…where he remains to this day, 10 years later. Meanwhile the courts could have cared less that they were dumping an ill woman and her two children both under the age of 10 out onto the streets, nor did they care that my ex's financial situation had miraculously improved while mine was in the toilet.

I moved the children, the dog, and myself to a rental home in a decent suburb of Milwaukee. I took a job as a Secretary to the Secretary-Treasurer of a Teamster's Union. The job was extremely demanding time-wise and moderately stressful but it afforded me the luxury of being immediately available for my children. Now they were only 20 blocks away at all times. However, I found myself having difficulty for the first time, with curbing minor irritations. Small matters which would not normally upset me, now seemed to cause a hair-trigger anger, which I struggled sometimes to control.

Perhaps it was because my ex was stalking me and my friends, and pulling stunts that involved the children, I don't know for certain, because stress levels were high. And I don't remember ever being overly angry at the children, (people around me said that I was not), but I am certain it made me less than patient with them to some degree, at times. In addition, I injured myself by hitting my head during this time period, and I suffered a mild concussion. I was sent to the hospital for X-rays and a CT scan, and I remember feeling very confused as to why the signs in the hospital were blank. (Once again there did not appear to be any lettering on them).

When I returned to work a day later, I honestly could not recall the events from the day before. No matter how hard I tried, it was as if my memory was wiped clean of that day's events. That was more than a little frightening, even when the memory did return some days later.

Stress continued at that job and in my personal life and I began to have problems calculating numbers, which was something I was actually quite good at doing before. One of my duties was keeping the (manual) accounting books for the Local, and I found myself making errors I wouldn't normally have made. This was a source of frustration and embarrassment for me. In addition, I began having difficulty sleeping at night, and I was up and down, all night long, and having trouble staying awake during the day. All of these problems were dismissed by my General Practitioner, who said I was "just under stress." I also noticed that riding on the back of a motorcycle during a Union public relations event, produced a sudden unexpected panic attack in me. I also kept bumping into things, or I would misjudge the distance it took to put my cup of tea on the desktop, spilling it. I would transpose words when typing, which was odd for me, after having been a master typesetter. At times my hands and fingers or toes would suddenly "fall asleep" and feel numb and then tingly and prickly without explanation.

Yes, it was true I was under stress, but many of my symptoms had been with me for years, and now I had new ones to boot, including difficulty concentrating, daytime sleepiness, trouble falling asleep, headaches, and light and sound sensitivity. I visited many doctors over the next few years in search of answers and found none that made any sense.

In 2000, my family and a male friend (who later became my second husband) went camping in Pardeeville, (central) Wisconsin. We slept in tents and everyone had a good time. Upon returning however, within a week's time I noticed that I had another red rash on my scalp, which did not itch, but the skin on the scalp felt somewhat painful to the touch. My doctor called it "dermatitis" and prescribed nothing for it. However, within the next few weeks, I found myself with a swollen left ear, and intense burning, tingling and itching sensations on my outer ear and cheek; vertigo, and a fever. In fact, I felt like total crap.

I returned to the doctor. He decided I had an "ear infection" and prescribed antibiotics. Over a period of the next 5 days, I had to see 5 different doctors, all of whom witnessed a bad case of Bell's palsy, with cranial neuritis and radiculoneuropathy. Nearly all of my facial nerves were affected. I lost sensation in over 3/4 of my face, and my sense of smell and taste were gone. My tongue felt numb, and my face drooped (eye, eyelid, cheek, mouth), making speech difficult and disfiguring my face. The remaining quarter of my face had some basic feeling, but it was exquisitely painful to the touch. My arm, neck and shoulder were markedly painful, numb, weak, and "frozen." To make matters worse, my balance was out of whack and I felt like I was perpetually walking on a slant.

I also had incredibly painful, red-hot poker-like stabbing pains that began at the top of my scalp and which traveled down the left side of my face, through my ear area, jaw, cheek, and chin. It continued down the left half of my neck, to my shoulder, into my back left shoulder blade, and into my side about midway down my rib cage. At work I would sit holding a heating pad plastered to the side of my face in an effort to try to quell some of the pain which the pain relievers did not touch. I was in agony for the better part of 9 weeks.

I would cry from the pain, and the antibiotics and steroids prescribed for me did nothing but make me feel even more ill. On around the third day of taking predinsone and acyclovir, I had a serious reaction to the medications (or perhaps a herxheimer reaction). I ended up at the hospital. In the car ride on the way, I nearly passed out. I felt like I was poisoned or had overdosed. My heart rate soared (over 200 in the ER), and I was hyperventilating and could not control the spasms forcing me to breathe rapidly. My lips were numb from breathing too fast and it took some time before my body returned to normal. I was advised not to take any more medication.

The 5 doctors I saw in 5 days at the onset of my symptoms "diagnosed" me with an ear infection, cellulitis, bug bites, and shingles of the cranial nerve – despite there not being any lesions of any kind on my outer ear, which was swollen and red. This made my appearance at work very embarrassing and people would shrink from obvious disgust when I would talk to them. They did not seem to know how to react. Was it rude to stare or better to look away?

I had to cover my face when I laughed because my expression was hideous, and eating was extremely difficult, not to mention that I couldn't smell or taste anything. I would tilt my head to the right and chew the tasteless food with the good side of my mouth while holding my lips together with my fingers so the food wouldn't fall out of my mouth, which I couldn't close properly. Swallowing was also difficult and I felt hideous, like a circus side-show freak.

It was very tough being this ill, and only 10 weeks before my wedding to my second husband was scheduled. I threatened not to marry him if my symptoms did not improve. At my bridal shower my face was paralyzed. I got more than a few weird looks from friends wondering what was going on with my health. If I could just be better so that I could smile on my wedding day, I thought. That day came and I actually could smile a little bit, but I already had neurological damage to the face, which changed the way my smile looked, and my face functions, to this day. While I worked very hard to smile, as evidenced from photographs, I was actually not smiling in most of the shots. That is the funny thing about the residual effects of Bell's palsy in my case. I might *think* I am smiling, because it *feels* like I am smiling, but in reality I have to work *extra hard* in order to be able to have a smile physically *appear.* Many of our wedding photos show my face markedly grim-looking. People who did not know me well wondered why I looked so upset on what was supposed to be an otherwise happy day.

During this time I was going back to my regular doctor, who kept ignoring my symptoms, even my huge, inflamed ear! He actually told me he thought I was depressed because his nurse had asked me questions and I had been staring at the floor while responding to her. (Note, I was hanging my head because it hurt my neck to look up). She wrote that I refused to make eye contact as a "symptom" of depression. Had I known she was testing me, I would have stared her down. The doctor prescribed an anti-depressant, Zoloft, which I ripped up because I knew I wasn't depressed. I was angry that he would not take my symptoms seriously. What a joke this man is as a "doctor," I thought to myself.

Any sadness I eventually legitimately experienced was brought about by the fact that I was feeling so poorly and couldn't get any credence whatsoever from my doctors. This same doctor ignored me when I described new bloating, cramping and specific abdominal pain, and simply referred me to a Gastroenterologist instead. He had the audacity to say to me, "I'm not going to hold your hand every time you think you have something wrong with you," and suggested again that I seek "help" with a Psychiatrist or a Psychologist. I was livid and I began to cry. In fact, I left his office in a huff, in the middle of the visit. My patient charts, which I obtained at a later date, said something like, "patient abandoned the visit." How about the *truth*, which was more like **"doctor abandoned his patient."**

I visited the Gastroenterologist and was disgusted by both his bedside manner and his personal hygiene. He was a senior citizen who had no ability to relate to his patients. He questioned me extensively about why I thought I had a gastro issue, and after about 15 minutes he told me that he didn't think I had any gastro issues and referred me to a GYN after actually criticizing me for "wasting his time." As if he had more important things to do! I ended up writing a letter admonishing the clinic for this doctor's behavior, to which an actual letter of apology was sent to me in response, but not by the doctor, from the clinic director, big deal.

I went to the GYN and told her that being intimate with my husband was suddenly painful and had been impossible for weeks, and that I had pain and pressure in my abdomen along with new bloating, cramping and heavy menses. She did an exam which was very painful and said that there was "nothing" wrong with me, even after I audibly yelled in pain during an exam. I told her that I thought I might have Lyme disease, and she said, "Oh, I know all about that, I used to have Ehrlichia, but I was treated and I'm fine." She wouldn't talk about the possibility of Lyme disease at all, and suggested I allow her to do a hysterectomy instead. "Why would I want you to do that?" I asked. "Well, you're too old to have any more children..." (I disagreed, I was 39 at the time), "...and you have painful periods, and this would certainly take care of the problem." (Okay let's just yank out whatever organ hurts rather than try to determine what is causing the pain?) I quit that GYN and found another one who was more interested in helping me than perhaps making her "Mercedes" payments. Just six years later I would learn that this GYN who "had" Ehrlichia when she was in residence in a New Jersey hospital, had to abruptly end her practice due to health "issues." One can only wonder what issues those might have been, but my guess would be chronic, improperly treated tick-borne illness.

One of the doctors I had been seeing suggested that due to my new chest pains and heart palpitations, that I have a "heart scan" in a state-of-the-art CT-type scanner that (naturally), my insurance wouldn't cover. I don't remember how I scraped together the $800 it cost to have the test back then, but I did. It was a fairly easy test that did not require any fasting or any dyes. You essentially lay down and are passed through the unit in one piece and it takes various images of your entire body.

The results of the scan showed that I had absolutely no arterial plaque build-ups and that my heart and circulatory system appeared "excellent." But it did show some areas of white "lesions" which they felt were noteworthy that appeared over my liver area on the scans. (Years later I would learn that Lyme often affects the liver, causing lesions and other problems). I was put on a Holter monitor for a month's time, which was difficult because it seemed like it was used all the time. I had to push a button to register each time I felt my heart "skip" or do "flip flops" and I was pushing that button many times per hour. In addition, the sticky glue on the electrodes made me break out in terrible rashes. I had scabs all over my chest wherever the stickies were located, and I had to move them each day due to the intense itching. The results of the Holter monitor were only somewhat informative. They indicated that I had an unexplained AV node (heart) arrythmia, and I was sent to a Cardiologist for more testing.

The Cardiologist performed a series of stress tests, echocardiograms and I even had a type of tilt table test (but not Isuprel challenge). I also was injected with some kind of nuclear great-now-I'm-going-to-glow-in-the-dark thingy that somehow helped radioactive isotopes arrive at various organs to measure their function, like my liver and kidneys. All the tests said were that I was "healthy," except for a slightly leaky tricuspid (heart) valve that because of my "excellent" heart ejection fraction, wasn't a "problem." OK, I thought, then why did I pay for such expensive tests if you can't tell me anything other than I am okay, and why do I feel so sick?

Many hospitals, clinics and doctors later, it was the middle of 2001, and I finally convinced a General Practice doctor to test me for Lyme,

11 years after I remembered being bitten. All he offered me was a Lyme titer, which (no surprise), returned "negative" so the doctor told me I "couldn't possibly" have Lyme. He also said there was "nothing" wrong with me. This doctor authoritatively also told me that even if I "had" Lyme disease in the past, that my long history of being treated with many different kinds of antibiotics would have certainly "cured" me by now. I guess this doctor has a lot to learn with regard to tick-borne illnesses and the persistence of Bb in the body despite antibiotics.

In 2001, I was working as a director of Internet operations for a local manufacturer and distributor in Milwaukee. My job was stressful, but not in an out-of-the-ordinary way. Due to my work efforts, I was quickly promoted and given the highest merit bonus in the history of the company, during my first 6 months there. Obviously I was more than capable of performing my job. But somewhere along the line in 2002, things began to get dicey at work. The long hours and lack of sleep and stress took their toll on me. On a few occasions, I began suffering panic attacks at work. This made attending meetings most difficult because I could be sitting there just fine one minute, and suddenly the glare of the lights, the sounds of people talking and or for no apparent reason, my heart would start racing. I would begin sweating, a feeling of panic would ensue and I would hyperventilate. This was a horrible time for me and I worked hard to conceal my symptoms.

On a few occasions, I had what some might otherwise call psychic experiences which were very weird indeed. A person could walk by my office door, and suddenly I would "see" a flash of a picture, like a freeze-frame of a videotape, of something pertaining to that person in my mind's eye. It was really weird and hard to describe. When I would tell that person in confidence (boy was that a hard subject to approach), they would confirm that what I "saw" was in fact, a true aspect of their life. For example, with one man I saw "coins." He confirmed that he was a serious coin collector, certainly something I had no previous knowledge about. A girl had walked into my office and I suddenly saw what I described to her, and what she later confirmed to me, as the teacher for the new class she was going to be attending later on that same day. Talk about weird. I wonder if these experiences were "normal" intuitive thoughts which somehow intensified due to brain inflammation stimulating that area of the brain.

During this time, new problems were also surfacing. Because I worked on the third floor, I had to climb many stairs each day. My joints were feeling the burden of the added exercise and I would get very stiff if I sat too long. I was also becoming oddly paranoid and openly irritable. I was convinced that two of the managers were working together in the background to "oust" me from my position, (and in truth, they probably were, it would have meant greater responsibility for them and more money). But we got into frequent disagreements. Everything seemed intensely magnified and things less important became more-so. I was often conveniently left out of the loop, which caused repeated problems in day-to-day office dealings as I took everything as a personal attack.

I was also now struggling to learn new computer programming languages, which previously had been a piece of cake for me. I resorted to taking additional classes at college in an effort to figure out why I could no longer learn merely through the process of study and self-teaching, as I had done most of my life. My young son took my school attendance and time on the computer as something "wrong," and informed his father, (my ex), who apparently decided I was no longer "able to do my job," which he opportunistically would later try to utilize against me.

One day at work, I arrived in a foul mood, which had no apparent cause. I was very angry when I learned that one of the managers had deliberately gone over my head again on an important aspect of a project I was working on, that had nothing to do with him or his department. We got into a heated argument and he said something rude to me. In reply I remember for the first time in my entire life, telling him to go (pleasure) himself. Following that verbal release, I turned, packed up my things (I never kept much in the office anyway) and walked out on the job, and it was only 7 o'clock in the morning. I was so angry I only remember seeing red, and thinking that was *it*, I had enough of that place and all the crap from the stupid men managers there. I summarily quit that day with no premeditation or clue that morning that I would have ever done so.

I recall the shakes and a new, serious pounding headache, but I don't remember much else about the ride home that day. I did grasp that I was now unemployed and not feeling very well. And I remember a phone call a week later from my unemployment attorney who kindly informed me that my ex-husband had learned that I was no longer employed (probably through one of the children). Apparently he had actually contacted my former employer to tell them I was "nuts." He also incredibly offered my ex-employer the opportunity to use our then 10-year old son as a "witness" to my late-night computer studies, in an opportunity *to help them win their unemployment case against me!* Yes, that ex-husband of mine actually did contact my ex-employer, can you believe it? This fact came as a huge shock to me. My attorney had no way of knowing this information unless she had spoken directly to my ex-employer...who would have had no idea who my ex-husband was unless he had contacted them directly; which he had.

As it happened, after I found out about my ex's plans to manipulate my unemployment hearing, especially since he was offering to use our son to supposedly help my ex-employer deny me benefits, I was understandably confused, my mind was swirling, and I was *livid!* I became so angry at the kitchen telephone which kept skipping in and out with a bunch of static (it had problems), and that frustration along with what I had just learned, (and apparently my undiagnosed Bartonella which also causes rapid-onset agitation), that I stood there in disbelief and intense anger. I rationalized quickly about how I could dissipate the rage which was quickly welling up inside of me. I remembered a wonderful counselor whom I had seen years after my divorce first took place. She helped me to realize that many of the problems in my first marriage had been due to the selfishness of my ex-husband, and thankfully not largely due to my own issues. One way she had suggested that I deal with pent-up anger over the divorce was to find an inatimate object, and break it, and name the things while breaking the object, which were causing the anger.

So to me at the time, that seemed like one heck of a good idea. I summarily took the static-laden old phone off the wall, put it on the counter and set about trying to find something to smash it with. It was a lousy phone anyway, and believe it or not, I already had just bought a new one which I hadn't yet mounted on the wall. It was sitting patiently on the kitchen table waiting for me to make the switch.

I looked in the "junk" drawer, and could not find a hammer. So I had to go down into our basement, and rummage around my husband's toolbox. This took a couple of minutes. Eventually I located a hammer, and I returned to the kitchen and placed the phone on a stool and proceeded to murder my telephone. *BLAM!* "That's for being a piece of crap!" I said to the phone. *BLAM!* "That's for being a complete jerk of an ex-husband" *BLAM!* "How dare you try to hurt me using our child!" I said. I named each thing I was furious about and when I was done, I actually felt quite a bit better, cleaned up the mess and installed the new telephone, thank you very much.

I felt a bit foolish because that is not the ideal way to handle life, to go around breaking things, but in this particular application, it was all I could think of. So I figured it was a fairly healthy, one-time outlet. To make a point here, no one else was home at the time of this event. And when my children returned from school that day, they immediately noticed the new telephone and asked what happened to the old one. "Mommy killed it," I jokingly told them, and we all had a good laugh about the experience.

At this point, the stress of a newly filed court motion to reverse custody and placement of my children filed by my ex-husband was adding fuel to what was quickly becoming a blazing inferno. After 5 years, he suddenly wanted custody. He alleged many "incidents" of rage-filled behavior(s). There were now more than just the phone incident cited as he creatively invented many allegations in his bogus court motions. By all accounts, with the exception of the phone incident though, I wasn't exhibiting any rage-filled behaviors. But the truth didn't matter. According to his new claims, I supposedly also had *physically abused* my children. Of course no evidence needs to be provided to the courts to request a hearing, you only need to make accusations. You can say whatever you want just to get a hearing, and you don't even have to defend your motion verbiage once you get to court. I didn't know that, and that is abuse of the legal system; which was repeatedly done by my ex over the course of a decade.

You can well imagine that the stress of that one court action filed by my ex added a *considerable* burden to my already overtaxed stress levels and immune system – especially since I, my family, and everyone around me, knew that the accusations were completly unfounded and ridiculous. Nevertheless, when someone files a court motion for a hearing, you have to hire attorneys and defend yourself. Going to court is mandatory, not voluntary in this situation.

Unfortunately in family court, the entire phone incident was completely twisted by my ex-husband into an incident that never happened...and the courts would believe my ex's version of the "crime," and not mine. To his account, the children were supposedly present, were made to be afraid by my actions which they supposedly witnessed, and I was supposedly out of control with rage. These accusations, though left unproven, left a bad taste in the court's mouth as far as my name was concerned, because I openly admitted under oath that I smashed the phone, though not in the manner alleged. So in the judge's mind, if I was "going around smashing telephones," I *must* be a danger to my children – especially if those children had been present (but they weren't).

Nevertheless, despite the fact that my ex-husband hadn't even been present as a witness to the phone incident, and though he had lied and failed to prove his allegations, it didn't matter to the court! My ex-husband would lie, and he was believed. I told the truth and was called a liar. My attorney advised me after a hearing, "It's unfortunate, but a well-rehearsed lie is sometimes more convincing than the truth." Indeed it would be in this case, nearly each and every time we appeared before that court.

Some people are self-destructive and drink, hit others, and/or do drugs. Some unfortunate souls even commit murder. I smashed a broken telephone. Certainly it was hardly a "crime" worthy of removing children from me. But my ex had lied and that was just the beginning of the manipulations of the court system on his part, in his favor. I am saving most of the family court stuff for another book, because I want to focus on my Lyme and its symptoms and what that was like. In the future there will be a revealing look at the entire process by which this family was torn apart by both manipulation of a legal system, and discrimination of innocent people who simply have an infectious disease called Lyme. And though I go into some detail here for the purposes of telling this story, the focus and evidence of those aspects will remain in the future book where they belong. Nevertheless I must reveal some aspects of the events, because they tie into our collective illness on every level.

As I was now unemployed, I thought that perhaps the reduced stress of my former employment might help relieve some of my symptoms, but the opposite was actually true. My symptoms became more noticeably pronounced because I wasn't distracted by my work day. And the stress of an upcoming long court trial process intensified symptoms.

I noticed that I could not sit at the computer for longer than an hour or so, without my neck and shoulder (left side) feeling painfully "locked up" and unable to move. I was referred by my regular doctor to an Orthopaedist, who performed X-rays and a CT scan. He said that I had degerative disk disease in my cervical spine (C5-C7). He also said that I had an old compression fracture that had healed "oddly" and that one of my disks was herniated about 40% towards the front, and that was the cause of my seering neck and shoulder pain. I told him that in high school I had fallen from the uneven parallel bars (I was a gymnast), and landed on my neck and upper back, upside down, which probably explained the compression fracture. The Orthopaedist now ordered 6 weeks of physical therapy to try to loosen the frozen muscles in the area, but that did not explain why at age thirty-something I had sudden problems with my spine, with no apparent new injury.

Physical therapy for this problem was one of the most painful things I had experienced at that point (and I had two C-sections and many other major and minor surgeries.) The manipulation of the frozen shoulder area was horrible and all it did was make my already intermittent headaches turn into daily, non-stop headaches. Now I could no longer lift my left arm or use it to hold anything. My arm, hand and shoulder became numb and useless. I had to stop the physical therapy, as it seemed to be doing more harm than good. To boot, due to the neck manipulations and traction therapy also being implemented, the left side of my face had new-onset twitching and a loss of sensation in the nerve pathways. These were the same ones which had been compromised during the Bell's palsy. It seemed that the intense physical therapy was causing a flare-up of new, uncomfortable symptoms and a brief repeat of the Bell's palsy.

Now I could no longer do things like grocery shopping, because I only had the use of my right arm. Sometimes I wore an arm sling because I got tired of flinging my useless arm around all over the place. But the attention that caused was distracting to me. I had difficulty driving and learned to do everything with one arm. Getting dressed and doing my hair was an interesting challenge. I also had debilitating daily headaches which pain relievers did not help. One evening I had such a violently intense, head-splitting headache that I went to my bedroom to lie down. I told my husband that if I didn't wake up that he should call 9-1-1 because I probably had suffered a stroke. I don't know why he didn't just take me to the hospital, I really felt I was in trouble, it was that intense. I think he just didn't "get" that I was in so much pain. "I don't feel well at all" was probably all he heard and he did not take my comment about a stroke seriously. But then he never paid too much attention to my physical health or my complaints, probably because I tried to minimize them so as not to scare anyone. I think because I looked "fine," it was easier to believe that I was, than to believe my complaints of pain and dysfunction. Of course the ongoing custody issues combined with my health problems numbed him to a degree that he checked out of our relationship almost immediately after we were married. (He gets a ton of credit for honestly admitting this and allowing me to print it here).

I was too ill at the time to go to the hospital and the sound of my children and husband talking was excrutiating to hear. I yelled at my husband to please take the children elsewhere so I could try to get some sleep. I remember having a pervasive thought that if I went to sleep, that I might never see my family again.

I became so out-of-tune with severe pain from day-to-day that I felt like a walking zombie. When people talked to me, I was slow to respond, and I did not feel long for this world. I even put my affairs in order, from my will to letters to my children, and a letter of distribution of assets and how I wanted my funeral to be arranged. I virtually lived on my bed or our living room couch, with two heating pads attached to me at all times for pain management. One on my back/neck/shoulder area and one attached to either my face, my arm or my leg on the affected left side; wherever the most pain was at the time. Over-the-counter medications did very little to relieve the pain. Once after taking the maximum dose of Tylenol at one sitting, I realized that it wasn't helping me at all. I decided to just cope with the pain instead.

My regular doctor decided at this point, despite my intense headaches, gastro problems and problems with my left side, that I was "really" suffering from Fibromyalgia. Sometimes I had intense pain over some of the associated trigger points, but not most of them; only four that I can ever remember. This was around March 2002.

Around the same time, an incident during my ex-husband's visitation involved him "allegedly" attempting to run me over with his car (the truth), or I suddenly inexplicably "threw myself" in front of his car (his version). After which he lied about the incident and I was falsely arrested, but not in the typical manner. In reality I was simply driven (much later) to the police station by my current husband. I was never read my

Miranda rights, never told "you are under arrest," never hand cuffed, and always treated with respect, and differently than the others who came in after me. I maintained my innocence while an officer examined my leg swelling, and though photographed and fingerprinted. I was let go on $50 bond after being forced to sign a 72-hour "no contact" order, delcaring my ex-husband the "victim." No charges were ever filed, the case was dropped, and my ex of course, used the incident in court to help justify why he should be allowed to have custody – under a pretense that I was somehow now "dangerous." I cringed in fear when I heard his irresponsible attorney unbelievably allege to the family court commissioner that I would "kill my own children" if I was allowed to keep custody of them. Can you imagine how that must have felt? My mind swirled in disbelief at the idea that this could actually be happening to me, someone with no prior (or since) police record.

Never mind that I maintain to this day that my ex's actions at the time were *absolutely* an unprovoked and hateful attempt to run me over with his car. (Can you say "planned incident"?) Unfortunately for me, there were no witnesses and our two young children who were in the car with him at the time, were naturally coerced by him during his visitation to say the right lies at the right moment to the right people, which sealed my fate. The interesting thing about the case was that no proper investigation was done and that was admitted to in court by the attending police officers. Nevertheless, I was held responsible for the incident.

Later when the children were older, one of them recanted and told me the truth about the incidents and the lies. They were never to blame of course because they were manipulated and coerced, but it would have been nice if one of them had found the courage to speak up on my behalf at the appropriate time. But I well understand fear of reprisal. In fact it was main the reason I hadn't reported my ex-husband to the police in 1997 when he "allegedly" raped me just days before I filed for divorced.

The force of the car's impact, and my actions to avoid being hit by the front end of the vehicle (placing my hands on the hood and pushing my body to the right, over the hood and away from the car's nose), twisted my leg in the hip socket. In my efforts to avoid being run over, the movement stretched the ligaments and injured the soft tissues, causing new, unremitting pain and swelling in the affected right hip joint.

Every day for a week I walked with a limp and my hip was very painful. I begged the doctor to do a new MRI to find out why my hip hurt so much. I was also very bloated and painful in my abdomen and I was having a hard time walking, which I attributed to the hip injury. He ordered the MRI, and it revealed that I had a good-sized tumor; an adnexal mass the size of a lemon sitting on my left ovary, squashing my colon and rectum. (That explained to me why when I had a bowel movement it came out in a ribbon-like fashion, and also all the abdominal pain). I was also told I oddly lacked "normal" bone growth in both of my hip sockets – something that would ensure arthritis at an early age. (Note: Lyme *eats* bone).

When the doctor and I reviewed the MRI I brought in from the imaging department, I literally watched his jaw drop. "Now do you see why I have been complaining of pain," I asked him, somewhat indignantly as we looked at the tumor. I had worked for a few years at a hospital, and MRIs were not unfamiliar to me, so I already knew what we were studying. After a moment, he quietly said he was "very sorry for missing this" and that I had a large tumor and he would refer me to his wife's Gynecological Oncologist. I said "no thanks" to him and quickly decided to find my own. If this doctor couldn't diagnose a tumor in a rapidly distending abdomen, how was I supposed to trust him to give me a referral to a good surgeon? Incidentally, (and I kid you not), the pain in my hip dissolved into thin air *immediately* following the MRI test. God's intervention to help save my life as you will read, perhaps?

Now about this time, the court action stepped into high gear. Another reason my ex filed to remove custody and placement of our children from me was due to my remarriage and as he put it, he "was not going to allow some other man to raise [his] children." At one point the court ordered us to attend joint counseling sessions which they pretended would somehow "correct" our "communication problem." Of course the court's idea of "fixing" communication between us was entirely wrong, especially since my ex's hitting me with his car and lying about it leading to my false quasi-arrest made me rightly hostile toward him and the entire process. The communication problem was my ex's deliberate refusal to communicate in any productive manner, and his intention to harm me by whatever means he had at his disposal, in order to get our children away from me. Those issues alone when shown to the court, should have been sufficient grounds to keep the children away from him permanently, but things never seemed to go the way the laws were intended to in the Walworth county family court.

At our first trial, a number of witnesses testified that my ex would stand curb-side at visitation time and scream obscenities at me from the street, loud enough for neighbors to hear from inside their homes. The profoundly insensitive judge never once considered this behavior inappropriate, and neither did the court officers. Instead, somehow my ex charmingly convinced everyone that I was the culprit – despite witnesses to the contrary. *Are you kidding me? Can you tell me who paid off whom here?*

At the same time as these shenanigans, it was decided that I had to have immediate surgery to remove the tumor in my abdomen, which had now grown to the size of a small orange. At this point in time, I was immeasurably fatigued, had terrible pain and I was rapidly gaining weight in my abdomen. I felt miserable and had tremendous difficulty walking. The tumor's location was closing off my rectum from within, and squashing my reproductive system making elimination most difficult, and menses entirely painful. I was getting backed up inside; and as you can imagine, was feeling horrendously ill. Most days I felt so bad I thought I might actually die from whatever was inside me.

I was to undergo immediate surgery. I had a consult with the Gynecological Oncologist, because it was thought at the time due to the large mass and my symptoms, that the tumor might in fact be cancerous. Imagine having to deal with that issue at the same time your ex-spouse files false allegations of child abuse in a family court, while attempting to utilize anything against you to win placement of your children. (Even pressuring the children to lie for him, after "allegedly" hitting you with his car!) And all the while you are struggling with a mystery illness that absolutely no one will validate and which was quickly disabling you physically and cognitively.

I had to undergo surgery in secret without telling my children that I might be dealing with cancer, because I was so terrified of what my ex might do with that new tidbit of information. I didn't want to give him or anyone else any "ammunition" to take away my children undeservedly and I didn't want to scare the children with the thought that their mother might be very ill.

I cried tears of apprehension when I entered the surgical suite. It was not the surgery in and of itself that frightened me, as I had a dozen previous major surgeries and many minor ones. No, the fear came from not knowing what would happen, and if I was dealing with cancer, even though the doctor had given me "okay" odds. Was I going to lose part of my reproductive system or the whole darned kit n' kaboodle and then be forced to go through menopause and/or cancer treatments at age 41? What would the family court do, take away my children if it thought I was that ill?

Despite my concerns, I thanked the doctor and his assistants before the operation, for being willing to take on their challenging careers so that I could have the necessary surgery. The numerous concerned masked faces and the surgeon's compassionate comments brought grateful tears to my eyes. As it happened, this would become life-saving surgery, as apparently the tumor and my ovary had ruptured and I was bleeding into my abdomen. I was told I might have died had I not had the operation. I call that God's divine timing – even if He did have to use my nasty ex-husband to help find the tumor in the first place. (Remember the car incident led to the MRI which revealed the tumor and the subsequent surgery.)

Following the operation, recovery was difficult, painful and protracted. As was standard practice, I was discharged hours later under heavy sedation; a typical revolving-door outpatient surgery.The day after my surgery, I had a "reaction" to something, and I thought it was a complication. I wasn't feeling well of course, and barely made it to the bathroom when I was about to pass out. Since I was seeing "stars" and I felt like I was going to faint, I had my children tell the neighbor to call an ambulance and I was taken away. In the ER, I was given a lower GI X-ray despite having had surgery the day before.

At the hospital, the doctors thought I had developed a fistula. Well, I hadn't. "Nothing" showed up on the X-ray of course, and I was sent home hours later after the indignity of having an X-ray tech-in-training perform a clumsy barium enema on me while I tried to pose for her pictures despite my painful, fresh surgical incisions. As it would turn out years later, I would be able to identify the cause of the reaction which was actually a "leaky gut" food sensitivity causing a drop in blood pressure, and the associated symptoms of what the ER doctors would label an anaphylactic-type reaction.

[Years later I would be prescribed epi-pens and H1 and H2 histamine blockers to carry with me at all times, and told to "avoid" offending items causing the reactions. That is easier said than done with multiple food allergies. Unfortunately routine medicine's answer to medical issues is avoidance and masking symptoms, and not locating the cause and curing the patient.]

The abdominal surgery caused problems with the court-mandated counseling, because I could not attend the sessions at first (I couldn't walk). I missed a month and a half and in court. I was accused by opposing counsel for being "resistant" to counseling. I patiently explained the physical ordeal I was going through, and when I mentioned I had abdominal surgery including the tumor and half my reproductive system removed, my ex and his attorney both rolled their eyes skyward, as if I had made the entire matter up.

Once alerted to the circumstances, the family court commissioner at least gave me a whole 4-week grace period to heal…hardly sufficient, try 4 *months*. I was forced to go through the counseling sessions despite acute surgical pain, horrific headaches, new onset minor seizures, and symptoms of Lyme and brain fog. Then there was the intense anger I felt at my ex-husband's lies and the counselors' propensity to believe him and treat him like a colleague since he made them immediately aware of his Psychology degree. Naturally they looked at me with suspicion because I was the one who had the allegations filed against me. So of *course* I must therefore be guilty until proven innocent. Apparently they thought I was a mental case – in part due to my ex's allegations, and in part, because I wasn't physically or psychologically capable of handling being in the same room as him at the time.

In fact they were so obnoxious toward me that though we were ordered joint counseling sessions, the counselors (together with my ex I would learn later on), actually tricked me into arriving at a *single* counseling session, and tried to force me to allow them to question my two children. The court commissioner had previously made it quite clear about her position on whether the children should be involved or not in the counseling sessions. Her words were, "the children have absolutely *no business* participating in these counseling sessions." I knew because I had specifically asked her.

So naturally as a mother I wanted to protect my children. I questioned the counselor when she demanded that I bring my children in to talk with her (she knew they were with us each week). I asked her directly why she felt she needed to question them, because my children were already nervous about the situation and had asked me if they were going to have to talk to "these people," to which I had previously told them "no, of course not." Well, now the counselor was trying to force the issue, and I was worried she would try to manipulate whatever the children might say. (Remember how they had previously lied about abuse?) I told the counselor my feelings about the court's opinion, but she ignored me and pressed the issue. In fact, she became quite indignant, and I took that to mean that she felt I was not cooperative. Whatever I chose, I would look like the bad guy. If I refused the counselor, I was uncooperative. If I forced the children, they would hate mommy for "making" them talk. If I allowed the children to be interviewed, the court could be angry with me, and I ran the risk of them telling more lies to help their father, which would exacerbate the situation. I felt helpless and really did not know what to do.

I asked the counselor point blank again why she wanted to speak to the children. She answered me, "because I want to get their take on the situation." I did not think that either necessary or appropriate and my interests lay in protecting my children from manipulative family counselors (they weren't even Psychologists or Psychiatrists, just family therapists). So I replied, "Look, last year these children believed in Santa Claus and the Easter bunny. What makes you think they are old enough to have a mature understanding of the process here?" The counselor was now visibly angry with me.

I was put on the spot so I relented and allowed the children to come into the room. They sat nervously on the couch and looked at me, and refused to look at the counselor. "This woman wants to ask you some questions," I began, *purposely* softening my voice "Do you want to talk to her?" I asked them. They both shook their heads a definitive "no." "Okay, I'm sorry, they don't want to talk to you," I said to the therapist and the children were ushered out the door. In court the therapist would try to make it appear as if I had coerced my children on the spot to refuse to talk to her. I had merely asked them a simple question and they certainly gave her "their take on the situation," just as she had asked, which was that they didn't want to talk to her. Somehow it was all my fault.

Getting back to our joint sessions, of course I would cry from the pain and shake from the neuro Lyme symptoms, and be angry and openly hostile at the entire hateful process I was being forced to go through, as well as from listening to the overt lies being told about me. I cringed in disgust as I sat and listened to my exhusband fabricate entire conversations he claimed we had, which I knew very well (and so did he), that had never taken place. He was such a charmer and a good liar that he actually believed his own stories and so did everyone else except me, for I knew the truth.

I spent the majority of time defending myself against allegations of child abuse I knew had never happened. My ex told complex stories about how I hit my son and grabbed his arm and tried to shove peas down his throat, which was preposterous. It made me sick to think that this man whom I had been with for 13 years, would sit there and invent such hurtful stories to get what he wanted. He was vindictive and cruel and it made me sick to my stomach. Twice I got up and walked out in disgust – because the counselors kept telling me that *they needed to determine if abuse had occurred.* To which I would say "I am telling you that it *didn't* occur." And their reply would always be "but your ex says that it *did*." I reminded them that we were there to have *communication facilitated*, not to have them determine whether I was a child abuser or not, that decision was supposed to be for the courts. But neither of the counselors cared about what they were asked to do, they had their own agenda, and I had no choice but to be their scapegoat because they refused to acknowledge me. I find it more than vaguely ironic that the counseling center's name contained the word "credence," because I certainly never was afforded any.

The unprofessional nature of the sessions became a he-said/she-said battle zone, which was understandably non-productive, and we were eventually fired as clients, even though the court ordered the counselors to help us with communication. All the counselors did was complicate an already complicated mess, and one of the counselors would later further complicate our court trial by virtue of her irresponsible, unprofessional testimony.

Needless to say, I was in no shape whatsoever physically, mentally or emotionally to be able to handle this kind of "counseling" with a man who had "allegedly" raped me while we were still married, (I am told I have to say this because he was never arrested for it, tried, or convicted). I was even still quite visibly very afraid of him when forced to sit next to him. My insistence that I was innocent of all charges was summarily dismissed by everyone involved. Instead, I was harrassed, quizzed, methodically analyzed and microscopically scrutinized. From my perspective, it was apparent to me that everyone perceived me as if I was lying, or had mental problems, despite my insistence that I had surgery, and "some sort" of illness making it hard to concentrate, think, answer questions, be anything other than nauseous and irritable, and which made me a physical and emotional basketcase. Since I had no diagnosis, it must have been "all in my head" to them, I suppose.

There were other things going on at the same time as the counseling fiasco. The children had admitted to their own therapists that they were *openly lying for their father to help him win his custody suit.* (This counseling was not court ordered. They were seeing counselors at my request because I felt they were maladjusted to the divorce). The court officers, incredibly *ignored* that revelation although it was read into our trial transcript via a counselor's oral deposition. In fact, when the deposition was read into the trial transcripts, it was read by none other than the children's Guardian Ad Litem, who is the court-appointed attorney acting on behelf of the children's "best interests." He mockingly read the words into the transcript and to this day, has never given that information one ounce of credence. *He never considered that what he was reading into the court transcripts might actually be the truth.* No one wanted to believe my ex was capable of such a hateful thing, so they would rather believe that I somehow forced my children to lie to counselors when I was not even present during their sessions. They even revealed how they were "practicing what to say so they would get it right for dad" when it came time to report to the court officers. Even the children's counselor carefully outlined why they might indeed lie for their father. Yet the courts did nothing with this information – absolutely nothing.

To boot, our court-ordered counselor had spoken to me once, alone, about my tumultuous marriage with my ex-husband. At the time I revealed to her about how my ex had (allegedly) raped me and told her that I had never been in the same room with him since the incident. Even though it was (then) some 5 years later, I was still terrified of being in the same room with him. She dismissed those concerns but admitted in our trial that she hadn't done anything about that revelation, and that we *probably* should have addressed the issue before the joint sessions had begun. (You think?) She noted that she *should have* recommended that both my ex and I undergo individual counseling (me for the rape/fear issues, my ex for his noted anger issues), before the joint counseling could ever move forward.[185]

But those issues had not been addressed and everything was somehow falling onto my already overburdened shoulders. My attorneys could never figure out why, but each of them said that Walworth county had the reputation of being the worst county in Wisconsin to be facing in the family courts. They were accused of thinking they were "above" the law, and I heard, and read stories containing various allegations of corruption and attorneys in judge's pockets, which when I considered the course of our case, and the difficulty we had obtaining attorneys willing to practice in that county, did not surprise me in the least.

To make matters worse, the weekly trips down to the joint counseling sessions were two hours round-trip, and we had to drag the children along with us. My second husband thankfully took the kids for an hour to a nearby park during the sessions and we would all drive home afterward. This was tough on the kids as they hated the drive and the time spent waiting for mom to be done with something they did not understand, but the park visits helped. From the perspective of children, all they were aware of was that mom and dad were "fighting," and that upset them. They did not understand the cause of the conflict which was their father deliberately filing court motions and the effect of me being forced to defend myself without a choice in the matter.

I was still obviously ill with all my symptoms, and now dealing with additional vertigo, sinusitus, and intense nausea and motion sickness when traveling to counseling. We would have to stop the car at least once per trip so I could use the bathroom. I didn't tell my second husband that I was often drooling over the toilet in the restrooms trying not to puke my guts out every time we stopped. I just kept that lovely little detail to myself. All the way down I shook from fear of what was to come, and all the way home I would cry tears of pain, grief, anger and anguish. I found very little comfort in any words which might have been expressed in sympathy or empathy although I really don't remember hearing any. Perhaps there were some, but I was so absorbed in everything that was going on around me, that I felt as if I was being sucked into a black hole whereby I would never get out alive.

Once or twice following the outrageously upsetting counseling sessions, momentarily all I wanted to do was to open the car door and jump out onto the highway and die. In an instant of suspended reality, the thought that perhaps death would allow an escape from the horrendous court process and the pain and suffering of "some disease" that nobody seemed to know anything about, let alone acknowledge, might be better than somehow figuring out a way through it all.

In that moment of mental confusion and despair, practically the only thing preventing that from happening was the thought that I did not want to leave my children that way, or in any manner. If I hadn't been such a strong person, I might have succumbed to those fleeting, horrifyingly dark thoughts. It's "funny" how extreme stress plays with the Lyme brain, making you think things you would otherwise never consider in a million years. The court of course held my "attitude" at counseling against me and said I wasn't "cooperating" in counseling. But for God's sake, who the hell *could* under that kind of duress, even if they were *well*?

The opposing counsel made every opportunity to exploit my obvious physical and emotional incapacities in court, and made many accusations against me which were both theoretical and unproven. He even made suggestions that the irresponsible counselor nervously agreed to. For example, opposing counsel asked the counselor at our first trial if she knew what the symptoms of *borderline personality disorder* were; and if so, to please decribe them for the court. The counselor said, "Yes" and then proceeded to describe "inflexibility" as one symptom.

After her decription, my ex's attorney cleverly asked if the counselor noticed any "inflexibility" in me during the counseling sessions. To which the counselor readily replied, "yes." Of course no *direct* accusation was made, but the inference of the opposing counsel was that I must have *borderline personality disorder* (because I had been inflexible), *and therefore I must have a diagnosis of a mental illness.* And **the judge** that we had at the time, had heard him loud and clear and **was not intelligent enough to differentiate between a diagnosis or an attorney's wishful thinking.**

Incidentally, no diagnosis was given for either myself or my exhusband by the court-ordered counselors other than the working diagnosis of "adjustment disorder with anxiety" which was required by law in order to provide counseling in the first place, and we were asked permission to use that "diagnosis" for the purposes of initiating counseling. In fact during the trial, the counselor made it quite clear that she was not "out do to a heavy-duty diagnosis or anything"[186] (An interesting side note was that during the time the counselor was on the stand, although I was literally 10 feet in front of her, she absolutely *refused* to make any eye contact with me the entire time she was being questioned.)

And yet my ex's attorney's inference that I somehow had symptoms of "borderline personality disorder" became part of public record and permanent court *orders* which he also conveniently drafted (under objection I might add), and which still stand in public record to this day. In fact, he had a pattern of embellishing over and above what was actually said at hearings to help his client win on paper, even when those claims were simply untrue, much to my detriment. And this pattern of behavior would become the foundation of how our decade-long court case could have been so notoriously wrongly handled that it is somehow tragically comical.

At all subsequent hearings, the opposing counsel's accusations of mental illness and other things somehow always conveniently morphed into the *judge's final decision and orders* despite the fact that the judge never said those words at any time during our entire 10-year trial process. As time went along, the paper trail of slanderous claims against me grew to such magnitude that despite a lack of evidence, I was somehow painted as basically mentally disturbed, possibly violent, and not worthy of having my children around me. My 11 attorneys of differing caliber due to my lack of ability to pay them, case complexity, inexperience, and carefully designed allegations from the opposing counsel made things go from bad to worse on a regular basis.

This just goes to show you that even accusations, though unproven, can affect the outcome of court custody cases, even when no witnesses, medical records or evidence ever exists. In fact, in our case, evidence to the contrary was repleat within the process, and yet my ex and his attorney nearly always prevailed because they had so carefully set the stage with false allegations and a twisted interpretation of history, beforehand. (I suspect there were other matters which ensured their win each and every time they went before the courts, despite there being no evidence or witnesses whatsoever.) Once accused in family court, it is almost impossible to surmount those accusations, no matter the weight of the evidence, or lack thereof. In this family court at least, it seemed to me that the judge's perceptions or perhaps his acquaintances were always much more important than the actual evidence or the truth for that matter. As a matter of fact, it was related to me that one of my attorneys openly accused the judge and the opposing counsel of collusion while in the judge's chambers.

In my opinion, it was largely due to the prejudice and ignorance of the court officers and judges from which our case suffered, and accusations of mental illness as outlined by a corrupt, sociopathic man (my ex) and his wayward, manipulative attorney, and that attorney's close ties with the family court officers which caused my children to be removed from our loving home. Because at no time were any laws broken or any state statutes ever met which would have moved any other court to remove physical custody and placement from me. And at no time was there any activity or behavior on my part that would constitute reason for a judge to remove custody of children from my care. My symptoms of Lyme disease only became markedly noticeable to others in 2005, two years *after* the children were already removed from my custody, and not before. Sure, I had been an emotional (and physical) wreck following my surgery in 2002 and mandatory court-ordered counseling, but the fact that I was emotionally incapable of handling counseling with a man who "allegedly" had raped me and with the counselor's admissions that counseling should not have moved forward, never seemed to hold any validity. Instead, the responsibility of failed counseling fell upon my shoulders amidst false allegations of "child abuse" and "mental illness" that was never, and has never, and will never be, proven true – because they were, and are, absolutely FALSE.

My only "crimes" according to the court, were being physically ill with "something," being emotionally upset at counseling; and honestly admitting I smashed a telephone once in my life when extremely angry, when no one else was around. These so-called "behaviors" were added to previous statements from an inept social worker that I had a "face full of rage" (neuro-Lyme impairment) and that we lived in a "changing urban environment" (both opinion, not fact). These allegations were stupidly made by a social worker performing a home study and taken as gospel by a clueless judge. And because I had an ex-husband determined to remove my children from me and their new step-father using any means at his disposal, these situations combined very neatly with undiagnosed chronic Lyme disease as manipulated by him within the courts.

In truth, Lyme disease, whether diagnosed or not, irreparably affected my emotional responses to the horrendous situations I was repeatedly thrust into through no fault of my own. My inability to function at what the court considered a "normal" level, quite literally allowed the court and my exhusband to obliterate our family. Somehow in the entire process, I went from being a perfectly fit parent who deserved custody of two children according to the court, (and had them for 6 years), to being a suddenly "Lyme-obsessed," "mental patient" who has no custodial rights whatsoever and extremely restricted visitation; all built upon false allegations and the fact that I have chronic Lyme disease. Note it was something I had from 1992 to 2003, during most of my children's lives! An interesting side note here is that in 1997, my ex-husband testified that he had "no concerns whatsoever" about my ability to parent – and remember, I already had Lyme disease for 5 years at that time. But once I remarried, my ex suddenly slung accusations of "child abuse" and "mental illness" around, in a convenient, contrived effort to reverse custody and placement – and he succeeded, simply because I was physically ill from something no doctors would diagnose or treat at that time (hardly my fault).

If anyone would take the time and study the transcripts and the case history (if anyone wanted to), I assure you this case is a phenomenal travesty of "justice," and guide book on "what not to do" when going through two custody trials, at least eleven attorneys (on my side), a couple hundred thousand dollars, and an appeal process. We're not "done" yet, at this point we still have a year and a half to go before my youngest turns 18, and anything is possible with my ex, and I have a long haul reporting certain attorneys to the state oversight board.

Before you attempt to speculate on any of my possible contributory behaviors, I was examined closely on three separate occasions over the course of 9 years by three separate Psychologists, one of whom was paid for by my ex, using extensive psychological testing. All tests indicated that not only was I clearly *not mentally ill*, nor did I have an abusive bone in my body, but rather that I was of above average intelligence and that I was fully capable and responsible as a parent, with appropriate responses to our situations, even under extreme duress.

The two most recent evaluations later found me to be suffering from physical ailments, and not mental ones, which they attributed to Lyme disease (the last exams occurred in 2005 and 2006, respectively, *after* I was finally diagnosed). Prior to that, my ex was only evaluated once, in 1998 shortly after the onset of our divorce. In the notes which I wasn't supposed to be given but was, it indicated that my ex had problems with "inappropriate rage," and that his psychological profile was "invalid." Essentially I was told that he had lied so much that the Psychologist felt he was incapable of telling the truth. Because of his violent actions and mishandling of situations pre- and post-divorce, it had been originally recommended that he *not* be awarded placement of our children. I was granted joint custody with placement, which I held for 6 years before it was taken away from me under false pretenses.

Unfortunately for us, but lucky for my ex, the court actually ignored those findings six years later when we attempted to refresh the court's memory about my ex-husband's earlier actions. The court actually defended him by saying that they were somehow now "too old" and "irrelevant!" **People, when a party to an action has a history of bad behavior, lies, and violence, those records *never* become irrelevant and should be admissible in any related proceedings.**

When we requested for the court to allow us the same courtesy to psychologically re-examine my ex, our request was denied. Yet I was simultaneously forced to undergo a new psychological examination as demanded by opposing counsel, despite having two other studies independently done proving I was not mentally ill. After forcing me to undergo this again, the opposing counsel *never used or discussed the results in court* – because they had nothing "on" me, they had done this purely to harrass me and delay our proceedings another half a year's time.

In addition, the stack (sixteen inches) of personal medical record history I had to furnish under protest to the opposing counsel, my ex, and the court officers on three separate occations over the course of 2 years clearly indicated that *at no time was there ever a diagnosis of any mental disorder found, anywhere*. But none of that seemed to matter. Only one medical record was ever used in a trial by opposing counsel. It was a stool culture *parasite* test done at onset of my Lyme. He tried to pass it off as being a negative "Lyme" test, which was both comical and a tragic testament to the opposing counsel's own ignorance about the disease.

During the ongoing custody trial, I was now working again, at a new job, which had begun on September 10, 2001. Imagine your second day of work and the 9/11 tragedy happens. It certainly gives you a clear idea of how compassionate people are, and these fellas were unbelievably compassionate. As a matter of fact, I was very lucky that by August 2002, I was well thought of at my place of employment, due to hard work on my part. I can't think of any other workplace in the United States that would have been as flexible as these kind people were, when my physical health rapidly went downhill.

When I was having terrible symptom flares, they allowed me to use my vacation time to go to the doctor, have surgery and also to attend the countless numbers of unavoidable court hearings. They also over time, allowed me to tailor my hours to my health needs. As long as I did my main body of work, I was allowed to work part-time hours instead of full-time because that was physically the best I could possibly do under the circumstances. These people were unbelievably understanding and great (www.pwrtst.com). Though I was at a loss for a diagnosis or an explanation of what happened to me at the time, they did their best to deal with my complicated life by simply trusting me. I want to personally thank them here for their kindness. Compassion is always appreciated and never forgotten. I know I did the absolute best I could under most difficult circumstances and undiagnosed illness.

Over time, our court case developed into a full-blown trial, and the stress of that alone exacerbated my undiagnosed Lyme disease and co-infections. By this time, I was having great difficulty with daily function. Nobody knew how sick I really was, or if they noticed it, because I somehow held things together, it was difficult to put a finger on. And yet I spent more than a few moments in the bathroom, in the lunch room, hiding from the debilitating panic attacks that would suddenly hit me. I also had intermittent forgetfulness and new daily sleepiness, making continuity of work performance difficult. I found myself having to do things more than once, and it took longer and longer to do simple things that should not have taken that long to do. But nobody seemed to notice my cognitive issues except for me, or if they did, they certainly didn't say anything.

In time, I began to have bloody urine, (I found out later this was probably due to Babesia); extreme fatigue, headaches, and problems with my left shoulder and neck (again). I also had a new-onset tendonitis in my right elbow. I wore a brace on my arm which was supposed to help, but it did little. After a few months of one elbow hurting painfully, it would get suddenly better and then the other elbow would inexplicably begin a several month-long assault. Also, when I sat too long at the desk, when I stood up, I was painfully stiff and I would limp for awhile until my joints and ligaments got "going" again.

One day while at work and dealing with my pain and other symptoms, I was eating a pear at my desk for lunch, and I had a weird "reaction." It felt like anaphylaxis. I was having trouble breathing, my chest was tight and I was thrown into a state of panic. I suddenly felt very ill and I went into my manager's office and told him so. It was bad timing because just then he had salespeople he had to deal with, but he did say, "Don't go anywhere, I want to be sure you are alright." I did as I was told for a while, but felt it urgent that I seek medical attention. Against his advice not to drive myself, I went to the ER and was examined. They did not know what had happened but later discharged me with a diagnosis of an "allergic reaction," after doping me up with Benadryl. I couldn't work on that stuff, so I went home.

On my way home I stopped in at the doctor's clinic just two blocks from my house. In his office I was having another allergic reaction and was turning beet red without provocation. He did not know what was happening and strongly suggested that I stay off work until "we" could get to the bottom of what was causing these "reactions." He thought that perhaps the smell of ammonia from the blueprint machine might have caused the earlier reaction, but that did not explain what was happening now in his office. In addition, my blood pressure was out of whack and he took some blood and ordered me on bed rest. I was told not to return to work until further notice. In fact he advised me to quit my job on the spot.

This of course made things difficult, because how could I tell my employer that I was too sick to return to work – for "something" that my doctor couldn't explain? It sounded ridiculous to me, but in my blind panic and unclear thinking and Lyme brain fog, my fears were causing me to believe anything the doctor said (no matter how irrational), as the absolute truth. I did not know what to do, so I quit my job on the spot. This was a horrible thing to do to these guys and I regret that, but we are talking about someone who was not in their right mind at the time, and who was being horribly affected by a rampant, undiagnosed systemic infection. The reality was, by virtue of my illnesses, I was not responsible for any of my actions nor the blind acceptance of my doctor's conjecture.

So now I was home again, and once again, unemployed. Luckily my husband was working and doing okay at supporting us. But finding good medical care which could explain what was happening to me physically was nearly impossible. Instead I was sent hither and yon from General Practitioners, to GYN's, to Orthopaedists, to Osteopaths (for severe nerve pain which felt like "bone" pain), and to Gastroenterologists, Internal Medicine doctors, Allergists, to Infectious Disease doctors, Travel Medicine doctors, and Neurologists. One Allergist did a skin test and I reacted to nothing except the histamine control. He said I had no detectable allergies whatsoever, not even shellfish. And yet I had developed a new symptom that was increasing with a perplexing severity. I began having episodes of immediate, moderate to severe anaphylaxis to foods, medicines, and at times, even smells.

I also began hallucinating again at night time. A few times I awoke to see "someone" standing next to my bed, and on one occasion that "someone" actually "spoke" to me! Can you imagine how frightening that was to see someone you don't recognize, who is as solid looking as a real person, standing next to your bedside and speaking? Is this heightened perception or delusional psychosis? What if the brain can be rewired by infection-altered biochemistry to be able to perceive outside the realm of "normal" – thus allowing us to see what is perhaps really all around us, but normally imperceptible by virtue of "normal" brain chemistry and sensory skills? We know the nervous system becomes hypersensitive due to Lyme disease, why not the brain and sensory abilities as well? And yet I told no one about these incidents lest they be used against me in court.

I remember a strange incident where I had gotten a new set of *Ginsu* kitchen knives. I wondered how sharp they might actually be in real life as opposed to as shown on the television commercial. Without even thinking about what I was actually doing (because I was in such a state of brain fog), I ran one of the knife blades across my outer forearm, scratching it. I didn't even realize what I had done until after I had done it a second and a third time, trying to see if the knife was sharp enough to cut. How stupid! How "Lyme brain-like" and how frightening! I wasn't trying to hurt myself, I was just so disconnected from my own thoughts and actions that I didn't regard my own flesh as somehow a part of me! Fortunately, although the knife was sharp, I hadn't used very much force, and the blade caused only minor scratches. But what I distinctly remember about that incident was the thought, "Huh, not very sharp." I had no regard for the fact that I had just scratched myself or could have seriously injured my arm! And then just a moment later the full impact of what I had done hit me like a ton of bricks. I thought, "Oh my God! I could have sliced my arm wide open!" That thought of being unaware and on auto-pilot was extremely scarey to me and the first indication that something might now be seriously wrong with my thought processes. I didn't know what to do at the time but I was definitely scared. But no one knew about this incident except for me, because I never told anyone, and no one saw it either.

One afternoon I was feeling well enough to go outside to sit in my garden, which was something I loved to do. While making my way slowly to a bench, I used the wooden fence as a support to walk, and received a painful splinter in my right index finger, which I felt merely an annoyance. Once inside I washed the wound and tried to remove all traces of the treated wood. I thought I had gotten it all, but apparently I did not and it quickly became infected. Over the course of 24 hours, my finger swelled in size, and turned purple. I could not bend the joint and was rightly concerned. I went to the doctor who said to soak it and put some disinfectant on it and that it would be "okay."

I returned home and followed the doctor's instructions. But later in the day I began to have severe chills and a fever. I felt more unwell at that time than I think I have ever felt in my entire life. I thought I was coming down with a horrible flu. I went to go to bed at the usual time after sitting on the couch wrapped in 3 blankets, trying to keep warm to no avail. When I was undressing however, I noticed that I had red streaks beginning to form on my hand. Was I imaging it? I stared at them for a time and they seemed to be moving. I thought my eyes were playing tricks on me. Yes, they were indeed moving. I watched them advance like so many soldiers from my hand to my wrist, and from my wrist up my arm.

Though I had already laid down in bed by this time, I realized that I should probably go directly to the hospital. Somewhere in the dark recesses of my mind the word "septicemia" leaped out. We rushed to the emergency room where I was immediately put on intravenous Keflex (Cephalexin), which intrestingly enough, is also used for treating Lyme disease. The attending physician told me that if I had gone to sleep that night that I probably would not have awakened the next morning. I watched the streaks retreat in a 45-minute IV treatment, from my shoulder (they had gotten that far in the 15-minute drive), all the way back down into my hand. The drugs made me dizzy and feel like I had been hit by a truck, but the chills went away and I actually began to feel a little better.

> *[Author note: Septicemia or blood poisoning is a life-threatening condition that should be heeded at the first sign of problems. This is something about which many who have picc lines and ports installed, need to be on constant alert. Septicemia can and will, rapidly kill.]*

After the finger infection, I was switched to oral Keflex. That was one tough medicine to take and it gave me extremely painful migraines and made me feel very ill. When I took my medications, my mother-in-law would come over and monitor me because it made me so ill. She said I even looked immediately "off" when taking the medication. I was unable to continue after about three days, because the medication was affecting me so harshly. I now wonder if the reactions I had to the medication were severe herxheimers, which caused an increase of symptom intensity. For a brief while following the finger infection, I actually recovered a bit. Though I still had a myriad of symptoms, for about a month's time I felt much better than I had in quite a long time, especially cognitively. But shortly thereafter, the same symptoms crept quickly back.

When I was able to be out in public (usually accompanied by my husband as I could no longer drive), I would not be very reliable at functions. I could not stand still in one position very long because I had problems with maintaining balance. I took to leaning on a shopping cart or the counter if I had to stand in line for any length of time because I would feel weak or like I might pass out.

Sometimes the fluorescent lights would instigate panic attacks, because I could "hear" or "feel" the buzzing sounds eminating from them. I can't explain it but it would send me into a blind panic and the only relief from fluorescent lighting was to remove myself from the situation. (The high-pitched squeal of store security systems were a particular problem as well.) Sound and light hypersensitivity is a common issue with neurologically-affected Lyme patients. The central nervous system becomes easily over-stimulated, and hypersensitive. The slightest noise, movement, sight, smell or touch is like the irritating sound of nails on a chalkboard, but a thousand times worse.

I felt like there were bugs crawling under my skin, especially if I was tired. It would unbearably feel like I was being bitten by insects – shooting pains like a fly bite or a bee sting might feel, even when there was nothing causing it. I suffered jerky muscle spasms on my hands, arms, legs and face. In court, my attorney thought I was winking at him and remarked about my "winking" eyelid. In another court hearing, I sat holding my left shoulder in place because it was involuntarily spasming up and down as if I was shrugging my shoulder. That was particularly embarassing for me. At times I felt a "buzzing" sensation inside of my head, and there were times when my entire body would visibly shake or vibrate uncontrollably. It was as if I was sitting on a foot massager, and we did not know what we could do about it. Doctors shrugged their shoulders and dismissed me with indifference. I was told to get more sleep, eat better, stop worrying, and go talk to somebody.

When I got out of bed one day and my knees buckled and my legs wouldn't work, I decided that I should go back to bed and get more sleep. Since nobody believed that I had anything wrong with me, I started to believe that maybe it was "all in my head." Perhaps the extreme stress of the court hearings and subsequent trial were causing the bizarre range of symptoms. After all, stress does amazing things, doesn't it? But no matter how hard I tried to ignore that my body was not functioning properly, the more it told me that I was indeed ill. After all, my lengthy list of symptoms had been hanging around for over a decade.

I saw my cognition slipping in moments of clarity where I noticed that just five minutes before I had been doing something irrational. That was frightening. I would find things put in the pantry cabinet that belonged in the refrigerator. I would lose my car keys and find them in places like the underwear drawer. Sometimes I would drive some place and then "forget" where I was going and when looking around, would lose any idea of what road I was on or how I had gotten there. It was frightening and I would simply keep driving in the hopes that I would soon remember who I was and where I was going. I recall once pulling over to the side of the road, to take out my driver's license in the hopes that it would clarify what *state* I was driving in!

In fact, nothing I did seemed to make sense any more. I also could no longer lift a milk carton nor do housework, as I had no strength or stamina. I had to let things go that I would normally take pride in doing. Projects were left unfinished, and worse, nobody noticed or cared, not even me. That was not like me at all. Sometimes when I got up to walk into another room, by the time I would get there, I would have forgotten what I was doing. You might chuckle at the realization that this occurs with "old age," but I was far from old at the time and it was distressing.

And there were fleeting, pervasive thoughts of a subject matter which I would never otherwise think about – death. Suicide, while not normally in my personal vocabulary, would enter my head in an unguarded moment. I might be thinking about letting the dog out for a moment and then a thought of, "you should kill yourself" would randomly enter my mind. It took work to chase those horrible thoughts away, which were both disturbing and frightening. I prayed an awful lot during that time period. One day when returning from work (when I was still working and driving), I pulled into the driveway. I was very fatigued and rested my head on the steering wheel for just a moment after parking the car. In a flash of a moment, I saw in my mind's eye an image which frightened me terribly.

I "saw" what could be described as a freeze-framed picture of my oldest child, my daughter, lying on her back, dead on our kitchen floor with her stomach disemboweled. I shreiked and shook my head and hit my head with my hands trying to purge the horrid image from my mind. Where had it come from? What did it mean and why did I think it? I was too horrified to dwell on it and went into my house instead, visibly shaken. Just 2 years later of course I would actually learn the meaning of that "vision."

> *[Part of my daughter's story of "alleged" (meaning undiagnosed) neuropsychiatric Lyme disease is told in the book "The Singing Forest, a Journey Through Lyme Disease." For those who have not read it, it covers aspects of my family's life with Lyme disease, including my daughter's obsession with the ancient Japanese practice of Seppuku (ritual suicide where the victim is disemboweled and then beheaded). It also explains my viewpoint that my daughter is suffering from untreated neuro-*

psychiatric Lyme disease, with accompaning depression, and suicidal ideology. I will discuss her story in this chapter to teach people about what I believe to be issues of neuropsychiatric Lyme disease and how it is ignored in the family court system and within families themselves.]

Before the "vision," there was no way I could have known about any sort of fascination of Seppuku at the time because it wouldn't come to pass until nearly two years later, and there had been absolutely no indication of my daughter's interest in the subject matter, because she *didn't have any* at the time. This vision disturbed me so much that I even paid for a shaman to come into my house to perform a house clearing and a personal blessing ceremony. If it couldn't exorcise the "demons" in my mind, I thought that perhaps it would at least get rid of the bedside visitors who kept waking me up!

One of the stranger behavioral changes that began to present in me was a copious, sudden need to "count" things. This is a form of OCD, or obsessive-compulsive disorder, and was entirely new and perplexing to me. If I was in a car for example, I would find myself counting the passing telephone poles, or the road signs, or trees. It would happen more frequently when under stress (which was a daily thing at this point). I would have to consciously work to make the desire go out of my head and it was aggravating. Sometimes if I completed a task, I would feel doubts about whether I had performed it correctly and I would go back and check and recheck, several times to be sure. I would also wash and rewash my hands to ensure that they were meticulously clean.

Over time from around March of 2003, eating meals was becoming very difficult. I would often have sudden food reactions during a meal. I would have flushing, throat spasms, difficulty breathing, and my heart rate would soar. (It was measured over 200 bpm in the emergency room during one visit). Then a horrible chemical "dump" would occur within my body, which always felt like I was being poisoned. The chemicals caused argumentativeness, a state of confusion and panic, and my breath and body odor would noticeably change to foul. Following that I would shake uncontrollably for between 15 to 45 minutes, (an adrenaline rush I supposed), and then I would need to urinate and then be extremely fatigued. The whole process would begin instantaneously when exposed to the offending food, and take between 30 minutes to an hour from which to recover. It was truly bizarre. Depending on the amount of exposure to the offending food, the reactions would be either localized or severe. Many of them forced visits to the emergency room for additional support.

Unfortunately it didn't appear to be only one food causing the problems, so it was hard to pinpoint what were the causative agents. Therefore, I began to keep a database on computer, tracking every food item that I was consuming for every meal. If I ate it safely, I would add its ingredients to the "good" food list, and if I had a reaction, when I felt better, I would list every ingredient into the "suspect" column. Over time, a few things began to stand out and a pattern began to emerge.

I became "reactive" as I called it, to shellfish and anything that had shellfish in it. Sauces were a problem because if they contained clam juice or shellfish for flavor, that was a problem. Also teriyaki and worchester sauce and some salad dressings were an issue, as they used anchovies which was also a problem. To any kind of seafood, I was hands-down reactive. We found that ammonia was a problem, but only after we had a friend analyze an offending salad dressing in the food testing laboratory where she worked. She found large amounts of ammonia in the sample, which she said was probably a result of the cleaning agents used to disinfect the manufacturing equipment, and not an actual food ingredient.

[I wondered as I typed this, after seeing the correlation of my food "reaction" to my illnesses, if my "reactions" weren't in part due to being ammonia-toxic. If I am hypersensitive due to excessive levels in my body, perhaps any additional ammonia was setting off a toxic chemical overload "dump" which acts much like an allergic reaction. I wonder also if these very real "allergies" are reversible. If my new "allergies" are caused by infectious disease altering immune function, can other food allergies, (such as peanut), also be the result of a different infections doing the same thing? We know in "leaky gut" syndrome that food particles enter the body and are flagged by the immune system. It has been shown that Helicobacter pylori *causes ulcers. If Lyme/Bartonella/Babesia/EBV (my personal systemic cocktail mix, thank you Mr. tick) can cause my "allergies," who's to say that peanut or wheat or other allergies aren't caused by other infections which may in fact, be reversible and curable?]*

Since ammonia seemed to be an issue for me, I now had to avoid it including in smells, foods, and hair dye and perms, (which set off localized reactions like intense itching, flushing and difficulty breathing). Even the smell of baby diapers or seafood in the grocery store would cause a slight reaction. And chemicals on fruits and vegetables and certain preservatives were now also causing reactions. None of this made any sense at all, but I kept my lists going anyway, trying to pinpoint what was causing the reactions. It seemed that the list of "reactive" foods was growing every day. (I have discovered these reactions are a common situation in Lyme patients, and it seems related to our skewed body chemistry and inflammation levels).

Over time, because of the continued anaphylactic food reactions, eating became virtually impossible. As each food was eliminated one by one, I was physically starving to death and eventually unable to eat anything but white potatoes, corn, baby food bananas, water and white cheese. These were the only "safe" foods we could find which did not cause reactions. I hovered around 90 pounds at my lowest weight, (I'm 5'3" and usually weigh around 120 pounds). For several weeks it got worse and all I could eat were white potatoes and water for each and every meal. (Can you imagine that?) I accepted it nevertheless but cried all the time and at each meal. I looked and felt like a concentration camp victim.

My hair began to fall out and my gums bled each time I brushed. I had jaw and tooth pain on top of everything else. I didn't care if I died, and quite nearly did. My heart beat was irregular and caused several sudden trips to the hospital. My support person of my husband did not know what to do with me, so he did nothing except drive me whenever I asked him to, if and when I was sentient, that was. If I ran out of food to eat, it was up to me to either go to the store or give him a list of exactly what to buy, because he clearly didn't understand the allergy process or my dietary needs. That wasn't his fault, I didn't either, and eating for me, was like playing "Russian Roulette." If I wasn't clear about what I needed, he unfortunately would then leave me alone to fend for myself. Instead he buried himself in his work, often working late into the night so as to avoid the complications at home.

I think he did the best he could. In truth, few people are prepared to cope with the demands of a very ill, irrational thinking sick person. I don't necessarily feel his actions were entirely his fault, nobody else (including doctors) knew what to do with me either, and everyone pretty much ignored me and my "problems." It seemed that family members whispered about me behind my back and treated me like I only had mental problems. In fact, my children were the worst culprits because they didn't understand that I was ill or why, or that I did not choose to be ill. Often they would make fun of my surgeries, being sick "all the time," and my food "choices," which naturally came in large part, from their father. Of course he negated my illness to the children and continually called me "crazy" to them, so is it a surprise that they might echo his words?

This is probably one of the worst things that family and friends can do to an extremely ill person. Ignoring a problem or refusing to act will not make it somehow go away. We must become involved and help the ill person find the healthcare they need – after all, it may be you who is one day in need of assistance. I cannot speak enough about basic human compassion and empathy.

I had "friends" sever their friendships with me because I was, as they said, "unreliable" – meaning that when I made plans with them I often failed to show up because I was "supposedly" ill. They did not even believe that I was literally starving in front of their eyes because to them, I *didn't look sick.* Many patients have echoed similar issues to me. Their family and friends do not understand their illness so the sick patient is held accountable for behaviors and limitations that are beyond their control, even physical and cognitive disability.

The doctors did nothing for me except shrug their shoulders and charge me thousands of dollars. "Idiopathic" to me was synonymous with "idiot," and though it wasn't my fault I was physically ill, I *felt* like an idiot. Even as sick as I was, I knew it wasn't healthy or rational to be unable to eat anything except potatoes. We now have an inside "joke" about my now strengthened remote Irish heritage, not only by distant relations, but by virtue of my necessity-drive, massive potato consumption.

Mayo clinic in Rochester, Minnesota, where I spent 10 days in 2003 with many tests, was unable to diagnose anything. They would not listen to my hypothesis that I might have Lyme disease. Instead, they focused on gastrointestinal and allergy screenings designed to discover why I was suffering from anaphylaxis when I ate food. Of course even with their extensive serological testing, not a single allergy was detected. And yet because I reacted to medications, they had me undergo an upper endoscopy without a sedative.

Let me tell you there is nothing to compare with laying on your side for 25 minutes with the equivalent of a garden hose down your throat while the doctor tries to roto-rooter (biopsy) your stomach and you are involuntarily wretching the entire time. After he actually yelled at me because I "wasn't cooperating" (meaning hold still and don't vomit), I involuntarily (or voluntary, I'm not sure which), slugged him with my free arm in the stomach and he abruptly ended the procedure. (Ok, I had *enough* and he was torturing me. Make sure you get anesthesia if you ever have to do this.)

After spending 10 days at Mayo clinic in a wheelchair unable to walk from weakness, I was sent home without any answers whatsoever, and I expected *something* for a diagnosis. When they told me, "We know this is happening, but we don't know what it is, or what to do for you," I was shocked. I asked, "So I'm just supposed to go home and *not eat anything at all and starve to death?"* **The doctor's actual reply was, "Well, that's one way of handling it."** I knew at that point that if I wanted to live that I had to find my own way through this hellish illness.

> *[Note: I now not-so-affectionately call the clinic, "Hold the Mayo." This sentiment is sadly echoed in Lyme patients who cannot understand why the doctors there don't seem to comprehend that Lyme disease is endemic in the Midwest, including in Rochester, Minnesota where this clinic is located. Time and again patients report that their Lyme disease concerns were dismissed by this clinic. While it is doing excellent things for illnesses in other areas, Lyme patients want to know why such a major facility would seem to consciously ignore legitimate patient concerns about this disease in recent years. Update: in the past two months, a patient here or there has indicated that they are now <u>at least being tested</u> for Lyme disease, even if they are not being treated. But doctors are still misinterpreting the test results, and following CDC surveillance criteria. Now if we can only get these doctors to actually <u>treat</u> the illness longer than what a minority few and insurance companies are pushing as a "standard of care," which is neither standard, nor patient care-based, in my opinion, we will finally be making progress.]*

One morning I was so distraught about not being able to eat anything other than potatoes that I had called the *Sylvia Browne* prayer hotline to ask their ministers to put me in their prayer chain since I had been unable to eat food properly for months. Believe it or not I had already also paid out over eleven hundred dollars to a "medical intuitive healer" who said they would help me recover through regression and meditative long-distance phone "healings." Well the regression and past-life exploration was wonderfully interesting but it certainly didn't help me eat and I was out more than a thousand dollars and felt appropriately stupid when my brain fog lifted. When you are desperate and not in your right mind, you are willing to try anything to get an answer and become well.

So the next morning, with nothing left to lose, I promised God that if I did not have a reaction to a piece of toast that I desperately wanted to make and eat, and if He would help me to figure out what was causing the food anaphylaxis and make me able to eat again, that I would dedicate the rest of my life to helping other people who were in a similar situation. Whatever this illness was, I would help people deal with it if only I could be made well. I was very nervous of course, because just the day before, I had a food reaction to the very same bread. Yes I had tried to eat a piece of buttered toast the day before, but unsuccessfully. I instinctively knew that I would probably have another food reaction, but I was so tired of the potatoes and I did not want to die, that I put the bread into the toaster nonetheless, because I was desperately starving and I knew I had to eat.

I waited and prayed, and when it popped up, I said, "Okay God, here goes nothing" and I bit down on the plain, dry toast. It sounds so ridiculous now but when you are in a state where you are not thinking clearly because your body and brain have been starved of calories for months, you get to a place where anything and everything begins to make sense. I have touched that place in its quiet darkness, and I can tell you that it is one place I never wish to visit again, even briefly. As you can well guess, I did not react to the toast, and tears fell down my cheeks as I gleefully ate it. I made another piece and ate it and another and another until I had eaten half a loaf of bread. Thank you God! Thank you Sylvia Browne prayer chain! I said, excitedly.

Because I was "suddenly" able to eat bread "again," it got me thinking about what I had eaten the day before that had caused a reaction.

I realized that it wasn't the bread, it was what I had put on *top* of the bread the day before, which might have caused the reaction. Turns out I had used a butter which contained salt in it that (probably) had *Morton* table salt in it. When I switched to unsalted butter later, I could eat butter. If I ate the salted butter, I had a reaction – BINGO! This was of course, a huge revelation for me. Little did we know that the cause of many of the food reactions, had been a chemical in *Morton* brand table salt. I think it was an additive that could have been made from shellfish. Even if it was not, whatever was in the salt, was causing a definite, immediate and devastating reaction. And even *one grain* of Morton table salt could set off a fairly moderate reaction!

I had thought vegetables and then meat initially the cause of the food reactions. I reacted first to beef, then to pork, and then chicken. It seemed whatever I ate, became the enemy. In reality, it had been the *salt and/or butter* I was seasoning the food with that was causing the problems, but I didn't know any better. If I reacted, I eliminated the offending foods. So now I was finally making progresss and I could eat again but I had to be careful to avoid salt. Some manufacturers use Morton brand table salt, and some do not, but there was no way to know which by reading labels. Every meal became an experiment with tough and sometimes frightening consequences. And iodine cross-reacted, so I ate local foods from organic markets grown in iodine-depleated soil, a feat easy enough since we lived in Wisconsin, (an area with iodine-depleated soil.)

Over time I saw that I reacted to iodine, shellfish, anything with Morton salt on or in it, certain smells like ammonia; and annatto and tamarind (spices). This made my diet shrink to a few, dismal choices. I also had to avoid the organic foods which contained sea salt, since it also caused a reaction from shellfish contaminants. I could no longer eat out at restaurants or people's houses, because we had to be cautious about what ingredients were in processed and prepared foods. That was depressing and embarassing, to say the least, and very hard to explain to other people who have not experienced this less common aspect of illness. I could readily identify with people who have severe food allergies, only this seemed much worse, because it involved multiple triggers, and not "just" one. Let me tell you when you have suffered a hundred or so bouts of anaphylaxis, the fear alone of having another reaction is enough motivation to make you live vigilantly and be protective of every single food item you put into your mouth, whether you want to or not.

I took to carrying all my food around with me at all times. Every meal had to be prepared beforehand and carried with me if I was going to be away from home. This made travel very difficult as you can imagine, and long-distance travel, impossible. If I was going to be gone for more than a few hours, I had to carry with me enough food to last however many meals. But at least I was able to begin to eat again, even if my "diet" was very restricted. Thank God for my ingredient lists and that piece of toast, because without it, I might have continued to spiral downward into starvation.

By the end of our court trial in 2003, child abuse was finally proven not to have occurred, but the GAL and the judge thought "something" was "odd" about me. The GAL accused me of nothing more than "possible physical or emotional issues" which were "not being addressed" – something which had not even been discussed in court. If I had issues (and obviously I did), they were hardly my fault since no doctor would diagnose me for more than a decade at that point. We know that the court and counselors wouldn't give me a break to recover from surgery or past trauma, nobody would listen to the truth, and nobody counted the three abdominal surgeries in 18 months or all my doctor visits as attempting to address "issues." I don't know what else I could have done at the time! I don't recall ever seeing "possible issues" within the Wisconsin state statutes as a reason to remove custody, as no substantial change of circumstances were ever brought up, discussed, or proven.

The GAL somehow felt it appropriate for my youngest child, (my son), to go live with his father, even though it was known that he had lied for his dad. In the court's opinion, let's not punish my ex for wrongly filing false allegations against me, let's punish *me* because my coerced son was telling everyone he wanted to go live with his father. The stupid social worker who claimed we lived in a changing urban environment felt my child was "screaming" out to go live with his dad, and the sleeping judge just went along with the suggestion, without considering what was in the best interests of everyone. No one was able to grasp the fact that my children were being manipulated to lie for their father.

Something about my son's inability to adjust to the current situation was mumbled about, but I was no longer paying attention at that time.

I don't know what that could have meant, he was always a straight A student, with friends, who liked his school and had friends in the neighborhood. Why he would suddenly do better in a new school with no friends and no neighbors (in a rural area), with a father who manipulated and lied didn't make any sense to me at all. By this time I was already growing furious at the stupidity of it all.

In stark contrast, my oldest child, (my daughter), was allowed to stay with me, and as it was explained by the court, "she could cope" with the arrangements. My attorney tried to argue our case including the fact that why should one child have to "cope" and another be rewarded for lying, but to no avail. I couldn't see why the GAL thought it better for my children to be split apart and raised separately. In my opinion, what a shortsighted dunce!

Against my better judgment, I painfully put my own needs aside and unselfishly allowed my daughter to go live with her father along with her brother. I felt it vital that the two of them stay together while I attempted to right the terrible wrongs being perpetrated on our family by a manipulated court system. There was no way those two children deserved to be split apart because of an ignorant system and a vindictive father. But I thought that I stood a chance of recovering my children – if I could just get the court to hear the truth and listen.

In hindsight, I should have kept my daughter with me regardless, because once you give up your parental rights for any reason and on any level, *you will never get them back.* I did not think it fair for the courts to stupidly split up my children, so I told them "over my dead body" would I allow them to do that. Children are not pawns or possessions to be divided. The judge said, "very well then," after the GAL "commended" me for making what he called the "most mature decision he has ever heard any parent make in his career." My thoughts at the time were "yeah right, like you really ever cared about me, what you were doing to my children or the fact that you left me with no real choice."

After the judgement and losing my children, I remember storming out of the court room ahead of my husband and everyone else. I began walking and didn't stop walking until I was about a mile out of town. I absolutely knew in that moment that if I didn't keep walking, that I could not be held responsible for anything I might say, and that would probably have been to my ex-husband and/or his attorney!

My spouse went to get the car while I stomped right through an intersection with cars on both sides. "Go ahead and hit me," I thought to myself defiantly, not really meaning it. At that point, I had lost everything because "they" had wrongly taken away my children, and I didn't feel anything except contempt. My husband found me about 10 minutes later and picked me up with the car. I was nearly out of town and would have kept on walking, I was so upset. I cried all the way home (about an hour) and I didn't stop crying until some months later. But when I did stop crying, it would be years before I would be able to cry again, that is how badly it affected me.

I felt truly and completely brokenhearted, knowing that my children were in the hands of a horrible monster who would think nothing of using them to harm me and manipulating them to get what he wanted. I truly felt at one point that it would have been perhaps easier on me if I had lost them through a tragic accident because "at least" I would know they were safe and loved with God. Being in the hands of my ex-husband, the man who had lied, cheated, manipulated and also who had "allegedly" raped and was abusive to me, was a fate worse than death for them, or so I thought. I knew that he would undo every aspect of their good upbringing, and turn them against me through ruthless, long-term alienation tactics.

Sadly, my daughter considered my decision that she stay with her brother as a form of complete rejection, and she plunged into a nightmarish depression shortly thereafter. She sadly lost her best friend thanks to the courts as well, and that was very hard on her, and changed her attitude profoundly. Later she would be further driven away from me through her father's alienation tactics and circumstances which forced me to make tough decisions to protect her.

Again, her story is told in the book previously referenced, but the removal of both of my children from my custodial care was the most devastating thing to have occurred in my entire life up to that point. It even surpassed my physical illness, and I admit that the two events combined nearly took me out of this world. I remember at one point being so exhausted by my illness and the stress of the changes that I prayed at night that God would please just take me.

My body felt like lead each day, and my eyes were always puffy from crying. I wore no makeup and barely kept myself clean. I cared about nothing and just went through the motions in every aspect of life.

I sank into the inky black pit of depression so deeply, I felt I would never get out alive. I was weary mentally, physically, emotionally, and on a spiritual level, but I hid it very well. Some days it felt like it was tremendous work just to breathe. I remember lying on the edge of the bed one afternoon once again after weeping, and closing my eyes to feel nothing but blackness. I think that was the lowest point of my entire life. It was right around the same time period that my diet had all but disappeared, and I was only eating potatoes and water. A shadow of myself was all that remained and at this point I felt I literally had to make a conscious decision of "do I give up, or not," to go on. I understood how someone could die of a broken heart, because mine felt absolutely shattered.

And yet in that moment of complete vulnerability, the tiny spark of myself that was myself, remained. I could "see" it in my mind's eye, and I knew that I didn't really want to leave this world. Somehow the recognition that my children needed me to fight for them, was all that I needed to find the courage to get up and deal with another day. I knew I could not live with the terms and conditions that had been thrust upon this family, and I knew that I had to fight them at any cost. That was enough motivation for me to put myself back on track, but it was hard work and it took me a long time to recover.

I can tell you from personal experience, that depression of that magnitude, is unbearable for most people. Am I different somehow than other people? I don't know, I wouldn't think so really. Perhaps it was because my earlier life had been quite difficult that I survived. Perhaps because of many negative experiences I did not write about here that I understood on some level that "this too shall pass." I know that at any given point I never truly wanted to die. But in my moments of profound illness, lonliness, grief, and despair, my only thoughts were not that I wanted to die, but that **I simply no longer knew how to live.**

My personal burdens were lifted by prayer and the knowledge that my children needed me no matter what. That was my motivation. Without that and my self-respect and my fighting spirit, in my twisted body chemistry, who knows; I might too, have "checked out." However we do it, we must help people to find *their* motivation to keep themselves functioning and to prevent needless tragedies. And so we must reach in and be the hand that guides the ill patient back to reality, before they ever reach that deep of a level of despair, so they aren't left to do it themselves – because sometimes they simply cannot.

I really did not have what most would call a meaningful support team behind me. Yes I was married, but my spouse was ill-equipped to support me emotionally. He admits he basically "checked out" on the relationship when it became too difficult, and went to work so as not to have to "deal with" the overwhelming sadness and problems which surrounded me (as if many of them were my fault). That was certainly a choice he could make, though in my opinion, was not a very good one. But family members will be who they are, and ultimately, the chronic symptoms and sometimes even the depression which can and often does encompass chronic Lyme patients, alienates many an otherwise decent spouse, child, friend or relative. When you throw factors like doctor dismissal and complicated custody trials and false allegations on top of the mix, the Lyme patient will sadly find themselves all alone when they need the most support – during the toughest fight of their life.

At this point in time, we were so in debt from my surgeries, treatment medical costs and attorney's fees that we had to sell our house and move to a less expensive one. We were never "rich," and we always lived modestly. We never drove new cars and our house sold for less than $150k, so you can see we were frightfully "average" people. The debt consolidation from selling our home at a miniscule profit was far less than we expected. We were left without much of a downpayment, and so we were forced to find a rental property just two weeks after we sold our home. Despite my symptoms, I set about finding something to rent. I located a house about 45 miles southwest of Milwaukee, and set about moving most of our belongings there. Despite the fact that it was an hour's drive one way, I loaded up the van to the ceiling and made many trips between the two locations, largely unaided.

The house we rented was on Lake Koshkonong, a good-sized lake located in the southern part of the state, just east of the capitol of Madison. It was a serene wooded collection of lake homes clustered on the banks of the lake, and there was a forest behind the property which teamed with wildlife, including deer. I never realized even at that time, that wild deer meant ticks. We would set out corn to feed the small herd of 11 that would bravely walk up to within feet of the sliding glass door in the kitchen to eat. At night when I could not sleep, I would sit in the kitchen and watch the wildlife outdoors. I found it peaceful and relaxing, even if my days were still filled with weird symptoms and food reactions, which though better because I could now eat more food, still occurred. Once we pinpointed the fact that the table salt, shellfish and certain common spices were the main triggers, I was able to resume eating fresh fruits and vegetables, meats, and dairy products. So I was gaining nutritional ground, but little else.

I was still dealing with horrendous arm/shoulder muscle and joint pain, and my left side was very dysfunctional. I was no longer able to work, and I had difficulty with vertigo and walking. Even my cognitive function was slipping into a foggy veil. I found my IQ noticeably dropping thanks to some tests I had taken. I even "felt" less intelligent – that is I had the keen awareness of mental dullness that was on a different level than my "typical" self.

Because I had lost custody of my children, I was home alone most of the time. My husband worked an hour away, and I had no one but the landlords to rely on, and they lived several miles up the road, and were rarely home. My solitude at the lake was interrupted only by the occasional visitation of my children. It was difficult to hear them loudly vocalize their unhappiness with the new arrangements. It was not shocking to hear that their father hadn't made good on the promises he made if they helped him win custody – like money, trips, and yes, even a puppy. As a result they felt manipulated and betrayed. And the truth of course, would never make it to family court. We were all now trapped within a situation not of our making with no choice but to do the best we could with what was left of our damaged relationship.

Also during this time period, we were still going through more court hearings, because despite gaining the children, my ex continued to torture me with whatever games he could invent. Once I was held in contempt of court for failing to pay for travel costs which were not clearly explained in the marital "agreement." I had to appear in court pro-sea (by myself without an attorney), and I didn't know what I was doing and was off-focus due to cognitive Lyme issues. So evidence that would have exonerated me that I should have presented had I been in good shape logically, went unpresented to the courts and I was ordered to pay $1100 to my crummy ex for something we never agreed to, or face jail time of 6 months. My second husband coughed up the money for me. Things like that repeatedly caused problems. My ex would file motions, and though he lost most of the subsequent motions, he enjoyed the process of trying to hurt me and make me look bad in court. And what a long paper trail he created. Since he earned a very good wage, he had no problem spending it, even for this petty foolishness.

To illustrate how poorly the chronically ill patient is treated in this family court, I would like to share a few events which happened during the course of our third trial, 2005-2007. First, at one hearing which was scheduled at 8:00 in the morning, I was very ill but had no choice but to be at court. Despite not being able to function very well and running between the bathroom and the court room several times, it was communicated to the judge that I wasn't "feeling well" that day. During discussion about a court-ordered psychiatric evaluation that was to take place, it was indicated that I could not attend a full-day session that was scheduled to begin at 8:00 a.m. I would need the session broken up into two separate appointments. This was due in part to the two-hour drive to the Psychologist's office, as well as the fact that my nervous system doesn't function well in the morning, necessitating a sort of "camping out" in the bathroom, due to diarrhea. Well, the judge took one look at me, and said, "well, you're here now, and it's 8 a.m., I see no reason why you need to have 2 appointments."

What he was saying was in essence, "you don't get any special treatment because you are right here in front of me and it's 8 a.m., disabled or not, and I don't believe you are disabled." What the judge didn't "get" was that there is a huge difference between being driven somewhere at 8 a.m. because you have no choice but to be there and all you have to do is managed to sit through a 15-minute hearing; and being driven somewhere where you are expected to function and perform tests and mentally taxing interviews for an entire day.

I had to go to the psychiatric evaluation appointment at 8:00 a.m. in the morning and as you can imagine, I wasn't functioning well. I spent the first 20 minutes in the bathroom, was hobbling about on my cane, my body was shaking and my electrolytes were off, so I was obviously ill. Over the course of the day however, as I explained to the doctor, my mental and physical function would actually improve. Though I was essentially useless in the morning, by noon I was functioning somewhat better. The Psychiatrist watched my nervous system correct itself, and was amazed at how different I was in the morning, from the afternoon. But that is the way of Lyme disease. By virtue of how it affects the body different times of the day, a patient can be two different people within the span of just a few short hours.

Another aspect of discrimination against ill patients in family court is illustrated by a judge holding me in contempt of court for being unable to work. He had been given letters from my doctors stating that I had to reschedule court hearings due to ongoing IV treatments. He even saw the picc line in my left arm during one hearing, but never questioned it. Then finally in one court hearing he said I "didn't look sick to [him]," and immediately following that hearing, while standing outside the court room, I collapsed in a moment of a mild seizure or a drop in blood pressure – we don't know which, with my head hitting the glass door and my body slumping into a sitting position on the floor, in a heap. My ex and his attorney witnessed it, and they looked at me and audibly chuckled – as if I was faking it. I was too ill to feel even remotely embarassed. A baliff rushed to my side and asked if I was alright. My attorney did nothing but stand there, impotent. My husband at least asked if I wanted to stand up. I couldn't, so I just sat there for a few minutes to collect my bearings while everybody stared. I guess I didn't "look sick" to any of them.

The most blatant example of the difference in accommodations provided to myself and "the other side" came as a slap in the face in March of 2007, during our third trial. We had already gone through two separate trial dates, and this was supposed to be our third, and final date. A bit of history: on trial date one, (January) the long day of sitting on the court chairs had wreaked havoc in my back and left shoulder, which were frozen from lack of movement. When I got home, I was absolutely unable to sleep at all that night, due to intense pain and muscle spasms which occurred all night long. On the morning of trial day two, I had been up for more than 30 hours and was physically exhausted. I also could not eat. We warned the court that I would be ill all day and unable to testify, and all the judge said was "well, then she [meaning me] can lay down on one of the court benches over there," pointing to the hard, wooden benches which looked like church pews, that observers utilize. In essence, his reply was "that's too bad, but we're going to have this hearing, sleep or no sleep." So I was forced to sit through another entire day, without food or sleep, and I can't really tell you to this day, how I got through it, but I did. I don't remember much about trial day two though, I can tell you that much.

On trial day three two months later, we prepared for court and arrived at the courthouse, and fortunately I didn't feel too badly. When we attempted to scan the docket however, which was usually posted outside the court room, it was not there and had been removed. Our case had been postponed from the docket and nobody had told us. The clerk of courts came out into the hallway to request that my ex and myself come into the hearing room. Since my attorney was not there yet (typical for him as the hearing had been scheduled for 5 minutes later and he was never on time), I informed the judge that my attorney was still on his way. The judge chuckled and said it "didn't matter." He explained that opposing counsel (my ex's attorney) had telephoned him the evening before, to tell him that he was out in Denver, Colorado, and that he had "missed his plane" due to "traffic." The attorney had called the judge at home on a Sunday evening (our trial was on a Monday) to tell him that he was taking a red-eye plane so he could arrive at our trial hearing at 8:00 a.m. the following day. But he had told the judge that his plane would be arriving at 2:00 a.m. Monday morning. Since that would have afforded the attorney only about 4-5 hours of sleep before having to spend an entire day in court, he had asked the judge if the trial hearing could be postponed so he could be excused and not "have to function" on so little sleep.

Well, the judge apparently found the request reasonable, and he postponed our trial hearing so Mr. World Traveler could get his beauty rest. Unfortunately for us, nobody had bothered to tell us or our attorney about this, not even the opposing counsel, who had my attorney's cell number. Instead, the judge and opposing counsel simply made us all travel the hour to the court hearing, and *then told us* about the change. Not only was this aggravating for us, this now pushed our March trial date (which we had been waiting for, for nearly a year), off to September, and there was nothing I could do about it. Remember the second trial day where I had to suffer through *no sleep* and lie on the hard wooden benches? I managed. Why couldn't the attorney manage on 4 or 5 hours of sleep? Yes the attorney was catered to, and he wasn't even ill. And yet the chronically ill patient (me) with no sleep whatsoever, was expected to (and did) tough it out on a hard wooden bench, which incidentally, I never utilized. What a painful lesson on discrimination that was.

Remember the abdominal pain I had at the onset of my tick bite in 1992? Well this had been going on for about 10 years by this time, and

I finally had enough of the painful episodes. Once again I went to the doctor, and asked if there was any way to determine what was causing the problem. The doctor ordered a Papida scan and determined that although I had no gallstones, my gallbladder function was only at 6%. He recommended we remove it immediately. At this time of course, I simply followed his recommendations, I had no idea that I had Lyme disease and that it may have been causing the sluggish gallbladder. If I *had* known I had Lyme, I might have been able to save the organ, but unfortunately it's now history.

Once again I had abdominal surgery and once again they attempted to ship me out of the hospital the same day. However this time, I could not be aroused enough from the anesthesia to be able to successfully sit up. I just wouldn't "come to" enough to be moved. At my groggy insistence, my husband had to fight with the day nurse and the insurance company, but managed to get the doctor to allow me to stay overnight at the hospital, to sleep off the anesthesia. What were they going to do, shove me into the car unconscious? (They tried to do just that!) Unfortunately, as soon as they tried to move me, I had a sort of seizure reaction which threw them all in a tizzy – and which felt to me like the anaphylaxis again. The nurses were very curious about the process, and we told them about the fact that I react to chemicals like preservatives. It was suggested that perhaps there was a preservative in the saline IV that might be causing the problem. They unhooked it and I recovered. I left the next day. When we obtained a copy of my medical records however, it was interesting to note that no one had recorded the "seizure" episode in the records, but *had recorded* the fact that my husband had gone to the nurses' station in the morning because he had smelled smoke (from the hospital incinerator) wafting through the windows of my room!

Though I suffered no real complications following the gallbladder removal, I was still having cognitive problems, and an occasional visual hallucination. One afternoon when I was bored and feeling low, I attempted to play the piano (I had long given it up because I could no longer remember how to play). As I sat and tinkered out a tune, I suddenly *felt* someone standing behind me! I turned around very quickly in anticipation of a household intruder, but nobody was actually there. This was very weird for me, and I figured after some thought, that maybe I had actually "picked up" on a deceased person. (After all, the house was built near ancient Indian burial grounds, and Fort Atkinson where we were renting was the center of some heated battles over a hundred years ago.)

Another time I was anxious to get to the bathroom and since I was home alone, I did not bother to close the door. As I sat upon the "throne," I suddenly *saw* a man walk by the bathroom door, smiling at me as he went by. Now I knew there was no one else home with me, so if I hadn't recognized the individual, I would have thought an intruder had broken into the house. However, what perplexed me was the man who walked by the doorway was the father of a good friend of mine, who had been deceased nearly as long as my father had been. Now what do you make of that? I certainly wasn't thinking of that person at the time, and he appeared as solid and "real" to my eyes as you or I might.

I was also having trouble walking, and was very stiff and achey in the joints. At times I used a cane to help me walk, in part for stability, and in part to take some of the weight off of my left hip which was giving me trouble. I would do my best to take the dogs for a walk whenever I could, which helped take my mind off my daily symptoms and the horrible emptiness left by my childrens' absence. Several times during these walks, I would return home only to find adult ticks crawling on my shirt or my sleeves. I would stay out of the woods after that, and yet they would still make their way onto my clothing. I supposed that they were somehow dropping out of the trees, but they were just prolific climbers. All the while during this time I would pray to God to please help me figure out what was physically wrong with me. Funny now in retrospect, it may have been in answer to my prayers that we had moved into a heavily tick-infested part of the state. And these tiny creatures which were now almost a daily occurrence were God's little hint at what was wrong with me physically. But I still didn't quite get the hint.

I attempted to find healing through many means after that. More rounds of physical therapy were painful and useless. I felt at a complete loss as I watched my abilities dwindle on a weekly basis until I could no longer do much of anything. I couldn't even keep up with the housework, the pets, or my ebay business which I was trying to operate to help with our income situation. We lived in the rental house for 8 months, with boxes stacked from floor to ceiling as we tried to set aside enough money to buy another home. I didn't have the energy to unpack and didn't see a need for it, so I just dealt with all the boxes because the situation was supposedly temporary.

One of the most essential and important things I did for myself during this time period was to completely change my diet. I guess in one way it was forced upon me due to the eating problems, but that was in fact a good thing. True, I had gained enormous ground just from being able to eat some foods again. I began eating only organic products, organic meats, and eliminated most sugars, all soft drinks, caffeine, and all processed foods except for cheese, from my diet. So I was eating only organic, raw or minimally processed foods. That was the single most important factor in rebuilding as much of my immune system as possible that I have done. It did take work but I have maintained a careful, structured diet for 4 years now except for an occasional *Dove* chocolate, as we all have our human weaknesses.

I also don't smoke or drink or take any drugs except what is absolutely prescriptively necessary, and I even balk at antibiotics. I prefer herbs, essential oils and "natural" healing alternatives. I have done acupuncture, accupressure, deep tissue massage, Reiki, and many other wonderful, and some not so wonderful, adjunctive therapies. With the exception of necessary surgeries, allopathic medicine had helped, but pretty much failed miserably to heal this illness at this point. I also tried naturopathy, NMT, and NAET. I tried the power of prayer. I had perhaps fifty or more different combinations of oral antibiotics over the past decades, and none alleviated my symptoms 100% at any one time, and nearly all caused herxing on some level.

I tried herbal remedies and essential oils. If shaving my head and getting it tattooed would have helped, I would certainly have done that as well. All of these things helped the symptoms in their own way, but did not completely address the underlying problems, which were multiple infectious diseases. Like many chronic Lyme patients, I had not yet found the right treatment therapies or doses, or even an accurate diagnosis, for that matter.

During one NAET treatment, my nurse practitioner was talking to a colleague who had entered the treatment room. I heard them mention a seminar they had attended where a physician was speaking out about Lyme disease. "Hey, wait – can I interrupt you" I asked. I requested the name of the doctor who had spoken, because I knew in the back of my mind that despite all the time that had gone by, that I probably still had Lyme disease, though nobody would acknowledge it. The nurse happily gave the phone number to me, and I called and made an appointment to see the physician for as soon as was available.

When the day of the appointment came, I waited in nervous anticipation. I had brought with me a stack of my medical records that rivaled most dictionaries. I was sincerely hoping the copious paperwork would not alienate the doctor. Fortunately he has been down this road with many of his patients. He patiently spent over 2 hours with me at the first consult and listened to my oral history, examined me, and then reviewed my medical records. His answer was "I am going to do some blood work, but based on your symptoms, medical history and history of rashes, I can safely predict that you probably have Lyme disease," he said. "I knew it!" I exclaimed, excited at the fact that what he said finally gave credence to my symptoms. I was not looking for the diagnosis *I wanted,* but I wanted a diagnosis that *fit my symptoms* and to date, not one of them had. I did not care what the disease was called, I only wanted to find the cause so it could be treated.

> *Just for clarity's sake, I am not married to my diagnoses. I don't give a rat's patootie what you call the infectious diseases raging in my body – but when you can see photos of the actual organisms, years after "treatment," it is impossible to argue against the fact that they are still in my body, no matter what some research does or does not say about persistence! And the body of scientific evidence proves persistence, by the way, and researchers know it, including all the hard-headed soap-box lunkheads who insist that Lyme patients invent their illness or somehow wish to be ill with a disease that "doesn't exist." Some of the research on the inability to detect antibodies, the lack of accuracy in diagnostic tests, and the truth about the persistence of Bb within the body was in fact, written by some of the currently harshest anti-chronic Lyme critics out there!*[187-203]

When I drove home after the consult, I cried from mixed emotions. I felt great relief that after all this time I *finally knew* what was wrong with me, and that it was called Lyme disease. But at the same time, I cried tears of sadness because it had *taken so long* to find out that I had Lyme disease, when I had been asking about Lyme from the very beginning. All this time had gone by and I had suffered so greatly that it was infuriating to me to know it had all been unnecessary and I could have had treatment and perhaps made to be well years earlier if only someone had listened to me.

When I was finally diagnosed in December of 2004 by this doctor, who supplemented the diagnosis with IGeneX labs (IgM and IgG Western Blot tests, Palo Alto, California), I was in very bad shape physically and rapidly declining (cognitively too). I was very hostile in attitude, toward everyone, because of brain inflammation. I had a positive IgM but a negative IgG Western Blot. The doctor explained to me that I had chronic, active Lyme disease based on my obvious symptoms, my medical history, medical records, and serology.

I also had positive tests from several other national laboratories indicating that I had Lyme, Bartonella, Babesia, Anaplasma, Mycoplasma, and EBV. I have had years of intermittent antibiotics, (yes even doxycycline), and several IV medications and combination therapies designed to knock out these illnesses. I have tried a number of "alternative" therapies as well, but the symptoms never fully disappeared before.

This doctor wanted to insert a PICC (peripherally inserted central catheter) line right away and I was agreeable to do this, but he admitted to me at the time, that Lyme disease was still new to his practice, and he wasn't really certain he could cure me. I took this as a sign to go looking for another doctor, perhaps one more experienced in treating the disease.

I tried about 10 more doctors in Port Washington, Brookfield, Waukesha, Neenah, in several areas of Milwaukee, Lake Geneva, Kenosha, LaCrosse, and Madison. Nobody seemed to want to acknowledge my Lyme disease. At the UW-campus, a Neurologist told me I had "MS" and not Lyme disease, despite the fact that I had a diagnosis of Lyme and she performed no testing. "You don't have Lyme" is what she flat out told me, and handed me a prescription for anti-depressants which I tore up. Another physician told me that he "didn't believe in neuro-Lyme." He was a Neurologist. A different physician told me behind his closed office doors that he is "not allowed" to diagnose Lyme disease and in order to treat me, he would have to "call it MS or something else." **He actually explained to me that he might lose his license if he diagnosed me with Lyme!**

After trying to get a second appointment following the initial consult, we decided that he was perhaps not a good choice. We did not understand the politics of the disease at that time, which forces doctors to treat patients "on the sly" thanks to the policies set by the insurance companies, overzealous medical boards, and restrictive treatment guidelines. At the time, my husband and I thought his comments oddly suspicious. We were very wrong. We were not yet aware of the political firestorm of controversy that the illness is mired within. This doctor was in fact, being truthful to us, and though he wanted to call my illness Lyme disease, he felt unable to do so due to some perceived threat...was it insurance...big pharma...government...what, whom or why?

I surfed the "net" and found a physician who was supposed to be an expert, highly-recommended Lyme-literate physician who was located out of state, and I got an appointment with him. It would be a 15-hour drive, one way. The plan was to travel down there as far as possible the first day, then stay overnight at a hotel when tired, or if we could do the entire drive, at the hotel across the road from the clinic and go to the appointment the next morning.

As I dealt with my symptoms, we packed the car, including the necessary foods for 3 or 4 days, and headed down south. The trip was long and hard on me physically. Fatigue set in around hour 6 and I desperately wanted to go home. I remember crying and feeling like the trip was a stupid idea. At that point I lost it and an intense mental struggle ensued. I cried and got very upset. My husband did nothing to help calm me down. I cried that I wanted to go home, so he abruptly turned the car around. When a moment of clarity returned, I asked him why we were headed back home, when we were supposed to be on our way to see the doctor. He would say "because you said to turn around." And I would argue from my foggy brain that we were going to the doctor no matter what. And so he would turn the car around once again.

This happened a couple more times, and each time I would get a little more panicked, and then a little more frustrated because "he" couldn't seem to make up his mind whether we were coming or going. In reality it was me who desperately needed the comfort and strength of some simple encouragement. Simply being supportive and saying, "it's all going to be okay," or "you can do this," would have made all the difference in the world, instead of being on auto-pilot or being detached. My anxiety and panic attacks were taking the lead over common sense when my husband should have looked at the situation rationally, instead of trying to appease me. Remember I was very fearful, very ill and not in my right mind. I was saying things like "I can't do this," and "I don't know why I am bothering to go through this, it's too far away." "This just doesn't make sense to have to go to an out-of-state doctor that is so far away." I was relying on my husband for moral support, but who at this point, had absolutely no idea how to be supportive.

Instead of comforting me and driving to the doctor no mater what, he kept turning the car around and back, trying to placate his by now nearly hysterical wife. If you have ever watched a movie where a woman gets slapped on the cheek and snaps out of it, that was precisely the state of mind that I was in at the time. I am not advocating slapping anyone, but my husband's repeated turning the car around only escalated the situation...because I could see he wasn't being supportive of me in the way that I needed, but I was unable to communicate effectively. Instead, he was just blindly following directions regardless of their illogic.

When we reached hour 14 of travel, I physically and emotionally could not take it any more and started crying uncontrollably. At that point we stopped at a bad motel and stayed over night. The heater smelled like burned rubber, and the bed was horribly uncomfortable. I had to listen to my husband snoring in the next bed while I lay fitfully tossing and turning all night long. I was unable to get even one hour's sleep and by morning I was a complete basketcase. I looked out the window and noticed that we were right across the highway from a hospital. I remember asking my husband if he thought we should just check me in there. He ignored my request, but probably should have done exactly that.

Instead, that morning I was too sleep-deprived to know what to do. I was physically and emotionally drained and though we were only 56 miles from the clinic, I asked my husband to cancel my appointment. Instead of understanding my exhaustion and encouraging me again, my husband simply did what I asked of him. He called the clinic and told them we were 56 miles away but couldn't "make" it – though we had already driven *14 hours*. Well, if he hadn't wasted an hour listening to his irrational wife and turning the car around several times, we might have made it to the hotel where we had originally intended to stay, down the street from the clinic. At that point we could have just gone across the street to the clinic and gotten me the badly-needed treatment. Instead here we were less than an hour away, and my husband simply would not "deal with" me and take me to the doctor. Instead, he called the clinic, cancelled the appointment, packed up our things, and we began the 14-hour drive back home. How much sense does that make? Absolutely none whatsoever to a rational person, and again, my brain at the time, was far from rational.

This makes no sense to me at all now, and I did fault my husband for not being emotionally strong enough to get me the last leg of the journey when I was a physical and emotional wreck. You would think that after all of that travel, that less than an hour away would have been easy to do. All it would have taken was some simple encouragement from him to *help me get to where I needed to be.* But like so many people who are the "support" people in Lyme patients' lives, my husband did not know what to do, and unfortunately for me, he was unable to help me when I needed him the most, in the manner in which I needed but could not communicate because I was ill.

His defense was that he "didn't know what to do." While I certainly sympathize with the idea that what I was telling him was probably confusing, I can't understand why he couldn't tell that I was as sick as I was, and that asking him to take me home was not making sense with the objective of the trip. I was very sick with Lyme (and other things), but he just couldn't figure out how to deal with it. As a result, he just did whatever I asked him to. As a result, I didn't get the help I so desperately needed. Thirty hours of driving and we were right back where we began. The trip had been absolutely pointless and a terrible disappointment. Imagine explaining "what happened" to family and friends...

A lack of support (whether valid or not), is unfortunately a common theme in many Lyme patients lives, (and in any chronic illness) and leads to a great number of divorces. Sometimes the people closest to us are ill-equipped to help, and they simply walk away or otherwise don't know how to "deal with" the patient. In the case of my husband, I give him a lot of credit, because he can admit that he simply did not want to "deal with" me or my illnesses. Of course that was not fair to me, but he didn't care at the time, he just didn't know what to do, and so he chose to do nothing. He already resented the garbage that my exhusband was putting us through, and when I got sick, he openly admitted that he resented me for that as well.

After the fiasco of the failed trip, I called a Lyme disease support group, but they refused to give me the name of anyone who might help me in my home state. Only after several phone calls did they determine that I was not "the opposition" (whoever that was, I thought at the time), and finally did I receive a phone number for a supposedly Lyme-literate physician in Milwaukee, only an hour away from our house!

I saw a doctor who was in his eighties, and he agreed that I had chronic, neurological Lyme disease. He ordered an MRI test which revealed that I had white matter "lesions" on my brain, which he explained were causing the MS-like symptoms, cognitive dysfunction and my erratic behavior. The treatment would be a gruelling 8 weeks of IV and oral combination therapies. He said it would be "rough" and that I must muddle through the "aches and pains," but that was the extent of the instruction he gave me.

The hospital's Interventional Radiologist inserted a picc line in my left arm and I began outpatient IV treatments a day later. At the time I was on IV Rocephn and oral Flagyl. Because I was so thin, the picc line was very uncomfortable at first. Over time it grew tolerable, and because it was 2 hours round-trip to the hospital every day, we turned to home infusions. Because my husband had to be at work, I was left to do the infusions by myself every day.

After two weeks I was becoming liver toxic and my skin began to grow yellow. I also began to pass out from too low of a heart rate during my infusions. I found out later that if I had been given IV fluids my blood pressure might not have dropped as this is a typical side-effect of the drug Rocephin. There were problems with the medication dose and we tried to get the doctor to adjust the dose lower, but he flatly refused. He insisted that my 3 grams per day were not too much for me, even though I only weighed just over 100 lbs and I had lost 12 pounds the first week of infusions from diarrhea. He argued that "all" his patients get the same dose and they all "do fine" on it.

In fact the doctor told me about one patient, a man, that he put on 6 grams of Rocephin per day, and *he* did well. Well I wasn't doing fine, and wasn't his other patients, but he didn't want to hear about it. I asked him if he could adjust my dose downward, because it seemed I would do fine on 1 or 2 grams, but by the time the third gram was in, all heck would break loose. He yelled "no" and actually hung up the phone on me. (Later I would find reassurance from other patients that I wasn't the only patient who had been treated this way by this physician.) I begged my husband to straighten out the mess, but he never quite found the "time" to call because he was working so many hours, and again, he just didn't want to "deal with" my illness.

This was frustrating for me, as I was dealing with my symptoms and was not equipped to handle anything more than what was already on my plate. Once again my husband left me to deal with the coordination of my own outpatient care, IV infusions, training, home nursing schedule, office visits, medications, side effects, medical equipment, drug shipments, equipment sterilization, infusions, side effects, meals, the housework, and health care. He absolutely took no time to learn how to infuse me or clean or change my dressings, nor learn about my disease or help me, not even with the insurance company when they refused to pay. I had to coordinate that with the insurance company and the insurance liaison at my husband's workplace. The only thing to my husband's credit that he did help with, was the physical driving me from home to the hospital every day the first week of treatment. But he would just sit in the outpatient treatment room, ignore me, and watch television. He simply would not interact with me, no matter how hard I tried to engage him in conversation. So I felt like I was this huge pain in the butt that he was being forced to deal with and he simply did not want to be there. Well neither did I, but I didn't exactly have a choice in the matter. I wasn't asking for sympathy or enslavement, but I wondered would it have been too much to ask for him to act even partly interested or get a little bit involved.

The lesson here is not to tear apart and expose my husband's shortcomings. I asked his permission to tell the story as I saw it, and he kindly gave it to me in the hopes it might help someone else understand this process. He admits that he wasn't there for me and that he should have been, but that he just couldn't "deal with it" at the time. I do give him credit for his honesty about that. But his treatment of me left me, (a very ill patient,) entirely alone to handle all aspects of my care, and I should not have had to. This was very difficult to bear as a patient and as a vulnerable human being, especially when I was physically and cognitively impaired. I thought that a decade of court hearings and losing my children was the worst thing that had ever happened to me, but the combination of that plus the being alone in my illness, was truly a test of inner fortitude. Fortunately I would somehow manage to get through everything, but I assure you that it was not easy by any means, especially without a support system in place.

We had moved to a different town by now thanks to a lucky break with a ramshackle two-flat and a special banking program which got us financing. We finally were able to buy a home for ourselves and move in. The village was nice, but I did not know anyone. The neighbors I met said "hello" and things like "I'll pray for you," but no one offered to help me out, even when asked. They knew I was sick, because I had mentioned it. I think people realize you are sick, but just like my husband, illness is depressing to be around, and most people just don't want to "deal" with it. So where does that leave a Lyme patient on IV therapy? Frightened and alone, and that is never a fun place to be.

To make matters worse, my children were repulsed by the IV line and all the medications, and were openly rude to me about it. I tried to help them realize that it was just medical equipment and a process. But they really thought I was going to die and it scared the heck out of them. As a result, they were not very nice to me and stayed away from me as much as possible during their visitation. They even made jokes about my not being well, and criticized me for being sick "all the time." This open rejection was not admonished by their stepfather, because he was so tuned-out throughout this process that he didn't pay attention to what the children said. The combination of their rejection and my spouse undermining my parental role was difficult, coming on the heels of my children helping their father win custody by telling lies about abuse that never happened. It was a very emotionally trying time for me as a mother, wife, and ill Lyme patient. I suffered cruel rejection by my children, my neighbors, my friends, my doctors, the courts, and even my own spouse – and there was nothing I could do about it. I was a sitting duck, and a lame one at best. Still, we must forgive others of their shortcomings, and forgive ourselves for being unable to parent, be a spouse, a sibling, or to function as a human being during severe illness.

Unbeknownst to me at the time, my insurance company and private disability company were harrassing my doctor's office for treating me with IV therapy. They were demanding copious records, and he found this very annoying and finally said so to my husband. And when I began to have problems, it was almost as if we had no right to complain about anything, because he was already annoyed by my case, even though the irritants were all external and beyond my control.

When I began the out-patient treatments he had told us to alert him to anything "odd" including if I began passing out. In the hospital I was having allergic reactions to the IV saline flush. We tried to tell him that I needed dextrose instead, due to a preservative in the flush that I reacted to. This we had learned from the experience of my recent surgeries. He didn't listen and it caused some arguments between the doctor and myself. Finally after the third time this happened and a nurse witnessed it, he relented and agreed to prescribe dextrose flushes and the problem went away. I think he was angry that I was right and he was wrong, because he became rude to me after that. He did once say, "I'm the doctor, are you going to try to tell me how to practice medicine?"

When I was through on an out-patient basis and able to do the infusions at home, his nurse said to call the office if we have any problems. Well, we did call when I did have problems – the passing out during the home infusions, but he didn't listen nor seem to care. Instead he suddenly dropped me as a patient, citing his "busy practice" and not "having time" for my "silliness." It was not as if I was calling his office regularly, I called when there was a problem, like I had been instructed. He actually left me in the middle of treatment with a picc line that was beginning to become infected.

Once again my husband did not know what to do. The once-a-week visiting nurse said she didn't have the authority to pull the line. The pharmaceutical company endlessly shipped me the medications and could do nothing. We went back to that jerk of a doctor and I asked that he continue treatment, but he refused. He told me "I'll call you in a week after I take a break and we'll talk about restarting your treatment in the hospital." He said he was going to do in-patient care because of my blood pressure and liver problems but he never even bothered to *check* my liver enzymes or anything else. He told me to "wait" and he would call me with the day I should come into the hospital.

But a week went by and then two weeks, and I was sitting there with interrupted treatment and was flushing my line every day with dextrose and heparin by myself, to keep it clot-free. In addition, I had a small, but growing infection on my skin at the entrance of the line that I was worried about. I finally called the Radiologist who had inserted the picc and asked him if he would be willing to take it out, because the doctor had apparently dropped me as a patient (and didn't even bother telling me!) He said he couldn't do that unless the doctor requested it first. The doctor's office wouldn't take my calls. That was the end of June, 2005.

We had to drive to another hospital and ask them to take it out. They contacted the doctor's office but got no answer. Then they got ahold of the same interventional radiologist when I gave them his number, and he finally gave the okay to take out the line, so they did. Why he didn't do that before, I don't know! This left me without any more IV treatments. In all I had about 2-1/2 weeks worth, or maybe it was 3 weeks, I don't know; in pulsed Rocephin at 3 grams a day (because I took it 5 days on, 2 days off) and oral Flagyl at half a gram a day.

In a few weeks my skin looked better but I still could not walk across my living room floor. I was always very short of breath from the slightest exertion, and I would have to lie down. I felt I was useless as a mother, as a wife, and at times, as a human being. Surely I would need more treatments I thought, and once again I silently wondered if I was going to live through this illness.

I literally lived on the couch or in bed all the time. If the doorbell or the phone rang, I didn't bother to get up, because I couldn't. Visits with my children were of them playing by themselves while I rested as much as possible. It was the summer of 2005 and we hung up a hammock on the front porch so that I could at least lay outside for part of the day. We did not know our neighbors very well, and I had already heard comments from them about how easy my life must be, and how they would trade their life for mine, because all they saw was me in the hammock, day after day. Little did they know **I would have gladly given up everything I owned, to have a life without Lyme disease.**

By October of 2005, I was able to walk around the perimeter of my yard, and throughout my house, though I was still remarkably fatigued. I had been reading about Lyme disease since I was diagnosed, and learned that exercise was an important tool to recover strength and stamina in chronic Lyme patients. I also learned that the quality of life for Lyme patients was worse than that of congestive heart failure patients – and I can tell you *that* is an understatement!

By this time, many of my cognitive issues were slowly resolving, and many of my physical symptoms lingered but were significantly reduced. At least the horrible pain had lessened to every other day or sometimes every few days, making life more tolerable for the first time in years. For the first time in a long while, I began to feel like I was on the beginning of the road to recovery.

Since I loved horses ever since I was a small child, and we had moved to a house in a part of Wisconsin where there were many farms including horse farms, I thought I would see if I could find an equine therapy clinic somewhere where I could horseback ride to regain my strength. As luck would have it, there was one about 20 miles from our house, but I wasn't able to drive and with my husband working, it would be nearly impossible for me to get there each day. So I decided to see how much it would cost to *buy* a horse, and perhaps board it nearby. Maybe I would even be lucky enough to find a place that would give me lessons again (I had them when I was younger), and teach me everything I needed to know about horse ownership.

Well, I bought a horse, and I found a barn only 3 minutes from our house. Yes they gave lessons, and yes I learned much of what was needed to know about horse ownership. At the time I brought the horse there, I was unable to walk it across the indoor arena, because I didn't have the strength or stamina to do so. The challenge of learning to ride again and caring for a horse, seemed daunting and foolish. But in life, challenges never stopped me before. Nevertheless over the next year and a half, every day I could get there, I worked very hard and pushed my abilities a little bit further.

I still had problems with balance, so that made riding a bit dicey. But my trainer worked with me on my disabilities and helped me to learn how to ride safely. It took work to grip the reins or lift myself into the saddle. Even saddling up my horse was exhausting the first few months. My love for my horse and the bond that was built during those days became very strong. I think my horse instinctively knew when I wasn't feeling well, because she would never "try anything" on the days I wasn't feeling myself. Eventually we were able to get some additional ponies and then horses, and my strength and abilities improved greatly as I retrained my body to function more normally.

I gained improved muscle tone, range of motion, flexibility and weight management. I also increased my ability to balance, my stamina, energy, and my hypersensitivity to motion, noise and even horse hair improved. When it came time to worm the animals, in the beginning I couldn't even hold the box that the *Ivermectin* wormer was in,

I was that reactive to chemicals. If they were anywhere near my personal energy "field," my body would react, I had no control over it. Over time when my body chemistry and immune function improved, worming no longer became a problem, as I was no longer chemically hypersensitive to Ivermectin or many other things.

Although things seemed to be improving somewhat physically for me, I was still ill and not doing very well. I had applied for social security disability in 2003 when I was first originally disabled, but at the time, I did not have a working diagnosis, so the disability people told me they wouldn't even accept my application.

I also had medical short-term disability through my employer at the time I had quit my last job, but they harrassed me *every single day with phone calls* and questions like, "When are you going back to the doctor? What did the doctor say yesterday when you saw him? What is he doing for treatment?" etc. I understand now that the disability companies assign a pain-in-the-butt case manager to telephone and harrass you into dropping your case and your insurance. They do this by design because it's expensive for them to pay you benefits each day you are disabled. By harrassing their insureds most people will eventually drop out and therefore, no more benefits will have to be paid. To me, the harrassment wasn't worth the lousy $7.00 a day benefit which took me over 3 months and many letters of appeal to get in the first place. They won, I lost; and I was too ill to fight.

Federal social security disability was a bit different. They requested my medical records from the previous 4 years so they could examine them. Fortunately for me, every medical procedure and symptom that I had experienced (due to Lyme disease) was carefully displayed in those records. But not one single diagnosis of Lyme disease until December of 2004 appeared. The claim officer and I had a discussion on the phone where I told him that I now had a medical diagnosis of chronic Lyme disease. My records showed all kinds of other diagnoses, like the heart arrythmia, the Chronic Fatigue, the Fibromyalgia, the Endometriosis, the Gallbladder "disease," the co-infections, etc. He said to me, "It doesn't matter that you have a diagnosis of Lyme disease, I am trying to find out what is making you disabled." I replied, "Yes it *does* matter that I have a diagnosis of Lyme disease, because *that is what's making me disabled!"*

In the end, I did receive full disability the first time around which is rare for Lyme patients. Unfortunately, they selected an arbitrary date of something like February of 2005 as the disability "onset" date. This was ridiculous, although the illness began in 1992, I was able to work until April of 2003, when I had to quit. Yet they chose February of 2005, and I have no idea why. They shorted me months of disability benefits, saving themselves money. My attorney told me not to bother fighting the onset date, but it would actually affect some of the family court rulings in the future, because the court thought I was only disabled as of the social security *onset date*, and not according to my medical history, or the testimony of my expert witness physicians or the date I had to stop working.

Nevertheless, by July of 2006, I received a lump sum for the previous months, and so did my exhusband for the children's benefits. Naturally he ran down to the nearest social security office and claimed himself as payee immediately upon the discovery that I had filed for it. He had been told that I was going to be payee and that I had a phone conference scheduled a week away. Still he ignored this and physically went to the social security office and filed so he would be signed up to be payee instead of me. Incredibly, the social security people told me, "too bad, he beat you to it." (As if it was some kind of a joke.) Well whatever, he now receives about $900 a month from disability for my two children, and neither of them see a penny of that money – it goes into their father's personal bank account, as expected. Of course he makes up all kinds of "expenses" he supposedly pays on their behalf, like a big-screen television set and video games; while the children go without shoes, clothing or even a warm winter jacket or medical care. But that is our social service system for you. There is no justice anywhere.

Now you have a clearer picture of what happened to me during parts of my Lyme journey. I haven't focused on the treatment plans as much as what it was like dealing with the other issues that were concurrently evolving. Now let's talk a bit about what my children went through and where that leaves us today, if you don't mind.

Beginning in the summer of 2003 following the reversal of custody which my daughter did not want to do, I watched as my previously loving and happy child began to write depressed and guilt-laden poetry which I discovered one afternoon on the floor of her bedroom as she and her brother and their step-father were out riding bicycles. Her first poem was a fantasy poem about a character who was devastated because he had lied and caused a situation in his life to become something other than what was promised him. The echoes of her personal life in that poem were easy to see.

I also came across some very sad but beautiful (she is very talented) drawings of herself, sobbing near a pool of water. And there were pictures of herself and her brother comforting her, with her brother wearing monster feet...as if to say that she considered him a monster (sibling rivalry) but that he was clearly trying to comfort her. I tried to talk to my daugher about her artwork when she returned from her bike ride, but she was angry and saw it as a form of "spying" on her. This made her feel that I could not be trusted. And yet I had only expressed my concern because I knew how angry she was about being forced to live with her father, away from her friends, and that she felt guilty for being manipulated by her father. Over time she grew distant, depressed, and no longer cared about her personal hygiene. She withdrew from the family and only wanted to spend time in her room, drawing or listening to music. This was somewhat typical teenage behavior, but there also seemed to be a pervasive cloud of darkness following my daughter around wherever she went.

On top of that, both children were now becoming openly aggressive toward one another. They also were beginning to use profanity, and when cautioned about that, I was informed, "Dad let's us swear at his house." Fighting a losing battle, the children were being taught disrespect by their father towards me. They openly told me "Dad says we don't have to listen to you," when they were visiting me. Anything I did to correct their wrong behaviors was perceived by both of them as "abuse" and they made no bones about reporting everything said and done "to" them, each weekend to their father – who took everything to court. It got so bad that I was verbally abused by my children on a regular basis, and my husband, the children's stepfather, would not know how to handle it so he just sat there and ignored it. In time they became abusive toward him as well. For a brief period when my son was younger, he was even known to kick my husband in the shins when angry with him.

The situation was very hostile for some time, and I began to feel as if maybe I didn't need to see my children any more, because they were no longer the same recognizable beings I had worked so hard to raise.

In a very short time they were dirty, rude, hostile, physically aggressive, inconsiderate, and would make fun of me and swear. It was as if my ex-husband was letting them run completely wild over at his house and undermining everything I attempted to teach them.

Many days one or the other of them refused to come to my house, and I know that was my ex's influence over them. A few times my son would arrive at our home, try to pick a fight by being verbally abusive, and when corrected, call his father on the phone to come and get him – which he of course, did. And when we would be back in court, detailed stories about the event would be woven by a man who was neither present when it happened, nor able to tell the truth. No matter what I did or didn't do, I was the "bad guy." Visitation was disappointing and it usually left me in tears, crying in my room alone. My husband was often nowhere to be found, when I needed comfort because again, he didn't want to "deal" with me. He often made excuses to be other places or work excessive hours. These weren't his children after all, and I am sure on some level, he didn't think it was his responsibility.

I realized that I had to work that much harder to reconnect with my children and set about ways to become closer to them, and I tried to find out what was going on in their lives, because they would not tell me. They often said "Dad says we're not allowed to tell you anything that is going on at his house." It was not like I was playing 20 questions, I would not see them for weeks, and I would be clueless about what was going on, and I would ask them questions like, "how was your week." Instead, I would be ignored or insulted, or both.

Still, I did what I could to reasonably parent them. I played with them and we took them places when I was feeling well enough to do so (and sometimes despite not feeling well at all). We tried to have some semblance of family over the short 2-day weekends. And I followed typical parenting styles when allowing my children internet access, like monitoring the children's computer use.

In the course of doing this, I discovered that my daughter was posting items on internet forums including suicidal and homicidal images and anti-social dialogues. She was very profane and clearly not the child I had once recognized. Since I no longer had custody and placement of my children due to my illness and ex-husband's deliberate escapades in family court, I was relegated to parenting my children's internet activities from afar, every other weekend. I purchased software which facilitated this process, which any smart parent will do who wishes to reasonably monitor where their children are going and what they are doing in this age of technology.

It's a good thing I did this because what I found was very disturbing. My child defended her postings as if they were some part of a comic book she was legitimately creating, but over time her true thoughts became clear when she admitted openly to her peers that she was depressed, "bipolar," or otherwise perhaps "mentally ill." This was no comic book or "research" for same as she stated. In her posts, she admitted that the line between reality and fantasy was blurring and that her real life was being portrayed in her expressive works. I tried to get counseling for my daughter through her father, but he ignored me and called me "mentally ill" to anyone he met, even people I did not know but who I would subsequently meet later on (and he even testified that he did this during one of our court trials as well).

In school, my child's creative writing teacher pulled her aside after seeing some of her homework assignments indicating what she also perceived to be suicidal and depressed themes. After asking my child about her concerns, my daughter joked about the teacher's questions on-line. Needless to say when I saw disturbing things on-line, and which were posted both from her father's house, and during school hours (and from school computers), I contacted the school but they pretended I did not exist, as my ex had already falsely told them I had "mental problems." My concerns were repeatedly ignored or invalidated by the school board and staff. By the way, the creative writing teacher never bothered to call me and tell me of her concerns for my daughter, even after I had specifically called and asked the school staff to be on the alert for signs of depression in my child. *Even after being asked specifically by me to report anything "off," the school refused to do so.* I had already tried to obtain outside counseling for her but was repeatedly blocked from that, by my ex.

I tried the social services route, but they routinely screened out my calls, refusing to take them seriously. I contacted my sister-in-law in California who is a social worker and who has experience sitting with suicidal patients in order to keep them from harming themselves or others. Her opinion of my daughter's situation was that I knew my daughter best, and only I could make the call as to whether she was crossing the "line" I thought she was. She did indicate to me however, that some of what my daughter was posting was not outside the realm of "normal," but she was working with children who were suicidal, and I wasn't going to take any chances based upon what I had been reading and seeing, which to me and others who saw it, did not appear "normal." I knew my daughter, and could plainly see that she was depressed. I felt she may also have Lyme disease, and I had been with her, her entire life; and remembered the tiny ticks I had removed from her legs. I knew her physical symptoms, and the psychiatric manifestations of untreated Lyme. The things she was doing, saying, and the ways she was behaving, fell in line with symptoms of neuropsychiatric Lyme disease and the depression which often accompanies it.

In time, my child, (when still a minor), began posting threats about killing people and/or herself, and she became obsessed with Japanese ritual suicide (Seppuku). She drew comic book scenes showing cartoon characters (named after herself and who looked just like her), committing the act. This she followed with many poems and works of art clearly illustrating obvious depression and disturbed thinking.

Attempts to talk to my child about her artwork were met with extreme hostility and denial. She had no insight into her own behavior, and I felt she was too far gone with neuropsychiatric symptoms to be able to comprehend much of what she was doing. She had lost all insight into her own behavior, and looked at me, and called me "crazy" – words which echoed her father's allegations.

I did not mention yet that I had both of my children tested for Lyme disease when I was first diagnosed. Their laboratory tests came back as follows. My daughter was fully CDC-positive for Lyme disease. My son was "equivocal," but he had positive Lyme-specific bands on his tests. My Lyme-literate doctor told me that both children, based upon their tests, their symptom history (which I had shared), and their physical symptoms, were probably also infected with Lyme disease and/or other co-infections. Their "regular" doctor also diagnosed both children with Lyme disease, and he wasn't even Lyme-literate. He determined this by the test results, their symptoms and clinical history. Since both kids had rashes similar to EM rashes, and I remembered pulling what I now know to be nymph ticks off of their legs, combined with their symptoms all these years, I have no doubt in my mind that they are both harboring Bb. And my daughter's behaviors are just one aspect of neuropsychiatric issues which Bb can cause to manifest.

Over time, my daughter convinced herself that I had never discussed the topic of her postings with her, despite her online posts revealing that we *had* indeed discussed the topic. In fact, she criticized me for doing so. Eventually when she posted artwork showing her cartoon character shooting up the school in the style of Columbine, (which also happened just days before the similar Red Lake, Minnesota tragedy), I felt that something needed to be done. Police were arresting children all over the country for just mentioning any threats of Columbine-type violence. I didn't want my daughter's artwork in a very public forum to be found and reported. This child obviously was crying out for help, and she needed both counseling, and probably medical attention.

She followed that artwork with several postings openly asking "who wants to shoot up their school," and made threats from wanting to go out in a "blaze of glory" after making a "cool speech," to wearing the offensive artwork on T-shirts on the last day of school with one of her friends. In everything that she was doing, regardless of her motivations, it was clear to me that my child needed professional help. This was not mere freedom of expression or "research," in my opinion, it was depression and obviously ill thinking, brought on by chronic, untreated neuropsychiatric Lyme disease and/or co-infections.

After a frantic letter to my ex went ignored but was openly mocked both to my children, and in court, my second husband and I went to our local police to ask for guidance on how to deal with my daughter's growing problem. We showed them the posts and artwork she had created. The police agreed that my child needed psychological help and intervention of some kind. Because they weren't in the same district as where my child lived, we were directed to 2 other police departments before connecting with my child's high school police liaison officer.

After describing the artwork and posts to him and offering him internet web links to her posts for review, he informed me that my child would be taken out of class and brought to the guidance office and questioned about her situation. I stressed the importance of protecting her rights, and that I felt she was depressed and needed counseling. Instead, without my permission or knowledge, they searched her locker and confiscated her personal property that to this day, they have not returned. They found some things in her locker that, combined with her school work, her internet activities, my concerns and her creative writing teacher's admitted concerns, they determined that she was legitimately worrisome.

The school decided to remove her on an emergency detention, and she was remanded to a psychiatric ward for 72 hours, without my knowledge or involvement in the process. There she was evaluated and convinced everyone there was nothing wrong with her outside of being "sad." The Psychologist wrote in the notes that she was clinically depressed and may be a candidate for an SSRI (an ani-depressant). Of course right away her father grandstanded and tried to blame me for the entire episode – despite my having no knowledge of it beforehand. As a matter of fact, a social worker initially telephoned me to inform me that my daughter was taken from school on an "ED" (emergency detention). I had no idea what that meant and asked her to explain it to me so I could understand what was happening. It was only then that I learned the full extent of what the school had decided to do with my child – without my input or permission, and it absolutely horrified me.

Once my child was admitted, my ex made accusations to the psychiatric hospital staff that I was "mentally ill," and was "just doing this to teach [our daughter] a lesson," all claims which were ridiculous and unfounded. He refused to cooperate at first, and tried to pin everything on me. He even alleged that I was trying to "bankrupt him" and was "doing this" (meaning throwing my daughter in a psych ward) to harm him! (Can you see sociopathic and narcissistic traits here...) As you can imagine, this defamatory information wasn't shared with me. I *wondered* why I was so patronized during the parent/child meeting.

It was only after I obtained my child's medical records that I saw these allegations in print. Only then did I discover the full extent that my ex-husband had assassinated my character and reputation, and for what purpose. He had worked overtime with the school administration, our daughter's Psychologist, therapists, and others, in conjunction with involving his post-divorce attorney in the process (not only inappropriate, but a conflict of interest on his part). Further, my ex filed a legal action against the school because they were considering expelling my child (again without my knowledge) *with his divorce attorney representing him in that matter as well*. They later settled out of court without even involving me, the other parent, in any of this process. His divorce attorney sat in privileged meetings with the school board that I as a parent, (and someone with joint custody), was not even invited to attend – because the board wrongly assumed that I had mental problems thanks to what my ex and his attorney had told them! I had to fight with the school for my right to be involved in the process at all points, and they only did under protest to shut me up. After that, they refused to answer my letters, email or even take my phone calls despite my legal joint custody! So even the school administration discriminated against me due to the false accusations of supposed "mental illness" made by my exhusband and his attorney against me. Of course the administrators never once bothered to inform me about his accusations – presumably because they simply assumed they were true.

My child went through a lot, but only indirectly because of my revealing her artwork and posts to the school officer. I had no control over what she posted, either from school or her father's home. True, my notifying the authorities brought it openly into the spotlight, but prior to that, no one would listen to me. I have explained that I had no idea what an "ED" was. I never dreamed she would be, or could be removed from school and sent to a psychiatric ward. I was very naïve I guess. And the school's police liaison officer had told me something *entirely different* would happen to her than what actually occurred. The long and short of the situation was that I was the only person parenting my child, and my daughter's direct actions, combined with items found in her locker and her homework assignments, were what led to her ED, not my attempts to help and parent my ill, depressed, irrational child.

We won't even go into how the appeal of our first trial failed or the second trial where I attempted to reverse custody back to the way it originally was, in part because of my daughter's escapades and my son's failing in school and failure to thrive. The court, though shown the evidence of what my daughter had done, and the lab tests which clearly showed she was positive for Lyme disease, dismissed my concerns and granted my exhusband sole custody, while claiming that I was "Lyme-obsessed" and that I had "issues," through more of the same ignorance and discrimination it had shown since the beginning of the process. The judge ignored the children's positive Lyme results.

For a time, my daughter refused to come to terms with her behavior, but made excuses and attempted to minimize and dismiss her actions, (supported by my ex of course). She openly blamed me for "my" behavior that "ruined" her life, and said she never wanted to see me again. Her silence lasted 8 months. A perceptible level of depression has remained in her however, and when I found admissions later that she had indeed felt like shooting up the school and/or harming herself, I felt a sad vindication, but knew I had done my job as a parent to the best of my ability in the circumstances in which we found ourselves at the time. She is slowly coming around and acknowledging the past.

Having to make such difficult choices is not easy for a healthy parent in the best of circumstances, and yet I did the best I could and somehow managed to protect my child from harming herself (at least for the time being), by exposing her behavior to scrutiny. That came at the very high price of losing permanent custody and placement of both of my children, which was terribly unfair to everyone, especially the kids. As you can guess, my ex-husband is in complete denial about our daughter's actions, and enables her to continue her negative behaviors. And to this day, she continues her activites, posting artwork and writing essays from a very negative, hostile place, and I worry that her attitude toward her future has not deviated much since 2005.

While my child didn't appreciate my actions at the time, I hope that some day she will both recognize and value my efforts which came out of my extreme love for her. I don't know if the decision to report her was right or wrong, I only know I always had the best intentions and tried to protect her from herself and other people when no one was listening to her cries for help. But with Lyme affecting me cognitively, how does a parent see or make the "right" choices? When panic, fear, depression and ignorance cloud the waters of choice, and when an ex and the court systems are working against a parent who has an illness they refuse to acknowledge, what is an ill person to do? The answer is the very best we possibly can under the circumstances, and to accept the best we can do. In the end, absolutely none of these people would, or will to this day, acknowledge that my children might be sick with Lyme, and so this story is not ended yet.

My daughter suffers from sleep disturbances, dark circles under her eyes, droopy eyelids, mood issues, menstrual pain, extreme hostility, excessive profanity, weight gain and sugar cravings. At times, my daughter has exhibited bouts of both mania and depression, and described herself as "borderline manic-depressive" or "bipolar." She is niether. She was diagnosed "depressed" in the psych unit and she has pervasive ongoing anger, depression, and odd behaviors like an obsession with anarchy and all things negative.

Now my child is no longer a minor and attends a state University. Additionally, she is in complete denial that she might be Lyme infected. She has lost all insight into her own behavior, choosing to blame me for many of her problems. Her father worked very hard to alienate my ill child from me by blaming me for causing her troubles, and convinced her that I have "mental illness" which does not exist, and for which he has no evidence, except for his history of false accusations.

Yes I had some issues cognitively and emotionally when I was at my worst before treatment for Lyme. But that is not the same thing as "mental illness" in a standard sense. At no time did I ever act out toward any person, not even my children. Transient symptoms that affect mental processes and mood should not automatically label a person "mentally ill" and suddenly incapable of parenting. After all, I had raised those children their entire lives while dealing with Lyme and other co-infections. And believe it or not, my ex even stated at the start of our divorce in 1997 that he had "no issues" with my ability to parent our children. Suddenly 3 years later when I remarried, he felt completely different? Mental illness by the way, is merely illness of brain chemistry or structure, in my opinion. Illness is illness, there should be no stigma attached to any diagnosis. **And unless and until someone is convicted of a crime against others, parental custody and visitation should never be revoked on the basis of allegations alone.**

My ex has also managed to convince our daughter that all of her actions are "normal." She has convinced him and herself that she is merely performing "research." She says she wants to become a teacher to teach kids that "violence is bad." And that supposedly motivates her to continue to post online objectionable material that is profane, anti-social, at times anti-Christian, threatening, abusive and/or amoral. When asked why she continues to post negative things on-line, my child says "because it makes [her] happy." I certainly have to question that rationale.

"Research" is not what comes to mind while I see graphic artwork depicting a saddened, twisted soul, people committing suicide, or when I read posts wherein she described her "mental problems," depression and concerns about graphic dreams where she kills people and "feels" their deaths. I don't call it normal for my child to have researched the history of anarchy or drawing the circle-A symbol for anarchy in some of her artwork. I shuddered the first time I saw multiple photographs of my daughter posing with weapons, whether they were firearms or air-soft guns, it doesn't matter. I call this behavior anti-social and subversive (if she means anything by it), or at least disturbed and/or impaired if she just thinks it's "cool." Again, in my opinion she is a clear example of a child whose thinking is largely affected by both her situation and untreated neuropsychiatric Lyme disease.

My child continues to call herself "bipolar" and admits to symptoms that all fall under the category of "Lyme." She admits to depression, and is obsessed with death in all forms. She continues to post depressed and/or negative entries on-line. She appears to have learned little from her experiences except there are no consequences for her actions. She has also gained no medical or psychological assistance either, because no one seems to care about her or what she's doing, but me.

To hammer home a point that her behaviors are what most parents would question, a child who attempted to contact the deceased spirits of the Columbine killers via on-line séances and Ouija boards; and who wrote a sonnet to the Columbine killers, is *not* research, and I also personally feel, spiritually dangerous. I think a child who found it amusing to fabricate prayers and Christmas carols in the theme of Columbine, most disturbing. Inventing "Columbine the breakfast cereal," action figures, or ideas of Columbine field trips to "look for ghosts" is obsessive, and unhealthy, and not how I raised my child in a Christian home. My daughter exhibited interest in some of the darker "arts" and studied topics I shall not go into here, but are akin to what some might label as "hate" group curriculum. If she was doing this alone, I might believe her "research" theory. But combined with her words, deeds and other actions, and we see something else entirely.

I also think that a college-age child who lied about her activities and dressed as the Columbine killers for Halloween at school, complete with fake mortal head wound 2 years in a row, is abnormal behavior, gruesome idolatry; and should not be tolerated on any campus. I think drawing cartoons of people committing suicide and repeated images with demonic imagery abnormal. I believe that ongoing posts of thoroughly dark and depressing poetry and prose is an indication that there is something psychologically wrong with her. And I feel quite confident in stating that a detailed cartoon depiction of herself with a hypodermic needle stuck into the top of her head showing an exposed cranium with sarcastic remarks, indicative of depression and an angry disregard for authority. (This mocking artwork followed her incarceration at the psychiatric hospital).

My "normal" adult child should not be obsessed with all things dark, Columbine, death, violent, anti-social, or think it's "cool" to burn things or swear profanely at the drop of a hat. That is not comic-book creativity nor "research" into school shootings to teach kids how not to do those things. This is acting out and most assuredly abnormal behavior. Again, what I believe is happening with my daughter, are the neuropsychiatric manifestations of the spirochetes that infect her brain, which *absolutely and profoundly* affect her mood, functional logic, and her behavior. Although there is not a large body of scientific research to "prove" the existence of Lyme-induced psychiatric behavior, I assure you that to my daughter, and many people suffering from Lyme and other tick-borne illnesses, neuropsychiatric issues *are indeed real and pervasive.* Often patients are clueless about their own behaviors.

My daughter is clearly unconcerned that her behavior is shocking, negative, or even abusive. Her lack of empathy or concern for how she treats her own mother or how she is perceived by others might be astounding to me if I didn't understand the role that her "alleged" disease plays in her behavior. Her clueless father and the court system enables this behavior and undermines my parenting ability by entirely negating my role as her parent. In fact, she chooses not to associate with me in part because I don't enable her behaviors, and because I believe she needs to be tested further and treated for tick-borne illnesses. My crime has been in loving her and wanting her to be healthy. For that she feels justified punishing me by ignoring or mocking me.

To wit, I have been publicly humiliated and criticized cruelly on internet sites and in court for being a good parent to my child. Her "friends" have described in great detail how I am to be captured, tortured and killed to which she responds with laughter. She mocks my desire to love and support her, and yet she does not realize the extent of her illness and simply *cannot*, by virtue of it affecting her perceptions. I have been called "obsessed" with Lyme disease. Well, so be it, I am happy to be obsessed with trying to help my child become a healthy, better person when I know that she is ill – that is indeed my role as her parent. Some day whether she likes it or not, my child will have to deal with all of this, and I will be thre to help her, if she will allow me to.

Still I continue to try to reach her because I love her and if I am unsuccessful, I truly fear for her future. She may be able to conceal her dark thoughts from other people at will, but her posts and activities would indicate otherwise. All it would take is one difficult life issue for her to face unsuccessfully, and her entire house of cards could come crashing mightily down. We only need to review the numbers of Lyme-related suicides to find that it is one of the leading causes of death among Lyme patients. Ryan's story and others in this book series are tragic examples of this process. I am not saying she is suicidal, but I am saying the potential to become so, lurks in the shadows.

And for a certain Guardian Ad Litem who pretends that one or two or ten internet posts are my child's attempt to "bait" me, I personally invite him to review the over **2,000 posts** that I had collected from numerous internet sites during my child's darkest 2-1/2 year time period. Baiting does not occur in this huge quantity, across multiple web sites. You sir, in my opinion, are very naïve indeed, and have much to learn about children for whom their "best interests," you are supposed to determine. *You are simply <u>not</u> listening while you pretend to care.*

Of course there is the larger question of how my child's behaviors and this situation with my ex-husband denigrating me affects my son, who is nearly aged out of the system as well. We attempted to unravel and expose this situation through our third trial in 10 years in the family court that doesn't have a clue as to how Lyme affects the family dynamics. But that effort was ineffective in part, because the court refuses to believe anything other than the original false allegations of "mental illness." Instead it continues to deny that Lyme exists in this family, despite expert witness testimony from medical doctors stating for the record that it does. The court rather chooses to continue the status quo, even if it was ill-gotten at the onset, and calls me "crazy." Rather than admit to a mistake, it would rather see my life and the lives of my children destroyed, while my ex-husband laughs at us and the system which gave him the children on the basis of his lies and little else.

The court also conveniently overlooks my ex-husband's repeated perjorous statements during trials, and clear behavioral issues, even those the court admonished him for. It simultaneously acknowledges my very real concerns about my children, especially my daughter, but then quickly dismisses those concerns in the same breath and threatens me with monetary sanctions for "wasting" the court's time and forcing a new trial. How can a judge say that what my daughter did was "appropriately concerning" and "a parent's right to turn her in" one day, while at the same time further denying me custody and visitation, and calling me "obsessed" with Lyme disease on another day, when I never even brought up my illness in court – opposing counsel repeatedly did that for me.

If the opposing counsel wasn't (I have to say allegedly) in the pocket of the judge who presided over the bulk of our hearings, my family might have made some real progress. If the original judge had not been a week before retirement and had actually *known and practiced the laws*, we never would have been in this mess in the first place.

My recent attorney should have bothered to present crucial evidence before the court that he had been asked repeatedly to do, and should not have fabricated claims of a witness which did not exist; much to my consternation. He should not have refused to do his job, like failing to examine my ex on the witness stand. My legal counsel should not have spent recesses in the parking lot doing who knows what instead of consulting with me on breaks, (we found out about his drug issues and fired him). If anything in our case had gone correctly, opposing counsel wouldn't have mopped up the floor with my attorney (and me) and won the trial without any exhibits or witnesses whatsoever; just his conjecture, false allegations, and a judge making an obviously prejudiced decision.

The entire family court process in Walworth county Wisconsin is a tragic joke in my opinion, and our case is probably one of the best, clear-cut examples of a family court system gone wrong in the United States. The entire case reeks of legal malpractice but so far no attorneys in Wisconsin will address this ugly and complex of a case, so no one is held accountable for the way they destroyed this family. I am not kidding – you can see that when the book about our case comes out, including all of the court transcripts and documents to support these allegations.

My son currently suffers from varying physical symptoms and a bit of depression. One can argue that he is depressed due to the situation, and that is partly true, but he is also dealing with very real symptoms which can be manifested by Lyme disease. He understands that he is not feeling well when he is battling severe headaches, knee, wrist and other joint pains, daytime sleepiness, problems falling asleep, weird "allergic reactions," and concentration and anger issues. He also erupts into tiny hive-like bubbles on contact with certain things. He has difficulty breathing sometimes and is extremely sensitive to molds, pet dander and dust. He also freuently suffers from postural hypotension, a common problem in Lyme patients when their vagus nerve is affected.

In the past I have witnessed my son banging his head on the wall, having sudden fits of rage even when unprovoked, and an inability to concentrate as well as extreme impatience, and rigidity and lack of insight into his behaviors. He is afraid to say the words "Lyme disease" because his father has hammered him so much with those words. And yet this child now openly admits what really "went down" during the years preceeding the reversal of placement. He also admits he had been afraid to say anything against his father, even when it was the truth, because he doesn't want to deal with his dad's anger, which I understand. It is sad, but this child was unable to speak up and be honest about his situation, even though he desperately wanted to change it, and that cost me my custody and physical placement, and both childrens' happiness.

As a result, I was also ridiculed by court officers and vilified by a home study officer. One actually testified in court after one meeting with me, that I was "delusional" because I "believed" my son wanted to live with me (because that is what he had been saying for years), but that my child refused to tell *him* anything other than that he wanted to see me more but "stay with his dad." *Why couldn't the man grasp the concept that my child was legitimately afraid of what his father would do to him (and still is to this day) if he managed to find the courage to tell the whole truth and articulate his wishes? Why can't the man see the harm my ex was causing?* Instead it's easier to point the finger at the physically ill and accuse them of "mental" issues even when none exist. It's always easier to blame someone else than it is to spend time looking for the truth. With heavy caseloads, time is not a luxury apparently worth taking.

Even a person I consider a friend for many years, when interviewed by a social worker during a background check on me, stupidly agreed when asked if she felt I was perhaps a hypochondriac – only to later have me read that statement in the social worker's report. When I confronted her about why she would say such a terrible thing, she tearfully admitted that she didn't even know what that word *meant but chose to go along with it, because she thought that was what the social worker wanted to hear!* Understandably, this was devastating to learn both as a friend, and as a mother undergoing such detailed scrutiny for ongoing court matters. It just shows that "simple" but important errors such as a wrong word choice or unguarded thinking can unfairly be manipulated against someone during the process of determining custody and placement by individuals who do not know a family or the situation about whom they are making life-altering decisions.

Illness aside for a moment, in my opinion, the harm my ex-husband has done to our children (and me) is unconscionable and perhaps irreparable in many ways. His manipulation of private situations and our collective "alleged" Lyme disease in family court is heinous, and a testament to (again, my opinion), his warped character, or perhaps his own mental health issues. His attempts to block my ability to have my children properly tested and treated for Lyme disease are supported by what can only be described by me as a complacent court system that clearly doesn't understand the problem, and doesn't have our children's best interests in mind.

Accusations that I might try to "treat" my child with "experimental and dangerous chemicals" were unfounded, alleged but unproven, and ridiculous. One, I have never treated my children, physicians do that. Two, I would never do anything to harm my children, and I never have; and three, I would never treat children with anything I would not be willing to undergo myself first. All I ever asked for was a chance for my children to undergo additional testing to determine what was "going on" inside their bodies, with treatments appropriate for anything found, and family counseling to help them through the process.

And it apparently means nothing to the family court judge that there might be two children walking around harboring infectious diseases that are harming them on a daily basis. It means nothing to anyone that my daughter is donating her "allegedly" infectious disease-containing blood which she refuses to acknowledge might harm other people (because blood supplies are not screened for Lyme and some co-infections).

My son on the other hand, is intelligent enough to acknowledge that his "alleged" illness may indeed be real, because he is at a loss to explain his symptoms that he admits he experiences. But he is still too angry at the process he has been through and he vascillates between wanting more information about Lyme and residing comfortably within a state of denial of illness.

He admits that he lacks the motivation to get through the day at times, and he is just doing whatever he needs to do to "get through" this part of his life, and he is clearly miserable. Luckily he and I are very close and have a good mother/son relationship. On top of that, he alleges (and I believe) that his father is abusive and dismissive toward him, which is very hard on his self-esteem. I am aware of my ex's lies and abuse (from personal experience), and it is tragic though no surprise to me if he has been abusive toward our children. And yet the courts and their social workers refused to acknowledge my concerns about my ex, simply because my children wouldn't speak up against their abuser, which is common in abuse cases.

My son is so angry at his father's manipulations of him all these years that he can't stand to be around him any more. Now due to his fears to disclose the truth about life in his father's home, he is trapped within a process beyond his control. He is forced to live in an unsuitable situation for the next year and a half until he turns 18. He avoids contact with his father and is not doing well in school. This former A student now routinely has below-ability grades, ever since he went to live with his father in 2003. There is no excuse for his academic downturn except that he is in great emotional pain. He is depressed and angry and wants to run away. Meanwhile, my ex buys "things" in an attempt to placate our son, while the child ridicules him behind his back. He openly admits to losing respect for his father and "hating" him. He also admits to having physical symptoms mentioned previously, all well within the scope of the "usual" symptoms of untreated Lyme disease.

When he is with us, he is markedly better, laughing and feeling at peace, with regrets when it is time for him to leave. I do the best I can to help him make it from one visitation period to the next – and to give him hope that the future is a short time away, and at that point will he be free from the situation which has him quite literally pinned down. Only at that time can my son finally, truly be free and able to "breathe." And so I must ask who this situation has served? I answer, only my ex and the attorneys, and certainly not either of our children or their best interests, by any stretch of the imagination.

Because I have had custody taken away on unproven allegations, I no longer can treat my son with even an over-the-counter medication. I have been making healthcare and other decisions for him and his sister, all their lives. Suddenly, I am not capable of deciding if he can have a baby aspirin. I must treat him like the child next door – and go ask his father first. So as my son's health continues to decline, I cannot help him until he turns age 18. The court in essence, has relegated my son's health to the back burner, and is preventing him from getting healthcare that he may some day desperately require. **This is thanks to their refusal to even entertain the possibility that my children might have a real illness, even with positive lab tests.** (And yes, my ex routinely refuses our children proper medical care).

But based on allegations alone which never were quantified, I am relegated to being the "looney" parent who deserves only minimal contact with her children – all because I dared fight for their rights (and my own). This is a shining example of a flawed justice system which doesn't work for patients who have chronic illness not commonly "understood" by the general public or even court officials. If the word "Lyme" had been as mainstream as the word "cancer," I certainly would have been granted significantly more credence and perhaps even a little compassion. But the distinct lack of understanding of the illness of Lyme disease has led directly to ignorance-based discriminatory rulings, time and again over the course of 10 long years.

My son is intelligent and gracious enough to say to me that he never appreciated me before, but he now in fact, truly does and that he is sorry. He now clearly sees the picture of how he and his sister were used as pawns, and how cruelly we have all been treated. He knows I have done nothing wrong, and that I tried my best to defend the three of us over the past decade. That was wonderful to hear from a child who had been so cruelly manipulated by his father and afraid to speak up to tell people what he *really* wanted. It touch me to hear him say this and it brought tears to my eyes to know that he finally openly acknowledged me and all that I have done for him and his sister.

But sadly, it is too late for him now. We have to sit and deal with the next year and a half while my ex-husband files yet more petty court motions designed to force me to pay for more things he wants while he enjoys full custody and I struggle with limited visitation of every other weekend with my son. I now have a daughter who previously wouldn't return my phone calls or emails because she was alienated from me due to the court process and my ex's brainwashing of her. She has recently visited a few times, in part because of holidays and her wanting something from me – but even a few fractional hours are helping me get my foot in the door to begin to repair our shattered relationship. And she is beginning to respond, albeit in baby steps.

My ex is currently happy receiving the nearly $900 a month in child support from my disability for Lyme disease, (you know, the illness I supposedly fabricated). And yet he continues to harrass me by whatever means he can, trying to extort whatever he can from me. This is sick in my opinion and he clearly has no insight into what this does to our children to see their parents "fighting" – even if it simply means I have to defend myself repeatedly and nothing more thanks to his continued court motions and harrassment.

In all, it's hard to comprehend the "how and why" of my children's removal from my custody. The ignorant court appointees were not helpful to the process at all. The children's attorney (GAL) only ever infered that I had a "full plate." Of course the false accusations of child abuse and mental illness, though proven not to have occurred, hung around in the court's mind nevertheless, influencing the decision that I was somehow "unfit" to parent or that I failed to "communicate," when in reality it has been my ex manipulating events for nearly 10 years, and who was deliberately failing to communicate.

By the time 2009 rolls around, and my son turns 18, I will have spent more than a dozen years, and over a hundred thousand dollars within the family court system, trying to right the wrongs of ignorance and discrimination; a tremendous, uphill battle and a lesson of futility. We even had to file bankruptcy due to medical and legal bills which came about for little more than my being ill with Lyme disease. And my family is just one caught in social services and family court dealing with the ignorance swirling around Lyme disease, and who have children removed from loving, good parents due to an illness both poorly understood, and barely acknowledged.

I know personally what it's like to be accused of fabricating an illness, having "delusions" and "mental illness" that was not present, and was never diagnosed nor indicated on any physical or clinical evaluation. I have been disabled yet found in contempt of court for being unable to work, because a judge said I didn't "look" sick when the government's documented onset date of my disability differed from that of my personal medical history, which the disability people arbitrarily ignored.

I have paid thousands of dollars in fines to avoid jail time whenever my ex-husband wanted to find new ways to twist the screws of "justice" tighter yet so I would avoid being found guilty of some imagined crime I had not committed but for which I was falsely accused thanks to poor legal representation and discriminatory judicial practices.

My children are permanently affected by Lyme disease (and family conflict), and to date their "alleged" illnesses are untreated due to their father's and the court's denial. Additional factors include the brainwashing of the children that somehow mother made up her illness and is trying to force her "delusions" onto them. Combine that with the court system's current restraints against my parental authority to do anything for my children and you have a disaster waiting to happen with two depressed, ill children.

Now that our third and final trial is finally finished, I have been newly branded on paper as "delusional," "Lyme-obsessed," and a "mental" case who has apparently "fabricated" illness for myself and my two children. For what purpose did all of this serve I must ask? Legally my ex shouldn't have been able to do what he did to this family, but there certainly wasn't anyone stopping him, either. In fact, the courts wanted to believe the worst about me, because of its ignorance about chronic illness. It was easier to point the finger at the "crazy woman" than it was to believe that my ex-husband could have been so cruelly vindictive.

I can see hallmark Lyme-driven behavior in my ex-husband, who at one time, I magnanimously gave information about Lyme disease back when the children's tests were originally done. I suggested that he might also want to be tested because Lyme may be sexually transmissible in active illness, which I unknowingly had when married to him. Naturally he flatly refused, and instead choose to openly mock me to the children, his girlfriend, the court system, and anybody else with whom he came, and comes into contact.

Within the past year, I found it quite ironic that my children informed me that their father removed an attached engorged tick from his stomach. Shortly thereafter, he presented with "sudden" heart problems necessitating open heart surgery and surgical bypass, with complications. You may find it interesting that he had surgery in secret during our third court trial, and threatened the children if they told me about the surgery. When the court learned about it, they dismissed it as if it had no bearing on his ability to continue parenting – unlike what they did with my Lyme disease. Remember at the time the children were removed in 2003, I was neither diagnosed nor had I any clear symptoms that anybody actually saw, although like my ex, I had undergone major surgery, though not as serious as heart surgery. Yet his surgery was "not an issue" for the court, but mine (less serious), had been. To this day, he is suffering from health problems, and the court doesn't care about his ability to parent. It doesn't care that it made a mistake years ago by handing over my children to this horrible man – no matter what the evidence shown. The judge only cares that the court's decision not be reversed, whether it was correct, or in our family's case, miserably wrong.

My ex continues to take copious amounts of medications, and struggles with circulatory and intestinal problems and other health issues. I cannot help but wonder if he also has Lyme disease thanks to yet another Walworth county tick on his belly. Perhaps he is in for a long, hard lesson to learn about a chronic illness he not only dismisses, but openly mocked in his ex-wife and his own children for over a decade, and how ironic that would be if it proves to be true.

If he indeed has Lyme, perhaps the exercise here is in retribution or karma if you believe in that kind of thing. Despite what he has put the children and myself through, I can honestly say I still would not wish Lyme disease on anyone, not even him. Still the refusal to acknowledge something plainly staring him in the face (or maybe even from upon his own belly) may be the one issue that teaches him some of the most importnat lessons of his lifetime.

Personally, whether by a parent or a court system, I would call the refusal to investigate legitimate concerns about children who have potentially disabling Lyme disease (especially with our daughter's history of depression and our son's behavioral/anger issues and declining grades), a serious form of child neglect and abuse.

But gee, what do I know? I'm "lyme-obsessed" and "fabricating illness for myself and my children." The truth is the truth and one day my ex will have to deal with it, and sadly, so will the children. For them, they are like ticking time-bombs waiting to go off, and that is unfair but the court has tied my hands. The courts were carefully and successfully manipulated by a man and his attorney out to win at any cost – and that cost in our case, was my reputation and the health of two innocent children who were caught in the middle through no fault of their own. And when ill children are caught in the middle of adult matters that deny their illnesses, children are adversely and permanently affected.

So what can I say about our case, and my illness when the dust clears? Unfortunately, delays and events that cause rescheduling of hearings over years are very common in the family courts, especially from opposing counsel without a case but who wish to delay the process to maximize placement for their client. The psychological and financial burdens that come from being caught for years within a legal system that does not work have led to additional stressors that make recovering from chronic illness and financial devastation ever so much more difficult for all in this family. When one has to choose between purchasing medications or paying attorneys to continue a legitimate counter motion; or are forced to decide between delaying necessary treatments to attend endless mandatory court hearings, the line between personal need and lawful necessity quickly blurs.

Fabrication accusations aside, in conclusion, it is hard to argue with the incredible improvement of my overall health following IV treatments in 2002 and 2005, *years* of on-again, off-again oral antibiotics, herbal and nutritional supplements, and other so-called "alternative" treatments, all of which have restored much of the functionality I had lost. One simply cannot manifest bodily paralysis and cognitive dysfunction. Although I have improved considerably, my body remains actively infected with multiple organisms, and exhibits symptoms on a daily basis, although thankfully to a far milder degree than in the past. But even those symptoms wax and wane roughly in 30-day cycles, with total resolution always conspicuously absent. Each day I awaken with the anticipation of feeling as good as possible, with the keen realization that at any moment I might backslide out of remission with lingering mild symptoms into debilitation again, because I know I am not yet cured, but oh how I wish that I were and I am working toward that achievable goal.

I am sure that some people can readily see the effects of lingering neurocognitive issues even within the words that I write. Because life with chronic Lyme disease causes cognitive imperfections, it becomes at times, a challenge to communicate. Nevertheless, just as many other Lyme patients, I deal with symptoms daily and do the very best that I can. I consider myself worlds better than where I have come from, and years ahead of where I would have been, had I not received some of the treatments I have received in the past few years.

As most chronic (disseminated) Lyme patients can attest to from their own experience, I cannot recall a single day within the past decade and a half since I removed the tick on my back, when I have ever felt *completely* well. Not one, and neither can hundreds of thousands of Lyme patients walking, limping, wheeling, crawling or laying about in all parts of the world. I have been quite cognitively impaired and lived in a constant "brain fog" and had fleeting psychiatric "events" that defy explanation except in terms of brain inflammation. The loss of my children on top of all of this and the knowledge that my children are ill and being denied medical care at the hands of their own father and a court system, is absolutely heartbreaking to me.

Still, I have been not as ill as some who are permanently and irrevocably incapacitated, and certainly not as ill as those who have already left this world due to this disease – some who tragically died by their own hand.

Incidentally, in 1992 at onset of my illness, I did not receive the currently IDSA-recommended antibiotic doxycycline despite high fevers and multiple emergency room and doctor visits. Physicians did not know what to do with me, and simply guessed that I had "some sort of virus." Alas, any IDSA "recommended" treatment came *at least a full year after I was first infected* and exhibited the rash and systemic symptoms. By that time the organisms had already long disseminated into my brain, organs, and central nervous system. According to my understanding of the current guidelines, in my case since I wasn't diagnosed or tested within the timeframe I was originally infected, I therefore "might not have" Lyme disease, but instead I must have some other "syndrome." This thought process makes no sense to me. When one is infected with an organism that cannot be proven as "cured" by any amount of antibiotics, especially when symptoms persist, it is dangerous and irresponsible in my opinion to pretend that one or two or three weeks, months or treatment courses should be sufficient. And yet medical societies are repeatedly exerting heavy pressure to try to convince the masses that our illness does not persist when much research (including their own), and thousands of patients prove that it in fact, does persist.

Like many Lyme patients, I have had doxycycline (the typically recommended drug of choice) and many other drugs *multiple times*, over a *decade and a half,* always without resolution of symptoms. I also had a long list of other somewhat more effective oral and intravenous antibiotics, as well as natural, herbal and so-called "alternative" therapies, none of which have completely eradicated Bb or co-infections (yet), but they have done a good job of knocking down my overall viral load. I would be much further along of course if I could dedicate my entire days to nothing other than becoming well, but so far that just hasn't happened due to many factors, including ongoing custody issues and a lack of financial and emotional support, not to mention the tremendous difficulty of locating doctors willing or able to treat Lyme.

In reality I am like so many other patients who were denied testing, diagnosis and treatment, and we have fallen through the very wide cracks of the narrow CDC case definitions, and diagnostic and treatment guidelines. Hence we have developed what is now called "chronic Lyme disease." None of us have chosen to be placed in this position, and each of us would give up anything to be cured.

I personally have made my way through the bulk of this illness with a little luck, the grace of God, hard work, fluke connections, an odd mix of traditional and alternative treatments, and being in the right place at the right time. Through Lyme disease, I was led down a difficult path that would change my life forever before intervention would steer me back onto a road of relative (though incomplete) wellness. I don't know what the future holds for me, as I am still infected with Lyme, Bartonella, and Babesia. The last two were revealed in a micrograph (photo) and despite current tests saying I "did not have" these infections, (and one saying that I did), clearly the infections are present, based on the photographs and my symptoms.

The same holds true for Lyme disease. I have never had a resolution of symptoms though I am functioning at about 75% capacity. And new things turn up daily. My hormones are skewed in part from the Lyme, and now I have new health issues with which to deal, and am facing difficult medical choices. I still have a modified, restricted diet that forces me to limit my travels to how much food can be carried with me thanks to a severe allergy to a chemical that is in Morton table salt (which is used all over the world and in many foods). I cannot socialize at restaurants because it is important to avoid anaphylaxis and most foods contain table salt. This complicates my complicated life to no end. My hard work at exercise and proper diet and stress reduction have been difficult (especially the stress), but I do the very best I can and I have come very far. Rebuilding my immune system and erradicating even subclinical infectious diseases like mold, Epstein-Barr virus and Candidae (yeast) are also very important.

I wanted to share with you that living a full life (relatively speaking) with Lyme disease and co-infections is actually possible. At one point in my illness, I was cognitively impaired to the point of not easily recalling my own children's names, or remembering where I lived. I also was unable to walk across the living room floor, brush my hair or even pick up a milk carton. I have had repeated bouts of paralysis on the left side of my body and my face, and have walked with a cane. Fortunately I only spent 10 days in a wheelchair. Though I have not been as sick as some people with Lyme, I certainly have had my share of problems. I want people to know however, that despite the symptoms that we endure, whether transient or chronic, it is possible to become well enough that life can continue in a fairly normal manner. In truth, I feel my illness is in a state of semi-remission, though all symptoms are not gone.

My immune system is still skewed, and I am very vulnerable to illness and cancers. I continue to remove lumps, bumps and growths from all parts of my body, inside and out, and my last CD-57 (natural killer cells) count was at "2," which is thought to be indicative of relapsing, active Lyme disease. I still have pain, visual problems, mild impairments, horrendous allergies, and digestive issues. My circulatory system is taxed and I have new tissue growth in my reproductive system.

I still am co-infected and have to undergo more treatment, and my illnesses will probably relapse and remit for a time, if not the remainder of my life, because *we simply don't know if Lyme is 100% curable*. Ah, if only someone had listened to me when I first suspected Lyme disease. How common a theme for so many people, and how horribly sad we have gone ignored. Yet I greet each new day with humble appreciation for the tremendous gift that is my life, and I work to help others see their blessings, and not their losses, which our disease brings.

I hope that you take inspiration from the nearly 100 stories in this book series. Despite overwhelming odds, many of us have gone on to feel significantly better and a some feel they are well on the way to being cured, or are actually cured of Lyme disease and other infections. Most however, are aware that their illness is probably completely incurable, especially since when they have gone untreated and undiagnosed for so many years, and much damage has been done.

As Lyme patients, we know that at any moment, our lives can easily be cast back into the oblivion of uncertainty that comes with chronic illness. Yet we work hard not to dwell on an illness none of us want. We take comfort in the simple things in life, in a renewed spirituality, and the knowledge that life offers us no guarantees but to live it fully, and without reservation. Through chronic illness, we learn that love, patience, and understanding are the most important aspects of life. Lyme patients learn their lessons well. Life is precious, and health, a blessing. Take nothing and no one for granted, after all, you may be next, though we sincerely hope this disease gets the recognition and credence it deserves so you don't have to go through it as we have.

There is no reason that people should continue to make disparaging remarks about Lyme patients who **are, but do not wish to be ill.** We are not a conglomerate of depressed people who have nothing better to do than to fabricate health issues. The medical establishment knows this yet continues to pretend that chronic Lyme doesn't exist. Research and patients living with illness proves our illness is real. Why people refuse to acknowledge us is beyond our comprehension.

Had Lyme disease been acknowledged two decades ago, most of the people whose stories appear in this book series, wouldn't be available for you to read, because they might have been "cured" of Lyme. My family might not have had to go through much of what it did due to Lyme because our situation wouldn't have been able to be manipulated within the court system due to ignorance about Lyme disease.

And some people might still be alive today if Lyme had not been swept under the carpet. Because of ignorance, denial and improper treatment, each of us went on to develop what is called "chronic" Lyme disease, and a few of us are no longer here because of it.

Thanks to years of on-again off-again antibiotics, and especially IV antibiotics when I needed them most, I am now markedly better, even on "bad" days.

I still have residual Lyme, Bartonella and Babesia which can be seen in micrographs from peripheral blood smears. I am choosing to treat these illnesses through alternative, as well as traditional antibiotic therapies, for as long as it takes, until all symptoms are gone.

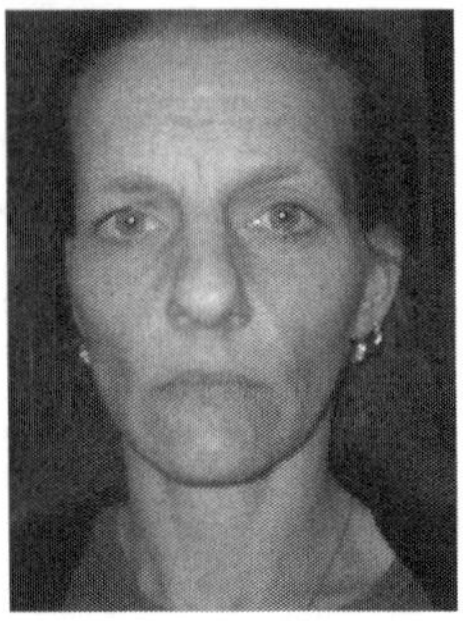

Right: a photo of me in 2005 during IV therapy which took 13 years to receive. My skin had a yellow-hue and my eyes were vacant.

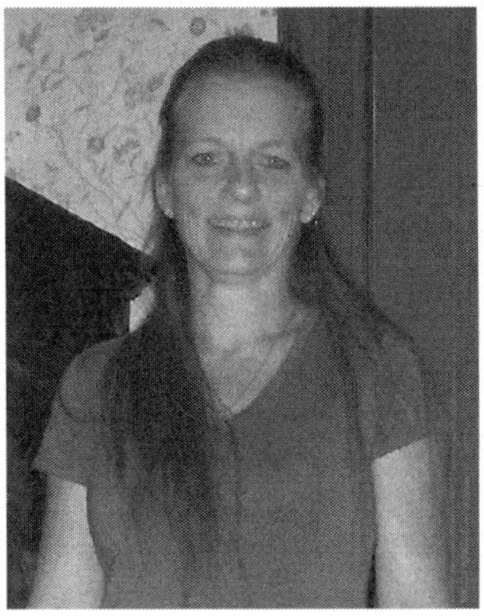

Left: A picture of me, October 2007, two years after IV treatments for a disease some doctors still pretend doesn't exist. At the time of my treatments, I was rapidly and seriously declning.

I hope we live to see a day where the words "Lyme disease" will mean a single curative pill, a warm handshake, and a "see you next year doc." For now however, living with Lyme disease and coping with the ignorance surrounding it is the best we can manage to do. But even with disability, we somehow manage still to "live." **But how much better it would be rather…to actually be cured!**

I do know this – that in time, and with continued treatment, and proper acknowledgement of Lyme by the medical establishment, I will become well...and so will you.

– In light and health, PJ

❖ ❖ ❖

A Student with a Clearer View of the Lyme Disease "Map" Than Most

Megan M. Blewett, Madison, New Jersey

I am a student researcher who *does not have Lyme disease,* and I confess from the beginning that I never intended to study Lyme. I now have one of the largest Lyme incidence datasets in existence and am distributing it to other researchers and patients. In the eighth grade, I began researching multiple sclerosis (MS). I did not know anyone with MS, but I felt studying the disease would be an interesting scientific endeavor. Most researchers believe MS is linked to an environmental trigger, and I decided to try to elucidate this trigger by mapping the incidence of MS.

After I had produced several nationwide and statewide maps, I noticed some interesting trends. Marine regions had particularly high incidences of MS, and Connecticut's incidence was disproportionately high. I considered why these trends were occurring. While looking at MS incidence in my home state of New Jersey, I realized a town next to mine was a hot spot for MS. I remembered that several of my classmates from that town had suffered from Lyme disease, and the prevalence of Lyme in this town was abnormally high. I hypothesized that perhaps MS and Lyme are related geographically. I knew that I would need advanced statistical methods and mapping techniques to definitively prove any co-occurrence.

As I shared my hypothesis with others, I found evidence warranting further investigation of an MS-Lyme connection. Several people revealed to me that they, themselves, or loved ones had been diagnosed first with Lyme, and then with MS. One judge at a local science fair told me he knew the symptoms of MS and Lyme to be quite similar. I re-read several MS textbooks that I owned, looking for any mention of Lyme, and I again found evidence linking the two diseases.

This emerging connection transformed my view of MS. I had previously believed that if an environmental trigger were involved in MS, it was viral. This was and is the most widely accepted etiological hypothesis. However, many of the viruses being implicated are ubiquitous viruses. These are viruses for which a large percentage of the population tests positive, and thus it is difficult to link these specifically to MS patients. Some of the viruses being proposed also did not occur in the geographic regions that showed the highest incidence of MS.

From my spatial statistical background, I reasoned that if an environmental trigger is linked to a disease, it should co-occur with high incidence of that disease. Thus, many of the viruses implicated did not agree with my scientific findings. However, the focus of my research is less on disproving other hypotheses than providing evidence for bacterial involvement in MS.

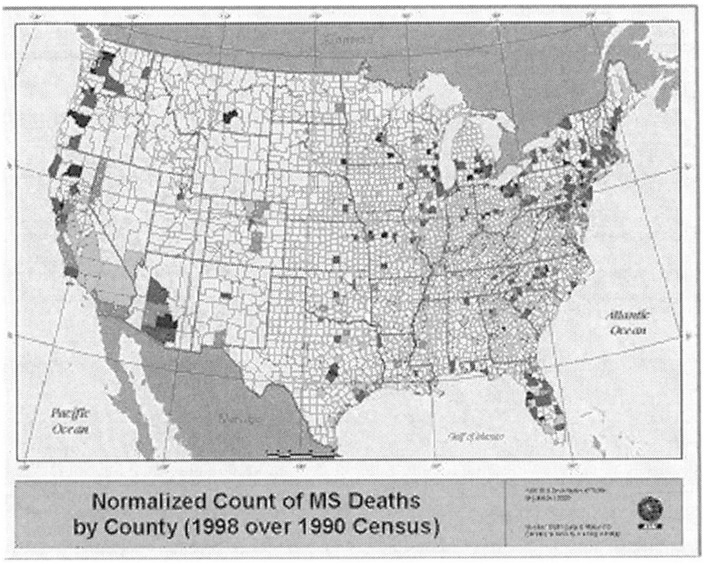

The map of MS incidence (above) is visually very similar to the map of Lyme incidence (below). The CDC classification for Lyme disease is "Other Specified Arthropod-Borne Diseases," or (OSABD). Maps courtesy and copyright of M. Blewett[1]

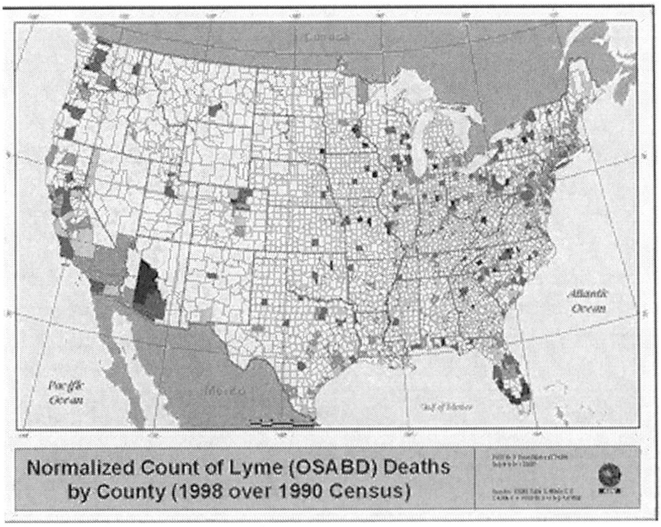

When I mapped the distributions of MS and Lyme, visually they were very similar. The spatial statistical results substantiated their co-occurrence – areas of the United States with higher incidence of MS also have higher incidence of Lyme.

After nearly six years of researching MS; and, in particular its distribution, the presence of an environmental trigger in MS still makes a great deal of sense. As our current view of Lyme is changing, its symptoms and long-term effects resemble more and more those of MS. In fact, late-stage Lyme looks very much like MS, resulting in memory deficits and even demyelination.[2] In Lyme though, researchers know that a stealth pathogen is present, and that demyelination is a result of a combination attack by *Borrelia burgdorferi* bacteria and by the immune system as it tries to combat these bacteria. In MS, the demyelination is often considered a result of a grave failing of the immune system resulting in an attack of "self" material.

Autoimmune diseases today are still not well understood. Sometimes what appears to be an autoimmune error is actually proper functioning of the immune system in response to a stealth pathogen. In the 1990's, Fiona Powrie et al. of the *DNAX Research Institute* (Palo Alto, California), introduced a T-cell culture lacking T-regs, (or developed T cells), into mice which were void of an immune system. The result was a serious inflammatory bowel condition. When the T cells met the gut bacteria of the mice, they attacked even to the extent of damaging the gut.[3] A similar malfunctioning of T-regs, and a similar pathogen, could explain the demyelination in MS.

I was fortunate enough recently to speak with acting Surgeon General Kenneth Moritsugu about the possibility that such a stealth pathogen is at work in MS. He mentioned two Australian researchers (Barry J. Marshall and J. Robin Warren), who made headlines in 2005 with their discovery that peptic ulcers are caused not by stress, but by the bacterium *Helicobacter pylori*. For their work, Marshall and Warren received the Nobel Prize in Physiology or Medicine.[4]

However, the road to the Nobel Prize was not an easy one. In order to convince the medical community, Dr. Marshall deliberately swallowed a culture of the *Helicobacter pylori,* which he and Dr. Warren discovered. Indeed, Dr. Marshall's symptoms were indicative of an extreme case of ulceration. His wife described him as being "dreadfully ill" and eventually forced him to get treatment.[5] Convincing the medical community that this common condition should be entirely reclassified, was not simple. A similar reclassification may be appropriate for MS and related demyelinating and autoimmune diseases.

Current research suggests that the future may hold many more paradigm shifts in medicine. Alonso et al. of the *Harvard School of Public Health* found that people who had taken penicillin within three years of the index date had decreased chances of developing MS.[6] Another Harvard study found that higher levels of vitamin D are associated with a lower risk of MS.[7] Vitamin D is one of the few natural antibiotics. These studies point to bacterial involvement in MS. The exact role of viral factors, including avian retroviruses, has not yet been elucidated. Further research must be performed to determine whether viral or bacterial factors, or both, are contributing to the progression of MS.

By now, I have touched on some of the science behind bacterial involvement in MS. Though researchers may disagree in this area, all should be united with regards to the social implications of their work. The common goal of all medical research is ending suffering. Lyme is not the "curable" illness I once thought it to be; long-term effects can persist among patients. The effects of MS are widely accepted to be chronic. Thus, the importance of medical research in these areas cannot be overstated.

Over the course of my five years of research, studying MS has become much more than an interesting scientific endeavor. My work is now motivated by helping patients. To a teenager, the revelation that a significant percentage of the population is bedridden or handicapped from incurable diseases, is shocking. These sufferers form a hidden community whose members are many but often receive little publicity or support.

Though MS was first diagnosed six hundred years ago, no one knows for certain what causes this disease. MS is a six-century-old medical mystery. We are now at a unique vantage point; and with new technology, we can better investigate the elusive mechanism and etiology of MS. Should prevailing evidence be found that the causative agent in MS is a virus or even purely a glitch in the immune system; I will, as a scientist, change my current viewpoint. However, when people's lives rely upon new scientific findings, I find it imperative to investigate every theory. As a student, I have the liberty to follow the hypotheses I feel to be most valid and sensible. I have found enough evidence for bacterial involvement in MS in order to dissuade me from my original acceptance of viral involvement. The bacterial hypothesis holds the promise of saving lives and ending suffering. The benefits far outweigh the risks, though the risks are many.

A short time ago, my English teacher's sister died of MS. She was fifty. Before she died, she was almost completely paralyzed and possessed only enough motor coordination to mouth her prayers. This is the sad state of MS. Situations like these can be found among chronic Lyme sufferers.

Curing these diseases will take a great deal of ambition and perseverance, though **these traits should be prerequisites for all medical researchers. The researcher should work at least as hard as the disease; if a patient must suffer, a researcher must work.** For me, though my work has been difficult, it is far from painful. In fact, one of the most fulfilling parts of my life is doing research. My work has proven to be both a cognitive challenge, and a source of great inspiration.

To conclude, I recently presented my research at a local Board of Education meeting to encourage student involvement in science. I ended my presentation with the quote by Teddy Roosevelt: "Far and away the best prize that life has to offer is the chance to work hard at work worth doing." Indeed, this is work worth doing. Millions of people around the globe suffer from MS and Lyme, and now more than ever, researchers may have the technology and the opportunity to give these people their lives back.

Megan's References:

1. Blewett M. A Geostatistical Analysis of Possible Spirochetal Involvement in Multiple Sclerosis and Other Related Diseases. http://www.canlyme.com/megan_geostatistical_analysis2.html. Accessed April 20, 2007.
2. Filley CM. The Behavioral Neurology of White Matter. New York: Oxford University Press; 2001.
3. Fehervari Z, Sakaguchi S. Peacekeepers of the Immune System. *Scientific American.* October 2006:57-63.

4. The Nobel Prize in Physiology or Medicine 2005. http://nobelprize.org/nobel_prizes/medicine/laureates/2005/index.html. Accessed April 20, 2007.
5. Sweet M. Smug as a Bug. *Sydney Morning Herald*. August 2, 1997.
6. Alonso A, Jick SS, Jick H, Hernan MA. Antibiotic use and risk of multiple sclerosis. *Am J Epidemiol* 2006;163(11):997-1002.
7. Munger KL, Levin LI, Hollis BW, Howard NS, Ascherio A. Serum 25-hydroxyvitamin D levels and risk of multiple sclerosis. *JAMA* 2006;296(23):2832-2838.

❖ ❖ ❖

Finding Our Collective Voice

Shortly after my dozen-and-a-half year wait for a diagnosis of Lyme disease, and at 2 a.m., I began typing away on my laptop computer because I could not sleep. I decided to list all the symptoms I had experienced in the course of my illness. I then reflected on comments that other Lyme patients had shared with me through my offering phone support to them, and from the 2 patient web sites I operated, and added those as well. At the time I was diagnosed, the only support group in my regional area was closing down due to its leader's disability and I felt that since I was still physically able to do *some* things, that my offering support web sites was a small way in which I could contribute to the cause and to raising awareness about living with this horrible illness called Lyme.

Through months of listening to patients discuss their health problems, a common denominator became apparent, which was that many Lyme patients feel as if they are all alone. Most of them feel invalidated in the medical world by their doctors, insurance companies, social security disability, and often even their own friends and family members.

A significant problem occurring in Lyme patients' lives is the toll this illness takes on their interpersonal relationships. Families, friends, spouses, co-workers and even their physicians fail miserably to comprehend the extremes in their symptoms, emotions, behaviors, moods, and abilities.

Temporary fits of rage, elevations of voice, mood, irritability, or even in the sudden use of profanity or insensitive remarks normally censored, are taken as personal attacks rather than as symptoms of a brain infection. The fact that fatigue and restorative sleep as well as diet play an integral role in the Lyme patients' ability to function from day-to-day (but is not curative), seems to escape even the most understanding of persons. In fact, very little clear understanding and true compassion are afforded Lyme patients, whose only crime is that they are suffering from an illness no one seems willing to acknowledge or sometimes treat – and at best, is egregiously misunderstood.

So with that thought in mind, I assembled my symptoms into a more appropriate vehicle which might more cohesively express the consensus of our collective opinions. Some may have already seen this work as I sent it out over the internet through my local Lyme support network in 2005. It was well received and continued to travel all over the country, or perhaps even further. Many have requested reprint rights of the poem to offer it to patients in clinics, therapy groups, support groups and between individuals. I offer it to you here.

"The Forgotten"

I am not crazy
This is not all in my head
I am not making any of this up
I am not a hypochondriac
I do not seek attention or fame
I do not have "borderline personality disorder"
I don't need a Psychiatrist or a Psychologist
Why do you admonish me,
  when it is *you* who does not understand?
None of this is my fault
How can you say that my disease does not exist?
Why do you say it is not in my town?
Hush, keep it down or panic will ensue
People might move away
Or worse yet, never come and visit
We can't have that, can we?
I stand here before you as a testament to my illness
I am a helpless victim of a cruel disease
And an even crueler system
Your misdiagnosis is designed to render a pill so I go away
You choose to ignore me and I will go away
Eventually I will die of a disease called ignorance
If the illness doesn't get me first
Some die by their own hand out of desperation
Many have tragically lost hope
You see the dark circles under my eyes
  and say that I must be tired
You have no idea of my tiredness
Not half as tired as I am of hearing that I don't exist,
That I am invisible,
That I am nuts,
Or that I do not matter
You say you don't believe in my disease

But it believes in me
Let's take stock of all my imaginary illness has given me
The gift of my experiences and the toll they have taken
I am allergic to most foods, and many medications
But not really, my body just thinks it is
I am not a basket-case, but I feel like one
I have seen 10 doctors, or 20, or 50, or 100
None will give credence to me
I have every illness known to man except that which
  I truly have, According to them
I don't smile because my face has nerve damage
You interpret it as looking mean instead
I try to communicate but it is work for me
You think I have an attitude problem
I can eat only 5 foods for months at a time,
  or sometimes only one,
But this isn't a diet
You don't understand and you make me feel bad
  about my food "choices"
I run screaming out of the store because the light bothers me
There is terrible bone pain
I can no longer use my limbs
I have no sex life
I suffer panic attacks and palpitations
I have a heart block, an arrythmia, or chest pain
Fatigue so profound I feel like the walking dead
"Hello" you say on the phone in my moment of silence
Did I hear what you said? Forgive me I'm quietly seizing
Blanking out, momentarily ceasing to function
You hardly notice, you think me not listening
I wear sunglasses in the daytime not to be fashionable
I can't stand sound at any volume or I cannot hear at all
Motion sickness plagues me, my stomach my enemy
Turn me in circles and I get confused, disoriented, dizzy
I struggle to regain my physical strength
Desperate for human connectedness
A kind word, an understanding heart
Save me from this isolation I feel
An unwelcome blanket of silent uncertainty

You say I want for attention
Tumors appear in me for no apparent reason
My organs are failing while you call my blood work "normal"
My ears ring incessantly;
My eyes no longer work or I can no longer see
My head hurts worse than any migraine I have ever had,
Even my hair "hurts"
I wince when you touch me, when you kiss me
I need reassurance but your embrace is painful to me
Or I find none at all, feeling your rejection from lack of support
Because I am too much work
Because you are tired
Or you have had a long day
You walk out on me
I have no value to you
Because you cannot relate
Strange sensations, odd tastes; smells that are not really there
I have lost my hair and not from bad hair genes
Lost weight, wasting away as nourishment escapes me
Or I look like a balloon, larger than life, you cruelly call me fat
I feel biting, stabbing and jabbing pain in my body.
Nails of fire are burning my skin, a red-hot poker
Bugs crawling on and under my skin
They bite me relentlessly but I cannot see them
I am being eaten alive, from the inside out
Excuse me while I die, one cell at a time
My immune system is thwarted by something I cannot control
My brain manipulated, my body stressed
This thing controls every aspect of me,
I see the world through a filter
My thoughts are dark, sometimes suicidal, you call me insane
Or elation, roller-coaster mood swings which have no meaning
I am so cold, hypothermic,
Or feverish, wet from night sweats or chills
My joints and muscles hurt, ache, throb, burn, and are swollen
Who are these people I am hallucinating?
I know they do not exist
Yet I see them before me, standing there, threatening me
I am paralyzed, I am incontinent,

I am a shell of the person I used to be
I can't breathe, or eat, and I can't think straight
Words fly out of my mouth that I did not choose
I am dyslexic, I am speech-impaired, I cannot speak at all
I forget where I am going, what I am doing, and who I am
I am confused and frightened
I lose my temper from nothing at all, and I fight with everyone
For reasons I can't explain
The night hours are long and I cannot sleep,
Or I sleep longer than I should
I fall asleep in the daytime and need rest throughout the day
I am afraid of slumber, nightmares disturb my sleep
I stumble along, knock things over and fall
You tell me to be "careful"
I have no perception of myself in time and space
I cannot control my own movements
I am called disabled by some; others refuse to label me that
You accuse me of crimes I have not committed
Like failure to work
Failure to pay child support
Failure to show up places
Argumentativeness
Impatience
Like it is really a choice I would make
You reject me because I am unreliable
Because you don't understand
I am sorry I missed your family function
Or dinner party, or funeral, I was too sick to attend
You say I am not sick and my disease is but my imagination
I have rashes on my body that are hideous and uncomfortable
I cannot eat; my toilet is a valued friend
I am hyperactive, or a slug, laying about each day
I have trouble learning new things
Or remembering them
When you poke me with a needle, my blood won't flow
I am so tired of the tests, the needles and the drugs
The home remedies, the sure-fire cures
And emptiness of the unknown
I am spastic, I twitch, I jerk, I tremble, I shake

I can't lift a milk carton, or dress myself, or comb my hair
My teeth hurt, my gums and nose bleeds
I have bruises all over my body and I don't even know why
When I look in the mirror, I no longer recognize the image there
The person I was is now a shell of my former self
I have lost my children, friends and family
Because they just don't understand
Maybe I can no longer work, uncertain how I will survive
I've lost my livelihood, my home, my finances,
my health, and my future
I cannot get disability because my illness is not on the list
Or maybe I have disability but it still doesn't help pay the bills
I have filed bankruptcy or live on the verge of it
I cannot get insurance because I am ill,
but no one will say that I am
I cannot go to doctors because they don't want me there
Or I have the wrong insurance
Or worse yet, none at all
Family courts have punished me
Taking away my children
They tell me I am playing games
Because I cannot work
Because I endlessly reschedule hearings
Because I struggle with my memory on the stand
You accuse me of heinous crimes
You ridicule my supposed disease
And chide me for not having proof
And take advantage of me
To get what you want, my children
Because you can and they let you
Because I am ill
Maybe you found me wandering in the street
Speaking insanity, out of my mind
You accused me and put me away – Shame on you
Yes I am still sick
Is this taking too long for you? I am sorry
I don't know if I can be cured
No there are no tests to see if I am well
I cannot find a doctor to treat me

or diagnose me, or care
This never should have happened
It could have been avoided
If you had just listened to me
And tried harder to help
I can no longer drive, walk, think, write, or function
What is a normal life?
I have a service dog
Or maybe I can't afford one
I can't stand up or walk straight, or walk at all
I am depressed, I am alone
I am lost in a sea of despair because no one sees me
I am invisible though I stand before you
You close doors in my face and send me away
Because you don't want to deal with me
Because you say three weeks is enough,
and I should be cured
Or 10 days or 30 or 100
Or worse yet you experiment on me
without knowing what or why
Because you are afraid of being a doctor
Of losing your license to practice
Hesitant to being compassionate
Or afraid to pass a Bill
To take governmental control
To assist your constituents
Because no one wants responsibility
To be forced to acknowledge that I am ill
Like it is some sort of a crime
I did not choose this disease – It chose me (oh lucky me)
To you I don't look sick, but I assure you that I am
Outside I look fine, but inside I am screaming
I am angry. I have a right to be
Let me explain,
I am the Forgotten
I have Lyme

❖ ❖ ❖

In this book I also wanted to include several items which were sent to me by patients, some of whom had stories published herein and others from Book II of this series, *"It's All In Your Head," Around the World in 80 Lyme Patient Stories.* These and other heartfelt poems; prose, and words of inspiration are found sprinkled all across the internet; in Lyme forums, on newsgroups, and on support group web sites. They all serve as emotional inspiration for thousands of ill and suffering people all over the world. Many people utilize poetry and prose in order to cope with, and articulate their feelings about having to deal with such a controversial illness, when they may be unable to effectively communicate those same feelings in other ways. For some, expressing their emotions through this very personal medium is sometimes literally all they have to cling to as they fight for cognitive clarity through what is known as Lyme "brain fog." All items are reprinted with permission from the authors.

❖ ❖ ❖

Thoughts on Lyme
by Brin King, Yorkville, Illinois

[Written in 1994 when he was going into his fourth year of Lyme]

Lyme Disease is devastating as we all know who have this disease. For I, in which I have had Lyme Disease now for the past four years, yet seems like eternity, as I am sure many can relate to! It has been a nightmare.

Lyme Disease has taken its toll on me and given me some pretty rough knocks and has put me down many many times, but I always manage to somehow get back on my feet, a bit weaker, a bit more confused and hurt and filled with a few more questions than the last time in falling.

Lyme Disease...has taken my mind, my soul and my health, as well as all of life has to offer me! But-it hasn't taken my spirit, my want and effort in trying, my will to go on though it has tested me, oh so many times, but I will be darned if I am going to quit. It hasn't taken away my effort in pursuing the many answers I and so many seek!

A CURE!

It hasn't taken away my love for life, my love for people and it hasn't taken away the compassion I have within, for everyone with this devastating illness.

I will continue to Hope. I will try the best I can, in obtaining somehow, the answers to the many questions asked.

Lyme Disease has hurt me bad…so very bad and the tears at times, more often than enough, seem endless. Falling down, seizures, pain and discomfort and the many questions asked, all bring tears to me!

So much loss, so very much, there is no scale to measure the loss of this proportion. But – I am going to go on, for whatever it is worth, for wherever it may lead and for whatever it may take.

Lyme Disease takes away other things too, besides your health, it takes away dreams and plans, relationships, friends, family, relatives, employment. Goals that at one time were within reach, now a distant far-going thought!

Let it take it all but my dream to know somewhere deep within you, that you are going to get better, maybe not today, maybe not tomorrow…not next month, or perhaps not next year, but hold onto that dream, for there is nothing else but to Hope and with that, we can, we will go on, somehow, some way.

My dreams live within the **Blanket of Hope** project and all of you are keeping that dream alive in your participation. Something so strong inside, I know that I and you – that all of us, can make it!

[Information about Brin's Blanket of Hope, and his personal story about Lyme can be found in Appendix A of this book, and in book II of this series, respectively.]

❖ ❖ ❖

From Glenroy Wolfsen, New Jersey

"For Julie"

The stately mansions of cold
Have set their pillars
Solid among the grains of sand
And the sweet juniper needles

Where she used to play
But the sun remembers
The brilliant days
Her tiny hands heard angels
In the songs of birds
And quiet shores watched
As at evening, with the gulls
She learned to fly away

❖ ❖ ❖

From Karl Odden, Connecticut

"A Period of Life Taken, Never Returned"

Unbeknownst to those near and afar
  my heart is pained.
In a world of its own tumult, I know not why.
For my hands are not part of my body,
  for only mere gasps of connectedness...they are not mine.
For, I, they were the strongest;
  ruthless in the battles of years passing...
  present...they are not mine.
Unbeknownst to the world
  my head...my mind is in captivity
  lost without reason,
  pained as my heart.
  Only, its world lies between the times
  purely of happiness and truthful grief,
  onto which my heart aches deeply
  amidst tight embracing emotions...
  Sweet memories in the days and nights, until slighted.
  For my Daughter so delights the apeasing ache
  to ease the time
  amidst the grief and her new hopes
  shine through my darkened eyes.
So, I dream for the life prior with all my physical wealth
  to keep her hopes and joys of what Father means.
Unbeknownst to those near and afar
  I am weak of mind and body, pushing each by the hour...
   ...and the glimpses of happiness do continue....forth.

For, they give me hope charging through the losses
and I strive to steady myself...again...
inside the unbeknownst...

❖ ❖ ❖

More From Glenroy Wolfsen, New Jersey

"A Matter of Time"

Sometimes you can see
The little events
Fall into place
Like pieces of a puzzle
But myopia keeps us
From a vision of the whole
Where life is guided
By an unseen hand
Only by a careful look back
Over the trail our feet have left
Can we sometimes deduce
That indeed there was a plan
If this then
Can become a parcel of our faith
When in trouble, worry or sorrow
It will only be a matter of time
We will know without a doubt
That accidents and fate
Were Divine Providence in disguise.

❖ ❖ ❖

"Leaves"

Showing their tops above the stonewall
Running along the river
The fragile branches poke up
With thirteen green-yellow leaves left
Before the snow falls tomorrow
Through beginning clouds
Light and thin,
The afternoon sun shines through the fine leaves
Making transparent with inner veins

Spreading out from stem to leaf ends.
The paths of nourishment
The fibers of life
That made them what they are.
So they stand this afternoon
Revealed in a golden oriental beauty
Soon to fade in the setting sun.
Could I so find the grace
To evoke such delicate truth as they
So transparent as they
That all could know the fibers
That have made me what I am.

❖ ❖ ❖

"This Fool"

I remember
When my day light
Seemed like night
Where each time
There came a point to try
Only left-over visions
Led the way.
Forward was an illusion,
Yet even a hope
But more a dream
That a fool kept beside him for comfort.
Here tonight I dream again.
This time I don't even hope
For another hand holds the light
As I decide to walk where it leads me
In the darkness.
Invisible –
Tomorrow waits and this fool asks:
Can I accept
Whatever the gift,
Whatever the light reveals,
Whatever becomes
A destiny?

❖ ❖ ❖

From the Ryan Guerin Family, North Carolina

"Homesick"

There was a soul – in Heaven once
Eternally happy, with no wants.
The Love of God filled his needs
But compassion called from desperate pleas.
There were others who left – by choice to be
What God needed on Earth – You see
But temptation was great – it created hate
And caused some souls to choose a fate
That put God last – and bodies first
Causing spirit hunger and homesick thirst.
One sould of many asked our Lord,
Can I please go to renew your word,
To help just one to be restored, to life eternal with You, O Lord.
Amen My Son, as You Request,
  but here is Home and do not resist.
When your journey is over and you hear My plea
Come home my "Ry," I want you with Me.
And so this soul – a body born, his name is Ryan, a gift to all
For he gave himself – to stop the fall
Of those who wanted only good,
  But weakened in their earthy call.
He chose addiction as his thorn,
  Amazing grace found him reborn,
To help so many drowing in scorn.
Disease attacked with crippling pain,
  he fought the evil till sick and lame
But his selfless Love was always plain.
He was kind and gentle and made us laugh,
With his boat and hat and cigarette pack
His nephews and nieces will all agree
What an Uncle he was – and now he's free.
We are blessed to know he was a sainted gift
To family, friends and those adrift.
But as time grew near – for Ryan to pick
He choose God's lap – he was just homesick

❖ ❖ ❖

After Word from the Ryan Guerin Family

Do not insulate yourself,
Do not isolate yourself,
But instead, demonstrate your need to seek help
And you will lift yourself and those around you,
By your quiet example,
To a higher level of compassion and spirituality;
Therein, you will discover
The infinite and intimate
Love of God.

❖ ❖ ❖

The Author Comments

Tick-borne illness has taken its toll on my extended family, children and friends, jobs, homes, marriages, finances, health, credit, reputation, trust, and so much more. I know what it feels like to get out of bed and fall to the floor when legs won't work. I have struggled to hold a pencil and write my name or remember where the keys are on the piano or the computer, even though I have been playing and/or typing for years. I have driven my car and forgotten where I was going, but drove on in quiet panic, attempting to jog some memory which seemed to sit stubbornly beyond the grasp of my reach like an obstinate child. I struggled for the right words in conversation, have written words and transposed them, or read words on a page that suddenly disappeared, making the pages appear blank. I have re-read the same paragraph over and over until frustration and momentary lack of comprehension forced me to abandon the task. I have read and re-read street signs, each time transcribing a different phrase as my brain struggled to make sense of the jumbled letters.

I know how it feels to misjudge distances when I can't see well, and I have hit the garage door with my car while onlookers laughed at my "inability" to drive. I have had the embarrassment of trying to get into the wrong vehicle because I have forgotten which car I took to the store and assumed the first green one was mine; and when my mind cleared, I saw the car wasn't mine, nor the right model or color, for that matter. I have tried to open my back door with a house key that was really the garage key, but when selected, it certainly looked like the house key to me. I have struggled to recall my children's names or my telephone number when those are things that should be permanently etched in my brain. And people have said "are you there" to me on the phone in a moment of quiet to check if I am still there, when my brain had quietly seized for a moment, transporting me to a distant void of "blankness" momentarily prohibiting perception of both thought and sound.

I have listened to physician after physician tell me my illness is ***all in my head,*** or any of a number of misdiagnoses which shamed and humiliated me into submission for a period of time because I thought "doctor knows best." Fortunately I have come to realize that doctors are human beings, and we are all fallible.

I have prayed, screamed, cried, pleaded, and begged God for assistance and mercy; to "take" me or to cure me – and received what seemed like very little in reply at the moment. And in quiet surrender I finally said, "God, not what I will, but what thou will for me." I have spent many days in bed unable to eat, drink or bathe because I have been so ill that I felt I was in a hole so deep I would never get out alive. I know what it's like to require a wheelchair or a cane, though fortunately the former was only a short-term assignment due to intractable fatigue. I know how frightening it is to have no bodily movement at all from the neck down, or be ambulatory and suddenly unable to walk across the living room floor. I have experienced failing mental faculties and the bewildering fear that comes from knowing you knew something yesterday but can no longer remember it today, when the next day things are strangely once again, quite clear.

I have felt the sting of embarrassment when nurses rolled their eyes at me because I demanded they wash their hands before handling IV equipment or to slow down the infusion pump because the medication flow rate was "too uncomfortable" inside my heart. I have passed out during home infusions with no one to help me when my blood pressure fell too low. I have awakened to find several hours have passed and the infusion pump beeping at me to disconnect. I have had neighbors make rude comments about my "lounging around in my hammock all day," instead of being at work at a "real" job when I can barely eat, walk, sleep, or function; and they have no clue how ill I truly am because I "don't look sick." I have felt humiliated when major medical centers have told me "we don't know," and then sent me home, literally starving to death.

I know the difficulty of combing hair (even when falling out), brushing your (bleeding) teeth or dressing yourself when you have unremitting pain and cannot lift your arms without tears. I have struggled to function with horrible head pain that I would gladly trade for the world's worst migraine. When my face was paralyzed and I struggled to speak slurred words in public, I felt the sting of embarrassment as store clerks averted their eyes from my disfigured face. I have felt the humiliation of trying to find a hospital willing to pull an infected picc line from my arm when my physician dropped me in the middle of IV treatments after feeling threatened by the insurance company.

I have suffered the indignities of lost bladder or bowel control and having to excuse myself from family functions for illness that I was at a loss to explain in short, palatable detail to those who would never understand. I have heard "are you still sick" from well-meaning relatives who dismissively compared their symptoms to mine. I have listened to comments like, "I know someone who had that 'Lyme's' disease too but they're all better, how come you're still sick, can't they give you something for that?" I watched countless doctors scowl, and relatives' eyes glaze over in indifference when I try to explain my illness or symptoms to them. I have watched my children deteriorate before my eyes and have been powerless by virtue of the court system and jurisdictional and other people's intellectual impotence, to help them. I was humiliated before a court of law many times over a decade because it vehemently denies my illness, and instead, prefers to ridiculously label me as "Lyme-obsessed, delusional," or a "Munchausen's By Proxy" mother, when none of that is actually true nor do they have any evidence whatsoever of same.

I know the devastation, isolation and loneliness that comes from having Lyme disease and tick-borne illnesses in an arena where credence is restricted or nonexistant and illness is denied for political and personal agendas. I can tell you without hesitation that having Lyme disease is no relaxing walk in the woods – which for many of us, is how we became infected in the first place. My sense of isolation in this illness was what originally drove me to reach out to others, and found support groups and web sites for Lyme patients, but also to find for myself, some comfort that I and my family were not alone.

During that journey which began following my diagnosis in December 2004, I began collecting Lyme patient's personal stories and published them on the web site, *www.lymeleague.com*. That effort grew into hundreds of stories from ill people all over the world – the unacknowledged epidemic, collectively on the same journey, with a most uncertain destination.

Lyme disease, and any chronic illnesses for that matter, are a journey of the soul. From being chronically ill, many of us have learned a better sense of self, a greater spirituality, a better acceptance of our limitations and of others, and pride in our collective ability to withstand the continued onslaught of so many intrusions, (medically, personally, financially, etc.). I thought I had patience before, but I find that illness requires *extreme* patience, despite a vulnerability to irritation (though thankfully for me much less frequent than in the past). I have gained knowledge in many areas, and friends I would never have known on a journey that has enriched my life in more ways than I can possibly quantify, though it has been a true test of inner fortitude.

It is for the hundreds of thousands of people who struggle with this common, growing, and unacknowledged **global epidemic** that continues to motivate me (and others) to assist in any way possible. If the collective "we" can utilize the knowledge gained from our personal struggles to **illuminate Lyme disease from the patient's perspective**, then perhaps doctors will begin listening to their patients at the onset of their illness, and offer treatments which can prevent or minimize disability.

Maybe governments, agencies, societies, academicians, and pharmaceutical and insuranec corporations will finally, intelligently and compassionately review their policies and practices and change them in favor of the very ill masses over the highly financially-motived, self-interested few. Perhaps legislature will be enacted to protect patients' rights as well as their treating physicians, who are courageous enough to treat, but who currently do so at great personal and professional risk. Maybe patients will finally receive the credence this illness deserves by opening the eyes of those who willfully and repeatedly, or perhaps innocently, refuse to see.

If within this process we can make one person's road to wellness just a little shorter or easier than we have found for ourselves, than the struggles we have endured, for most of us, will have been completely worthwhile.

❖ ❖ ❖

In Closing

From the perspective of many, we are only the patient, so what do we know? By clinicians and researchers alike, we and our symptoms are often referred to as **anecdotal evidence.** In truth, whether you choose to believe this or not, **patients are largely and keenly aware of what is going on inside of our own bodies.** And although we utilize mediums such as the internet and research libraries to help identify our symptoms and discover what is wrong with us, we base our quest for knowledge off of **real, and not imaginery symptoms.**

If you found that this book effectively communicated stories on behalf of these patients, then we invite you to learn more about this illness. Book II in this series, titled, *"It's All In Your Head, Around the World in 80 Lyme Patient Stories,"* is available and takes an intimate look at living with Lyme disease from the perspective of 80 patients from 23 U.S. states, 5 Canadian Provinces/Territories, and 11 countries abroad. Book III of the series, *"The Baker's Dozen and the Lunatic Fringe – How 'Junk Science' Shifted the Lyme Paradigm,"* is an intimate comparison of the history of Lyme disease and how scientific knowledge and academicians have changed the way we perceive this unrealized epidemic infectious disease.

We collectively hope these stories create an impact on your knowledge of Lyme disease and how patients are subjected to untold cruelties and ignorance from the very physicians and systems they look to for guidance and treatment. Indeed the very mention of the words "Lyme disease" in many doctors' offices brings immediate denial and dismissal; and sometimes, even outward aggression toward patients. Fortunately for Lyme patients, there are physicians who remain steadfast in their willingness to treat us, and they are the ones who are saving countless lives.

Patients are keenly aware of the firestorm of controversy surrounding the current CDC Lyme disease *surveillance* guidelines, and the recently published revised IDSA diagnostic and treatment guidelines for Lyme disease. We are aware of other parties' unseemly interests in keeping the words "Lyme disease" swept neatly under the carpet and who work to ridicule patients and their treating physicians alike.

We are aware of the use of scare tactics such as threats of investigation, government monitoring of IP addresses and internet access, and human "trolls" on Lyme newsgroups and support boards, who have individuals paid to enter those mediums to disseminate false and misleading information and discredit advocates. We have seen continual denigration of doctors and patients, especially through manipulation of the media and through medical board proceedings.

We are aware of certain people keeping tabs on who publishes articles "for" or "against" them, and of the media sources which write seemingly heavily-biased articles in support of a few powerful individuals who want Lyme disease patients and their doctors silenced. And we wonder where is the justice when physicians die under "mysterious" circumstances; or for patients who receive death threats just for talking about Lyme disease. Or perhaps for physicians who lose their license to practice due to medical boards who for "some reason," seem overly focused on ousting innocent doctors when they themselves do not appear to understand either Lyme pathology or human compassion.

We watch helplessly as those in power arrest people who attempt to bring the truth about Lyme to light and cringe as we watch social services remove custody of children from Lyme parents in retaliation for outspokenness, or worse, (as in my family's case), merely *having that illness in the first place.*

We witness women (especially) tragically being accused of being "delusional," having "stress, menopause," or "hypochondriasis" or "Munchausen's By Proxy" if they attempt to obtain Lyme treatment for themselves or their very ill children. And we rally together to protest the refusal of certain members of medical establishments who refuse to acknowledge that our illness is real and that patients deserve to be treated and not dismissed.

The stories in the book series should prove that Lyme Disease is not merely a knee or rash problem that subsists after 30 days treatment; or some autoimmune disorder which persists after "proper" treatment in a subset of people. The people in these books have circumstances which reach outside the margins of the current case definitions and treatment guidelines, and are proof positive that the larger picture of Lyme disease illness has yet to be addressed as epidemic numbers increase.

We are dismayed and frustrated as we watch members of state and federal legislators kill Bills meant to deliver important research dollars into the hands of those who might help find a cure for our illness, or protections for our Lyme-treating physicians. Some of these individuals seem to support the protection of the insurance and pharmaceutical machines over their constituents. Perhaps some of these same individuals help keep the veil of ignorance safely concealing any possible government or research academician involvement or private agendas which may run contrary to healing thousands.

We continually and actively protest the ill-treatment of our doctors whose only crime is one of stepping into the spotlight and daring to treat their very ill patients, something the hippocratic oath in fact, asks them to do. Perhaps we should remind certain people of portions of the words of that oath:

...To look upon his children as my own brothers...

...I will prescribe regimens for the good of my patients according to my ability and my judgment and never do harm to anyone...

...To please no one will I prescribe a deadly drug nor give advice which may cause his death...

...In every house where I come I will enter only for the good of my patients, keeping myself far from all intentional ill-doing...

...If I keep this oath faithfully, may I enjoy my life and practice my art, respected by all men and in all times; but if I swerve from it or violate it, may the reverse be my lot."[204]

I would like to suggest to certain researchers, members of world governments, medical board members, Lyme-denying physicians; pharmaceutical, insurance, disability, and legislative representatives, judges, social workers, psychologists, attorneys and members of society to consider the following:

If allowed to walk in the shoes of Lyme patients for just one week, you would immediately alter your opinions in favor of treating Lyme disease for as long as is absolutely necessary to eradicate it, and cause funding to be distributed for research and a cure. You simply cannot truly understand what it's like to lose your health, home, job, finances, friends, family, reputation and personal dignity from this disease unless and until you have been there, done that, and as one patient said, "got the T-shirt," yourself.

For Lyme-literate, and other physicians who *are* willing to treat patients with tick-borne infections, we extend a heartfelt **"thank you."** One patient specifically asked if I would ask all physicians to consider offering free patient care to those who have minimal or no medical insurance, for at least *one day a month,* or perhaps *a few hours a month.* This time might be dedicated soley to the diagnosis and treatment of tick-borne illnesses in patients who are otherwise unable to get help due to financial constraints. In this manner, you would be providing a tremendous service to very ill persons, many who are in financial dire straits through no fault of their own, all because they contracted tick-borne illnesses, and they have no other options.

We hope that these stories have helped shed light on this barely acknowledged, very misunderstood disease which, in the near future, will come to be known as the **largest and most prolific epidemic in the world.** And I hope that you take away from these books, several things. Compassion for the very ill, anger at the way the politics are preventing patients from being cured, and hope that the stories herein will illuminate the minds of those who are still in the dark about Lyme disease. This book series has been a collaborative effort to illustrate the plight of Lyme patients from all walks of life who say, "I dare to have a voice." Though many of us "don't look sick," we assure you that we truly are, and are sadly in need of understanding and credence – from our governments, our physicians, our researchers, our agencies, our communities and our family and friends.

The bottom line from the patients who are living with Lyme is this: **It is not "all in our heads." Tick-borne illness is real, and chronic Lyme exists, and we wish to be made well.** And despite a large body of evidence and research to support real illness, a select group of individuals choose to ignore it or slow-play the epidemic, instead. From the patients' perspective, when it comes to the current world opinion and medical guidelines for Lyme disease diagnostic and treatment purposes, we think we deserve so much better than that which we currently are receiving. After reading the stories in this book series, **wouldn't you agree?**

❖ ❖ ❖

My final statements regarding the issue of Lyme disease and the denial surrounding same are these:

- We are real people living with real disease.
- We need guidelines to assist us by allowing freedom of choice and open-ended treatment.
- We need on-going research and therapies designed to cure us, not to dismiss us.
- We need those in the medical community to acknowledge our illness and stop telling us "It's All In Your Head," because clearly it is not.
- We need to educate academicians who refuse to look outside of controlled studies and who dismiss the patient population and research that goes against their personal viewpoints or agendas.
- We need insurance companies (and disability) to be willing to pay for our medical ills without preferential diagnoses.
- We need to stop those who are trading human life for profit and self-interests – **that is the real epidemic.**

❖ ❖ ❖

Appendix A:
"The Blanket of Hope"
by Brin King

As many have heard and perhaps read about in the past along with information in this book, the "Blanket of Hope" project for Lyme disease, is a unified "voice" which reaches out far across this country as well as around the world. From large metropolitans to villages, suburbs to rural areas; it extends to the rich, middle class and to the poor. Lyme disease knows no boundaries, no religion, race, age nor specific country. The Blanket of Hope project was "born" in January 1993.

This project is a huge undertaking and an idea whose time has come. This was an idea by and through all people with Lyme disease. It is fabricated from my anger, from their anger, from our frustration and pain, and the many, many questions coming from experiencing the brunt of an illness called Lyme. Let it not be mistaken for anything less!

This project is to meet head-on, the ignorance, stupidity, and egotistical people from all walks of life who wish to close their eyes and ears and turn their backs and think that by walking away, they can shut out Lyme disease, and that it will eventually go away. It won't go away until we the people, the survivors, yell "I am a Lyme victim!"

This "Blanket of Hope" began with one piece of material, just as the smallest ray of hope is born and begins – one name, one state and date of when the disease was contracted, printed onto material. Each blanket panel is sewn together as a collectively large blanket (and voice). This blanket has grown and will continue to do so, from community to community, from small towns to large cities, from many states and countries. In this manner the many who suffer in silence as well as those who can speak, will be heard and will no longer be drummed out by rhetoric or empty facts and words. They will be replaced by research, by a strong and solid pursuit not only for answers, but for a cure, once and for all, for everyone who has Lyme – as well as the possibility of a vaccine for those who may still contract it.

I sincerely hope in the days and weeks, months and years to come, that the blanket will come to unite a world, and I firmly believe it will. For as we speak now, another person goes undiagnosed, is misdiagnosed, or has come to give up the fight in their struggle with Lyme disease.

Let us not die to be heard. Let us not cry in vain. Let us be one unified voice and a very big voice.

Every voice big and small will be heard at every lab, in every household, hospital, clinic, and every insurance office. From the mailman to the surveyor, to the housewife and the child on the playground, to the woodcutter and construction worker, the meter reader and the forest Ranger, to the hiker and camper, to the runner and the railroad yard worker. I pray as we all do, for a cure, but until then, all I ask for is direction to keep going forward and I will continue to hope and be a part of the "Blanket of Hope."

How to contribute to the "Blanket of Hope"

The blanket consists of 4 feet x 4 feet panels made of a material of your choice.

Each blanket panel contains the first and last name of the Lyme victim(s), and the date that Lyme was contracted, and city, state and/or country where contracted. Please allow a 3 inch border around the perimeter of the blanket which is used to join blanket panels together. You may add any designs you want to the blanket. You may sew, use markers, or anything you wish to record the information on the blanket panel and decorate it.

When finished, please mail the blanket directly to Brin where your panel will be joined with the many others already received.

Mail to:
Brin King
222 Mill Street
Yorkville, IL 60560

As Brin began to receive blanket panels, he sent this statement out to Lyme disease support groups, to doctors, and to businesses all over:

Let the word go forth. Let the word go out across the land, to every home, to every hospital and clinic, to every level of medical personnel far and wide, to every insurance company and their underwriters, as well as to every lawyer, pharmaceutical company and politician: "The Blanket of Hope," the unified voice of a nation on Lyme disease is growing in leaps and bounds and the drum beat is getting louder. No longer will we, those of us with Lyme disease, be ignored. No longer will we be silent on a rapidly spreading, devastating disease. No longer is it the voice of one person, of one support group, one town or city, nor one state, but now of every state! No longer is it the voice of one country, one nation, but the UNIFIED VOICE of the Blanket of Hope, coming together around the world.

The blanket's current size is estimated to contain over 9,960 panels and is approximately the size of **6 football fields**. In order to move and show the blanket, the costs are expensive, and it requires special permits, and an 18-wheeled flatbed truck. The blanket has only been shown twice due to the cost of moving it. Both showings were in 1995, with one presentation in Chicago's Grant Park, and the other in Washington D.C.

Please support this worthy project and send in your 4 feet x 4 feet panel to join with others to become part of the **UNITED VOICE OF LYME DISEASE.**

❖ ❖ ❖

About the Author

PJ Langhoff is a prolific writer, editor, and medical researcher for many books and articles, many on tick-borne illness. She is a columnist for the Public Health Alert newsletter, a medical on-line and print newsletter (www.publichealthalert.org). She also writes, edits and researches medical books, articles, and special projects for physicians and other parties as a ghostwriter. She operates a small press, and publishes books for herself and others in medicine and other genres. Her books are available at www.AllegoryPress.com, Lulu.com/lyme, Amazon.com, and other book sellers.

She is a mother of 2 young adults, an ordained minister, and has had (confirmed) Lyme disease for over a decade and a half. Her children both "allegedly" have Lyme disease and/or other tick-borne illnesses. PJ runs a Midwest region informational support group for Lyme sufferers, an international web site which collects patient stories, and performs limited prevention outreach services. She offers patient support (gratis) as part of her ministry services.

PJ is also active as an advocate for Lyme-treating physicians and meets with legislators to enact Lyme- and alternative physician-friendly legislation at the state and federal level. She is an active writer, designer, equestrian, gardener, painter, musician, and animal lover, despite being disabled by Lyme and co-infections.

With the proceeds of her projects, she will be contributing to a fund which will enable Lyme patients who cannot otherwise afford the cost of diagnostic testing, to be provided with funds to receive no cost, or reduced-cost diagnostic testing; and providing funds for other Lyme-related charities.

More books by this author:

**"It's All In Your Head," Around the World in 80 Lyme Patient Stories, Valid Reasons to Debate Current Treatment Guidelines* (Book II)

**The Baker's Dozen & the Lunatic Fringe: How "Junk Science" Shifted the Lyme Disease Paradigm* (Book III)

**The Singing Forest, a Journey Through Lyme Disease*

**Right Behind You, Spiritual Helpers from Beyond the Earth Plane*

*Available at: Allegorypress.com, Lulu.com, Amazon.com

Scientific Journal Articles by this author:

Schaller JL, Burkland GA, Langhoff PJ. *Are various Babesia species a missed cause for hypereosinophilia? A follow-up on the first reported case of imatinib mesylate for idiopathic hypereosinophilia.* MedGenMed**.** 2007 Feb 27;9(1):38. Available at: www.pubmed.gov.

Schaller JL, Burkland GA, Langhoff PJ. *Do Bartonella Infections Cause Agitation, Panic Disorder, and Treatment-Resistant Depression?* MedGenMed. 2007:9(3):54. Available at: http://www.medscape.com/viewarticle/562276.

The Author Recommends

A ground-breaking movie about Lyme: *"Under Our Skin, The Untold Story of Lyme Disease"* by Open Eye Pictures. http://www.openeyepictures.org/underourskin/index.html

Public Health Alert News – Investigating Lyme Disease & Chronic Illness Throughout the U.S.A. Available in print and on-line, with the latest information on chronic illnesses www.publichealthalert.org

The Use of the Herb Artemisinin for Babesia, Malaria, and Cancer, All the Practical Information You Need to Make Smart Decisions on Artemisinin, by Dr. James Schaller, edited by PJ Langhoff

The Diagnosis and Treatment of Babesia, Lyme's Cruel Cousin: the OTHER Tick-borne Infection, by Dr. James Schaller, edited by PJ Langhoff

The Lyme Times Journal of the California Lyme Disease Association www.lymetimes.org

Lyme in Rhyme and *The Flu and You,* two books by Geri Rodda, RN Available at Nmroddas@aol.com

Fighting my War and Keeping my Peace, by Paula Masso Carnes. Available at: www.PaulaCarnes.com

Coping with Lyme Disease: A Practical Guide to Dealing with Diagnosis and Treatment by Denise Lang and Kenneth Liegner. Available at Amazon.com

Death in the Air. Globalism, Terrorism & Toxic Warfare by Dr. Leonard G. Horowitz. Available at Tetrahedron Publishing Group, PO Box 2033, Sandpoint, ID 83864.

Helpful Links

www.ilads.org International Lyme and Associated Diseases Society. A Lyme-literate physician organization

www.columbia-lyme.org
Lyme Disease research at Columbia (NY) University Medical Center

www.openeyepictures.com/underourskin/index.html Open Eye Pictures Presents "Under Our Skin The Untold Story of Lyme Disease"

www.timeforlyme.org A nonprofit research, education and advocacy network

www.Canlyme.com Canadian Lyme Disease Foundation
Jim Wilson, President

www.bada-uk.org Borreliosis and Associated Diseases Awareness (UK)

www.molecularalzheimer.org A useful ollection of tick-borne images and research information

www.lymeleague.com International site to post your personal story about Lyme Disease, and read stories from other Lyme patients

www.sewill.org U.S. midwest region information support group (WI/IL/MN)

http://health.groups.yahoo.com/group/lyme_league/
Lyme League of North America Support Group at Yahoo

www.lymeblog.com For posting and reading blogs about Lyme disease

www.lymediseaseassociation.org Lyme Disease Association (LDA)

www.personalconsult.com Dr. James Schaller offers extensive free medical information on tick-borne and other illnesses, and excellent medical books on tick-borne illnesses and other subjects for a general and pediatric audience

www.lymedisease.org California Lyme Disease Association (CALDA)

www.lymenet.org Lyme support network

www.angelflight.com Angel Flight, Inc. People flying people in need of transportation (mainly the heartland region of the US)

www.chronicneurotoxins.com Information on chronic human illness caused by exposure to biotoxins

References

1. Godofsky E, Godofsky B. Performance of Clinical Trials in Private Practice. [slide presentation on the web]. Available from: http://www.idsociety.org/content/contentgroups/annual_meeting1/2004/presentations1/godofsky.pdf. Accessed 2007 Mar 28.
2. Steere AC, Coburn J, Glickstein L. The Emergence of Lyme Disease. J Clin Invest. 2004 Apr 15;113(8):1093-1101. Available at: http://www.pubmedcentral.nih.gov/articlerender.fcgi?tool=pmcentrez&artid=385417.
3. Carroll MC. Lab 257. The disturbing story of the government's secret germ laboratory. 2005. Harper paperback. [book].
4. Verdon R. Lyme Disease and the SS Elbrus. 2002. Elderberry Press.
5. Navokov VA, Sadovnikov AI, Uspenskii IV. Using a helicopter for dusting forest sources of tick-borne encephalitis. Foreign Technology Div. Wright-Patterson AFB OH. 1970 Feb 20. Access at: http://stinet.dtic.mil. Accessed 2007 Sep. 30.
6. Verdon R. Lyme Disease and the SS Elbrus. 2002. Elderberry Press.
7. Altman LK. Annual Exam Gives Bush Good Marks For Health. The NY Times. [web page]. Access at: http://www.nytimes.com. Accessed 2007 Aug 10.
8. Puhakka HJ, Laurikainen E, Viljanen M, Meurman O, Valkama H. Peripheral facial palsy caused by Borrelia burgdorferi and viruses in south-western Finland. Acta Otolaryngol Suppl. 1992;492:103-6.
9. Sauvaget E. Tran Ba Huy P. [Deafness of infectious origin]. [Article in French]. Rev Prat. 2000 Jan 15;50(2):150-5.
10. Cook SP, Macartney KK, Rose CD, Hunt PG, Eppes SC, Reilly JS. Lyme disease and seventh nerve paralysis in children. Am J Otolaryngol. 1997 Sep-Oct;15(5):320-3.
11. Walther LE, Hentschel H, Oehme A, Gudziol H, Beleites E. [Lyme disease-a reason for sudden sensoineural hearing loss and vestibular neuronitis?]. [Article in German]. Laryngorhinootologie. 2003 Apr;82(4):249-57.
12. Ishizaki H, Pyykkö I, Nozue M. Neuroborreliosis in the etiology of vestibular neuronitis. Acta Otolaryngol Suppl. 1993;503:67-9.

13. NIAID. Lyme Disease. NIAID Research: Transmission of Lyme Disease, 2007 [web page]. Access at: http://www3.niaid.nih.gov/research/topics/lyme/research/transmission. Accessed 2007 Mar 20.
14. Schwan TG, Piesman J. Vector Interactions and Molecular Adaptations of Lyme Disease and Relapsing Fever Spirochetes Associated with Transmission by Ticks. Perspective. NIH/CDC. [serial on the internet]. 2007. Accessed 2007 Mar 14. Available at: http://www.cdc.gov/ncidod/eid/vol8no2/01-0198.htm.
15. From CDC Image library photo #5968 caption. Available at: http://phil.cdc.gov/phil
16. Lyme Times. CALDA. Summer 2004;37-38:19.
17. Australian Department of Medical Entomology. [Web page]. 2007. Available at: http://meent.usyd.edu.au/fact/ticks.htm.
18. RedOrbit. New Tick Killers Avoid Widespread Spraying. 2005 Jul 30. Associated Press/AP Online. [web page]. Available at: http://www.redorbit.com/news/health/192283/new_tick_killers_avoid_widespread_spraying/index.html. Accessed 2007 Apr 3.
19. LDF. LDF Scientific Advisors (Current and Past). [web page]. Available at: http://lyme.org/ldf/advisors.html. Accessed 2007 Apr 3.
20. Alvey S. '4-Poster' Bait Stations Reduce Deer Ticks, Disease. U.S. Army Environmental Command. Environmental Update. 2006 Fall. [web page]. Available at: http://ac.army.mil/usaec/publicaaffairs/update/fall06/fall0610.html. Accessed 2007 Apr 3.
21. ALDF. About ALDF. [web page]. 2006. Available at: http://www.aldf.com/about.shtml. Accessed 2007 Mar 24.
22. Wormser GP, Dattwyler RJ, Shapiro ED, et al. The Clinical Assessment, Treatment, and Prevention of Lyme Disease, Human Granulocytic Anaplasmosis, and Babesiosis: Clinical Practice Guidelines by the Infectious Diseases Society of America. Clinical Infectious Diseases 2006;43:1089-1134.
23. Wormser GP, Nadelman RB, Dattwyler RJ, Dennis DT, Shapiro ED, Steere AC, Rush TJ, Rahn DW, Coyle PK, Persing DH, Fish D, Luft BJ. Practice Guidelines for the Treatment of Lyme Disease. Clinical Infect Dis. 2000;31:1-14. Access at: http://www.journals.uchicago.edu/CID/journal/issues/v31nS1/000342/000342.html. Accessed 2007 Mar 30.
24. LDF. LDF Scientific Advisors (Current and Past). [web page].

Available at: http://lyme.org/ldf/advisors.html. Accessed 2007 Apr 3.
25. Howenstine J. New Ideas About the Cause, Spread and Therapy of Lyme Disease. Townsend Letter for Doctors and Patients. 2004 July. Access at: www.samento.com.ec/sciencelib/4lyme/Townsendhowens.html.
26. Christian Gottfried Ehrenberg, From Wikipedia. [web page]. Access at: http://en.wikipedia.org/wiki/Christian_Gottfried_Ehrenberg. Accessed 2007 Mar 17.
27. Humber D. Piroplasms. [web page]. Access at: http://homepages.uel.ac.uk/D.P.Humber/piro.htm. Acccessed 2007 Mar 17.
28. Rawlings J, Burgdorfer W. 12th International Conference on Lyme Disease and Other Spirochetal and Tick-Borne Disorders, 1999 Apr 9. The Complexity of Vector-borne Spirochetes (Borrelia spp). Available at: http://www.medscape.com/viewarticle/429454.
29. Verdon R. Lyme Disease and the SS Elbrus. 2002. Elderberry Press.
30. Long River Winding Web Site, Available at: http://www.longriverwinding.com/polly_murray.htm. Accessed 2007 Feb. 24.
31. Murray P. The Widening Circle. St. Martin's Press. 1996.
32. Burrascano Jr. J. Advanced Topics in Lyme Disease. Diagnostic Hints and Treatment Guidelines for Lyme and other Tick Borne Illnesses. 15th Ed. 2005 Sept. Available at: http://ilads.org/files/burrascano_0905.pdf. Accessed 2007 Feb. 20.
33. Howenstine J. Lyme Disease Cause, Spread, Therapy. New Ideas About the Cause, Spread and Therapy of Lyme Disease. Townsend Letter for Doctors and Patients. 2004 July. Available at: http://www.samento.com.ec/sciencelib/4lyme/Townsendhowens.html.
34. MacDonald AB. The Molecular Link Between Alzheimer's Disease and Borrelia. [internet podcast]. Available at: http://www.medicalnewspodcast.com/media/stat071406.mp3. Accessed 2007 Mar 30.
35. MacDonald AB. Alzheimer's neuroborreliosis with trans-synaptic spread of infection and neurofibrillary tangles derived from intraneuronal spirochetes. Med Hypotheses. 2007;68(4):822-5. [Epub 2006 Oct. 20.] Available at: http://www.ncbi.nlm.nih.gov. Accessed 2007 Mar 30.
36. CDC. Lyme Disease Erythema Migrans. [web page] Available at: http://www.cdc.gov/ncidod/dvbid/lyme/ld_

LymeDiseaseRashPhotos.htm. Accessed 2007 Mar 15.
37. Burrascano J. Diagnostic hints and treatment guidelines for Lyme and other Tick Borne Illnesses. 2002 Nov. 14th Ed. From ILADS.org web site.
38. Burgdorfer W. From Penicillin to Mild Silver Protein An Answer to Lyme Disease Without Antibiotics. Rocky Mt. Laboratories, Div. Of NIH. Accessed at: http://www.xpressnet.com/bhealthy/burgd.html.
39. Fallon BA, Nields JA. Lyme disease: a neuropsychiatric illness. Am J Psychiatry, 1994 Nov;151(11):1571-83. Accessed 2007 Mar 14.
40. Picken RN, Strle F, Picken MM, et al. Identification of Three Species of Borrelia burgdorferi Sensu Lato (B. burgdorferi Sensu Stricto, B. garinii, and B. afzelii) Among Isolates from Acrodermatitis Chronica Atrophicans Lesions. Journal of Investigative Dermatology. 1998;110:211-214. Available at: http://www.nature.com/jid/journal/v110/n3/full/5602942a.html. Accessed 2007 Apr. 1.
41. Brzostek T. [Human granulocytic ehrlichiosis co-incident with Lyme borreliosis in pregnant woman – a case study]. [Article in Polish]. Przegl Epidemiol. 2004;58(2):289-94.
42. Goldenberg RL, Thompson C. The infectious origins of stillbirth. Am J Obstet Gynecol. 2003 Sep;189(3):861-73.
43. Maraspin V, Cimperman J, Lotric-furlan S, Pleterski-Rigler D, Strle F. Erythema migrans in pregnancy. Wien Klin Wochenschr. 1999 Dec 10;111(22-23):933-40.
44. Maraspin V, Cimperman J, Lotric-Furlan S, Pleterski-Rigler D, Strle F. Treatment of erythema migrans in pregnancy. Clin Infect Dis. 1996 May;22(5):788-93.
45. CDC. MMWR Weekly. Current Trends Update: Lyme Disease and Cases Occurring during Pregnancy – United States. 1985 Jun 28;34(25):376-8,383-4.
46. CDC. Lyme disease in pregnancy and in nursing mothers. Last update: 1999 Aug 1. Access at: http://wonder.cdc.gov/wonder/prevguid/p0000104/p0000104.asp.
47. Lyme Times. CALDA. Summer 2004;37-38:18.
48. MacDonald AB. The Molecular Link Between Alzheimer's Disease and Borrelia. [internet podcast]. Available at: http://www.medicalnewspodcast.com/media/stat071406.mp3. Accessed 2007

Mar 30.

49. MacDonald AB. Alzheimer's neuroborreliosis with trans-synaptic spread of infection and neurofibrillary tangles derived from intraneuronal spirochetes. Med Hypotheses. 2007;68(4):822-5. [Epub 2006 Oct. 20.] Available at: http://www.ncbi.nlm.nih.gov. Accessed 2007 Mar 30.
50. Steere AC, Coburn J, Glickstein L. The Emergence of Lyme Disease. J Clin Invest. 2004 Apr 15;113(8):1093-1101. Available at: http://www.pubmedcentral.nih.gov/articlerender.fcgi?tool=pmcentrez&artid=385417.
51. Galbally E. Warm weather means more ticks bearing Lyme disease. MN public radio [online]. 2001 Dec. 6. Available at: http://news.minnesota.publicradio.org/features/20012/06_galballye_ticks-m/. Accessed 2007 Apr 3.
52. Orloski KA, Hayes E, Campbell GL, et al. Surveillance for Lyme Disease – United States, 1992-1998. MMWR Surveillance Summaries. 2000 Apr 28;49(SS03):1-11. Available at: http://www.cdc.gov/mmwr/preview/mmwrhtml/ss4903a1.htm.
53. Howenstine J. Lyme Disease Cause, Spread, Therapy. New Ideas About the Cause, Spread and Therapy of Lyme Disease. Townsend Letter for Doctors and Patients. 2004 July. Available at: http://www.samento.com.ec/sciencelib/4lyme/Townsendhowens.html.
54. Surveillance for Lyme Disease—United States, 1992-1998. From MMWR Surveillance Summaries. CDC. 2000 Apr 28:49(SS03);1-11. Available from: http://www.cdc.gov/mmwr/preview/mmwrhtml/ss4903a1.htm. Accessed 2007 Feb. 27.
55. Seung-Hyun Lee, Bum-Joon Kim, Jong-Hyun Kim, Kyung-Hee Park, Seo-Jeong Kim, and Yoon-Hoh Kook. Differentiation of Borrelia burgdorferi Sensu Lato on the Basis of RNA Polymerase Gene (rpoB) Sequences. J Clin Microbiol. 2000 July;38(7):2557-2562. Available at: http://www.pubmedcentral.nih.gov. Accessed 2007 Apr 1.
56. Schwan TG, Piesman J. Vector Interactions and Molecular Adaptations of Lyme Disease and Relapsing Fever Spirochetes Associated with Transmission by Ticks. Perspective. NIH/CDC. [serial on the internet]. 2007. Accessed 2007 Mar 14. Available at: http://www.cdc.gov/ncidod/eid/vol8no2/01-0198.htm.
57. Mayberry LF, Canaris AG, Bristol JR, Gardner SL. 2000 Jan. Bibliography of Parasites and Vertebrate Hosts in Arizona,

New Mexico and Texas (1893-1984). Available at: http://www.museum.unl.edu/research/parasitology/UTEP-UNL/utep.pdf. Accessed 2007 Mar 24.
58. CALDA. The Lyme Times. Summer 2004;37-38:19.
59. CDC. Geographic Distribution of Potential Health Hazards to Travelers. 2005-2006. [web page]. Available at: http://www.2.ncid.cdc.gov/travel/yb/utils/ubGet.asp?sectoin=GHSection&obj=Europe. Accessed 2007 Mar 18.
60. Wilson, J. Canadian Lyme Disease Foundation. www.canlyme.com. Email communication. 2007 Feb.
61. Rodriguez I, Fernández C, Cinco M, Pedroso R, Fuentes O. Do antiborrelial antibodies suggest Lyme disease in Cuba? [letter] Emerg Infect Dis. [serial on the Internet]. 2004 Sep [2007 Mar 14]. Available from: http://www.cdc.gov/ncidod/EID/vol10no9/03-1048.htm.
62. CDC. Tick-Borne Relapsing Fever, What is it and How to Prevent it. [on-line pamphlet]. 2007. Available at: http://www.cdc.gov/ncidod/dvbid/RelapsingFever/Resources/TBRFBrochure1.pdf. Accessed 2007. Mar 25.
63. Yoshinari NH, Oyafuso LK, Monteiro FG, et al. Lyme disease. Report of a case observed in Brazil. Rev Hosp Clin Fac Med Sao Paulo. 1993 Jul-Aug;48(4):170-4. [Article in Portuguese].
64. Rawlings J, Burgdorfer W. 12th International Conference on Lyme Disease and Other Spirochetal and Tick-Borne Disorders, 1999 Apr 9. The Complexity of Vector-borne Spirochetes (Borrelia spp). Available at: http://www.medscape.com/viewarticle/429454.
65. Marvin S. Milner RM, Evans R. Chatterton JM, Joss AW, Ho-Yen DO. The use of local isolates in Western blots improves serological diagnosis of Lyme disease in Scotland. Microbiology Department, Raigmore Hospital, Old Perth Road, Inverness Iv23 UJ, UJ. J Med Microbiol. 2007 Jan;56(Pt 1):47-51. Available at: www.pubmed.gov.
66. Kyasanur Forest Disease Fact Sheet. CDC. Available at: http://www.cdc.gov/ncidod/dvrd/spb/mnpages/dispages/Fact_Sheets/KyasanurForestDis.pdf.
67. Schmid GP. The global distribution of Lyme disease. Rev Infect Dis. 1985 Jan-Feb;7(1):41-50. [Abstract]. Available at: http://www.ncbi.nlm.nih.gov.
68. Australian Department of Medical Entomology. Available at:

http://medent.usyd.edu.au/fact/lyme%20disease.htm#history.
69. Orloski KA, Hayes E, Campbell GL, et al. Surveillance for Lyme Disease – United States, 1992-1998. MMWR Surveillance Summaries. 2000 Apr 28;49(SS03):1-11. Available at: http://www.cdc.gov/mmwr/preview/mmwrhtml/ss4903a1.htm. Accessed 2007 Feb 27.
70. O'Connell S, Granstrom M, Gray JS, Stanek G. Epidemiology of European Lyme borreliosis. Zent bl Bakteriol 1998;287:229-40.
71. Grant AD, Eke B. Application of information technology to the laboratory reporting of communicable disease in England and Wales. Commun Dis Rep 1993;3:R75-8.
72. Trevisan G, Crovato F, Marcuccio C, Fumarola D, Scarpa C. Lyme disease in Italy. Zentralbl Bakteriol Mikrobiol Hyg [A]. 1987;263(3):459-63. Medscape Today. Available at: www.medscape.com/medline/abstract/3591098.
73. Steere AC, Coburn J, Glickstein L. The Emergence of Lyme Disease. J Clin Invest. 2004 Apr 15;113(8):1093-1101. Available at: http://www.pubmedcentral.nih.gov/ncidod/eid/vol6no4/smith.htm.
74. From CDC Image Library photo #3809 caption. Available at: http://phil.cdc.gov/phil.
75. Health Protection Agency. Lyme borreliosis in England and Wales: 2005. Zoonoses Lyme borreliosis 2005 data. Available at: http://www.hpa.org.uk/infections/topics_az/ zoonoses/lyme_borreliosis/Data_2005.htm.
76. Maraspin V, Ruzic-Sabljic E, Strle F. Lyme borreliosis and Borrelia spielmanii.[letter]. Emerg Infect Dis [serial on the Internet]. 2006 Jul. Accessed 2007 Feb 8. Available from: http://www.cdc.gov/ncidod/eid/vol12no07/06-0077.htm.
77. Ciceroni L, Ciarrocchi S. Lyme disease in Italy, 1983-1996. New Microbiol. 1998 Oct;21(4):407-18. Available from: http://www.ncbi.nlm.nih.gov/entrez/query.fcgi?db=pubmed&cmd=Retrieve&dopt=AbstractPlus&list_uids=9812324&query_hl=4&itool=pubmed_DocSum.
78. Trevisan G, Crovato F, Marcuccio C, Fumarola D, Scarpa C. Lyme disease in Italy. Zentralbl Bakteriol Mikrobiol Hyg [A]. 1987;263(3):459-63. Medscape Today. Available at: www.medscape.com/medline/abstract/3591098.
79. Sanogo Y, Zeaiter Z. Caruso G, et al. Bartonella henselae in Ixodes

ricinus Ticks (Acari: Ixodida) Removed from Humans, Belluno Province, Italy. Emerging Infectious Diseases. 2003;9(3):329-332.

80. Kruszewska D, Tylewska-Wierzbanowska S. Unknown species of rickettsiae isolated from Ixodes ricinus tick in Walcz. Rocz Akad Med Bialymst 1996;41:129-35.
81. Beltrame A, Ruscio M, Arzese A, et al. Human granulocytic anaplasmosis in northeastern Italy. Ann NY Acad Sci. 2006 Oct;1078:106-9. Pubmed. Available at: www.ncbi.nlm.nih.gov. Accessed 2007 Feb. 11.
82. Sanogo Y, Zeaiter Z. Caruso G, et al. Bartonella henselae in Ixodes ricinus Ticks (Acari: Ixodida) Removed from Humans, Belluno Province, Italy. Emerging Infectious Diseases. 2003;9(3):329-332.
83. J. Wilson. Canadian Lyme Disease Foundation. www.canlyme.com. Email communication. 2007 Feb.
84. Verdon R. Lyme Disease and the SS Elbrus. 2002. Elderberry Press.
85. Uspensky I. Ticks as the main target of human tick-borne disease control: Russian practical experience and its lessons. J Vector Ecol. 1999 Jun;24(1):40-53. Department of Biological Chemistry, A. Silberman Institute of Life Sciences, Hebrew University of Jerusalem, Israel.
86. Russia: South Urals prepare for tick encephalitis season. From Noviy Region, Russian Information Agency [trans. Mod.NP, edited] and received from ProMED newsgroup email (ISID.org). Accessed 2007 Mar 15.
87. de Sousa R, Barata C, Vitorino L, et al. Rickettsia sibirica Isolation from a Patient and Detection in Ticks, Portugal. Emerg Infect Dis [serial on the internet]. 2006 Jul. [Accessed 2007 Mar 14]. Available at: http://www.cdc.gov/ncidod/EID/vol12no07/05-1494.htm.
88. Wan K, Zhang Z, Dou G. Investigation on primary vectors of Borrelia burgdorferi in China. [article in Chinese]. 1998 Oct;19(5):263-6. [abstract] Available at: http://www.ncbi.nlm.nih.gov. Accessed 2007 Mar 25.
89. Ohashi N, Inayoshi M, Kitamura K, et al. Anaplasma phagocytophilum-infected Ticks, Japan. Emerg Infec Dis [serial on the internet]. 2005 Nov. [Accessed 2007 Mar 14]. Available at: http://

www.cdc.gov/ncidod/EID/vol11no11/05-04-7.htm.
90. Smith R, O'Connell S, Palmer S. Lyme Disease Surveillance in England and Wales, 1986-1998. CDC Emerging Infectious Diseases. Available at: http://www.cdc.gov/ncidod/eid/vol6no4/smith.htm.
91. Evans R, Mavin S, Ho-Yen DO. Audit of the laboratory diagnosis of Lyme disease in Scotland. J Med Microbiol. 2005;54:1139-1141. Available at: http://jmm.sgmjournals.org/cgi/content/full/54/12/1139. Accessed 2007 Mar 25.
92. Evans R, Mavin S, Ho-Yen DO. Audit of the laboratory diagnosis of Lyme disease in Scotland. Microbiology Department, NHS Highland, Raigmore Hospital, Inverness IV2 3UJ, UK. J Med Microbiol. 2005 Dec; 54(Pt 12):1139-41. Available at: http://med4um.com/about12405.html.
93. Zhang ZF, Wan KL, Zhang JS. Studies on epidemiology and etiology of Lyme disease in China. Institute of Epidemiology and Microbiology, Chinese Academy of Preventive Medicine, Beijing. Chung Hua Liu Hsing Ping Hsueh Tsa Chih 1997 Feb;18(1):8-11. Abstract.
94. Harris N. IGeneX Innovations. Available at: http://igenex.com/innovations1.htm.
95. [web page] http://www.lawestvector.org/erlichiosis.htm. Accessed 2007 Mar 5.
96. Holman MS, Caporale DA. Goldberg J. et al. Anaplasma phagocytophilum, Babesia microti, and Borrelia burgdorferi in Ixodes scapularis, Southern Coastal Maine. CDC Emerging Infectious Diseases. 2004 Mar 17. Available at: http://www.cdc.gov/ncidod/eid/vol10no4/03-0566.htm. Accessed 2007 Feb. 25.
97. Human Monocytic Ehrlichiosis. INHS Reports. 1996 Jan-Feb. [web page] Available at: http://www.inhs.uiuc.edu/inhsreports/jan-feb96/ticks.html.
98. Keysary A, Amram L, Keren G, et al. Serologic Evidence of Human Monocytic and Granulocytic Ehrlichiosis in Israel. 1999 Oct;5(6). [CDC web site.] Available from: http://www.cdc.gov/ncidod/eid/vol5no6/keysary.htm.
99. CDC. Geographic Distribution of Potential Health Hazards to Travelers. 2005-2006. [web page]. Available at: http://www.2.ncid.cdc.gov/travel/yb/utils/ubGet.asp?sectoin=GHSection&obj=Europe. Accessed 2007 Mar 18.

100. Human Ehrlichiosis in the United States. Signs and Symptoms. From the CDC web site. Available at: http://www.cdc.gov/ncidod/dvrd/ehlichia/Signs/Signs.htm.
101. Holman MS, Caporale DA. Goldberg J. et al. Anaplasma phagocytophilum, Babesia microti, and Borrelia burgdorferi in Ixodes scapularis, Southern Coastal Maine. CDC Emerging Infectious Diseases. 2004 Mar 17. Available at: http://www.cdc.gov/ncidod/eid/vol10no4/03-0566.htm. Accessed 2007 Feb. 25.
102. Schaller J, Burkland G, Langhoff PJ. Is Bartonella a Possible Cause of Agitation, Panic Disorder and Treatment-Resistant Depression? 2007. JAMA. Available at: http://www.Medscape.com. [Article in Press].
103. Sanogo Y, Zeaiter Z. Caruso G, et al. Bartonella henselae in Ixodes ricinus Ticks (Acari: Ixodida) Removed from Humans, Belluno Province, Italy. Emerging Infectious Diseases. 2003;9(3):329-332.
104. Bergmans AM; de Jong CM; van Amerongen G; Schot CS; Schouls LM. Prevalence of Bartonella species in domestic cats in The Netherlands. J Clin Microbiol. 1997 Sep; 35(9): 2256-61 . Available at: http://www.petalk.com/bartonella.html
105. Schaller J, Burkland G, Langhoff PJ. Is Bartonella a Possible Cause of Agitation, Panic Disorder and Treatment-Resistant Depression? 2007. JAMA. Available at: http://www.Medscape.com. [Article in Press].
106. Estrada B, Azithromycin and Cat-scratch Disease. Infections in Medicine. Infect Med 15(8):517, 1998. Cliggott Publishing, Division of SCP Communications. Available at: http://www.medscape.com/viewarticle/ 417381.
107. Regnery RL, et al: Lancet 1992; 339:1443-1445.
108. Brouqui P, Lascola B, Roux V, Raoult D. Chronic Bartonella Quintana Bacteremia in Homeless Patients. New Engl J of Med. 1999 Jan 21;340(3):184-189. Abstract. Available from: http://content.nejm.org/cgi/content/abstract/340/3/184.
109. Schaller J. The Diagnosis and Treatment of Babesia. 2006. Hope Academic: Tampa, FL. p. 17.
110. Herwaldt BL, Neitzel DF, Gorlin JB, et al. Transmission of Babesia microti in Minnesota through four blood donations from the same donor over a 6-month period. Div. of Parasitic Diseases, CDC and Prevention, Atlanta, GA. Transfusion. 2002;42(9):1154-

8. Available at: www.medscape.com/medline/abstract/12430672.
111. Schaller J. The Diagnosis and Treatment of Babesia. 2006. Hope Academic Press, Tampa FL. p. 13-14.
112. http://www.cartage.org.lb/en/themes/Biographies/MainBiographies/R/Ricketts/1.html
113. Chapman, AS. in collaboration with the Tickborne Rickettsial Diseases Working Group. Diagnosis and Management of Tickborne Rickettsial Diseases: Rocky Mountain Spotted Fever, Ehrlichioses, and Anaplasmosis – United States. MMWR Recommendations and Reports. 2006 Mar 31;55(RR-4). [web site report]. Available at: http://www.cdc.gov/mmwr/preview/mmwrhtml/rr5504a1.htm. Accessed 2007 Mar 23.
114. From Morbidity & Mortality Weekly Report. Tickborne Relapsing Fever Outbreak After a Family Gathering – New Mexico, August 2002. MMWR 52(34):809-812,2003 CDC. Available at: www.medscape.com/viewarticle/460740.
115. Schwan TG, Policastro PF, Miller Z, et al. Tick-borne Relapsing Fever Caused by Borrelia hermsii, Montana. Emerg Infect Dis [serial online]. 2003 Sept. Available from: http://www.cec.gov/ncidod/EID/vol9no9/03-0280.htm. Accessed 2007 Mar 25.
116. Dorsainvil PA, Cunha BA, et al. Relapsing Fever. 2004 Dec 22. Emedicine. [article]. Available at: http://www.emedicine.com/med/topic1999.htm. Accessed 2007 Mar 25.
117. CDC. Tick-Borne Relapsing Fever, What is it and How to Prevent it. [on-line pamphlet]. 2007. Available at: http://www.cdc.gov/ncidod/dvbid/RelapsingFever/Resources/TBRFBrochure1.pdf. Accessed 2007. Mar 25.
118. Schwan TG, Policastro PF, Miller Z, et al. Tick-borne Relapsing Fever Caused by Borrelia hermsii, Montana. Emerg Infect Dis [serial online]. 2003 Sept. Available from: http://www.cec.gov/ncidod/EID/vol9no9/03-0280.htm. Accessed 2007 Mar 25.
119. Dorsainvil PA, Cunha BA, et al. Relapsing Fever. 2004 Dec 22. Emedicine. [article]. Available at: http://www.emedicine.com/med/topic1999.htm. Accessed 2007 Mar 25.
120. CDC. Disease Trends. Epidemiology and Reporting of Tick-Borne Relapsing Fever. [web page]. 2004. Available at: http://www.cdc.gov/ncidod/dvbid/RelapsingFever/RF_Epidemiology.htm. Accessed 2007 Mar 25.
121. CDC. Cluster of Tick Paralysis Cases – Colorado, 2006. MMWR

Weekly. 2006 Sep. 1;55(34);933-935. Available at: http://www.cdc.gov/mmwr/preview/mmwrhtml/mm5534a1.htm. Accessed 2007 Apr. 3.
122. CDC. Southern Tick-Associated Rash Illness. 2006. Available at: www.cdc.gov/ncidod/dvbid/starti/index.htm.
123. Hayes E, Marshall S, Dennis D. Tularemia – United States, 1990-2000. MMWR Weekly. 2002;51(09);182-4. Available at: http://www.cdc.gov/mmwr/preview/mmwrhtml/mm5109al.htm. Accessed 2007 Mar 22.
124. MMWR Weekly. Tularemia—United States, 1990-2000. 2002 Mar 8;51(09);182-4.
125. U.S. Dept of Health and Human Services, National Institutes of Health, National Institute of Allergy and Infectious Diseases (NIAID) Contract RFP-NIH-NIAID-DMID-05-22 Tularemia Vaccine Development Team. 2004 Jul 13. Available at: http://www.niaid.nih.gov/contract/archive/RFP0522.pdf.
126. Hart MK. Absence of Mycoplasma Contamination in the Anthrax Vaccine. 2002. Emerg Infect Dis 8(1). Abstract. Available from: http://www.medscape.com/viewarticle/423543.
127. USPTO Patent Full-Text and Image Database. [web site]. Available at: http://patft.uspto.gov/netacgi/nph-Parser?Sect1=PTO2&Sect2=HITOFF&u=%2Fnetahtml%2FPTO%2Fsearch-adv.htm&r=13&p=1&f=G&l=50&d=PTXT&S1=5,242,820&OS=5,242,820&RS=5,242,820. Accessed 2007 Mar 21.
128. Scott DW. Mycoplasma The Linking Pathogen in Neurosystemic Diseases. From Nexus Magazine. 2001 Aug-Sep.;8(5). Available at: http://www.nexusmagazine.com/articles/mycoplasma.html.
129. Horowitz R. Lyme Disease & TBD's New Diagnostic and Treatment Protocols. 2005 Cervantes Productions. Available at: www.cervantesproductions.com. [video].
130. Hart MK. Absence of Mycoplasma Contamination in the Anthrax Vaccine. 2002. Emerg Infect Dis 8(1). Abstract. Available from: http://www.medscape.com/viewarticle/423543.
131. Stats taken from the Morgellons Research Foundation home page. Available at: http://www.morgellons.com. Accessed 2007 Mar 14.
132. Morgellons Research Foundation. [web page]. Accessed 2007 Mar 15. Available at: http://morgellons.com. Used with permission.

133. Schaller J. The Diagnosis and Treatment of Babesia. 2006. Hope Academic: Tampa, FL. p. 17.
134. DeVita-Raeburn E. The Morgellons Mystery. Psychology Today. 2007 Mar-Apr. Available at: http://psychologytoday.com/articles/pto-2000227-000003.xml.
135. Silver Colloids. 2004. http://www.silver-colloids.com/Pubs/herx-heimer.html.
136. Jarisch-Herxheimer reaction, or, Lucio's Phenomena. [web page] Available at: htp://www.earthtym.net/ref-herxheimer.htm.
137. Burrascano J. Diagnostic hints and treatment guidelines for Lyme and other Tick Borne Illnesses. 2002 Nov. 14th Ed. From ILADS.org web site. Accessed 2004, Dec.
138. Decker J. Immunology Tutorials. Cytokines. 2006. [Web page]. Accessed 2007 Feb 13. Available at: http://microvet.Arizona.edu/courses/mic419/tutorials/cytokines.html.
139. Mangin M. Observations of Jarisch-Herxheimer Reaction in Sarcoidosis Patients. JOIMR 2004;2(1):1. Available at: http://www.joimr.org/phorum/read.php?f=2&I=51&t=51.
140. Silver Colloids. 2004. http://www.silver-colloids.com/Pubs/herx-heimer.html.
141. Jarisch-Herxheimer Reaction. Road Back Foundation. 2007. Available at: http://www.roadback.org/index.cfm/fuseaction/education.display/display_id/91.html.
142. Sanogo Y, Zeaiter Z. Caruso G, et al. Bartonella henselae in Ixodes ricinus Ticks (Acari: Ixodida) Removed from Humans, Belluno Province, Italy. Emerging Infectious Diseases. 2003;9(3):329-332.
143. Munchausen by Proxy Syndrome. [article on the internet]. 2005 Mar. Available at: http://www.kidshealth.org/parent/system/ill/munchausen.html. Accessed 2007 Apr 4.
144. Wormser GP, Dattwyler RJ, Shapiro ED, et al. The Clinical Assessment, Treatment, and Prevention of Lyme Disease, Human Granulocytic Anaplasmosis, and Babesiosis: Clinical Practice Guidelines by the Infectious Diseases Society of America. Clinical Infectious Diseases 2006;43:1089-1134.
145. López-Andreu JA. Ferris J, et al. Treatment of Late Lyme Disease: A challenge to accept. J Clin Microbiol. 1994. [Letters to Editor] Vol 32:1415-1416.
146. Liegner KB. Lyme disease: the sensible pursuit of answers. J Clin

Microbiol. 1993;31:1961-1963.
147. Burrascano J, et al. The International Lyme and Associated Diseases Society. Evidence-based guidelines for the management of Lyme disease. Expert Rev Anti Infect Ther 2004;2(1 Suppl): S1-13. [66 references]. 2004. Available at: www.ilads.org.
148. Notice to Readers Recommendations for Test Performance and Interpretation from the Second National Conference on Serologic Diagnosis of Lyme Disease. MMWR Weekly. 1995 Aug 11:44(31);590-591.
149. Barbour AG, Tessier SL, Todd WJ. Lyme Disease Spirochetes and Ixodid Tick Spirochetes Share a Common Surface Antigenic Determinant Defined by a Monoclonal Antibody. Infec and Immun. 1983 Aug;41(2):795-804.
150. USPTO. US Patent Full-Text and Image Database. Bergstrom, et al. 1996 Dec 10. Patent # 5,582,990. Available at: http://patft.uspto.gov. Accessed 2007 Apr 6.
151. Lyme Disease Association (LDA). Conflicts of Interest in Lyme Disease: Laboratory Testing, Vaccination, and Treatment Guidelines. 2001. Available at: www.canlyme.com. [report]. Accessed 2007 Mar 22. Reprinted with permission from the LDA.
152. Barbour AG. Lyme Disease The Cause, the Cure, the Controversy. 1996. The Johns Hopkins University Press.
153. Wikipedia. Western blot. 2007. [web page] Available at: http://en.wikipedia.org/wiki/Western_blot. Accessed 2007 Mar 23.
154. Schaller J. The Dr. Jones' Approach to Reading Western Blots: A Common Sense Position. [article provided by author]. 2007 Mar 18.
155. Wikipedia. Immunoglobulin M. [web page]. Available at: http://en.wikipedia.org/wiki/IgG. Accessed 2007 Mar 22.
156. Wikipedia. Immunoglobulin G. [web page]. Available at: http://en.wikipedia.org/wiki/IgG. Accessed 2007 Mar 22.
157. IGeneX, Inc. Western Blot patient test results. 2005 Jul. Provided by IGeneX and belonging to the author.
158. Grier T. Western Blot Bands. Lyme Times. 2004. Summer. Vol. 37-38, p.24.
159. Notice to Readers Recommendations for Test Performance and Interpretation from the Second National Conference on Serologic Diagnosis of Lyme Disease. MMWR Weekly. 1995

Aug 11:44(31);590-591.
160. ASTPHLD. Proceedings of the Second National Conference on Serologic Diagnosis of Lyme Disease, Plenary Presentations and Workgroups. [supplement]. p.69. Available from: Association of Public Health Laboratories, 8515 Georgia Avenue, Suite 700, Silver Spring, MD 20910.
161. Markovits A. and Menefee BE. MarDx Diagnostics, Inc. Letter to FDA re: Attachment A – 510K Summary. 1996 June 5. Available at: www.fda.gov/cdrh/pdf/k950829.pdf. Accessed 2007 Apr. 24.
162. NYS DOH Wadsworth Center. Physician Office Laboratory Evaluation Program. [web page]. Available at: http://www.wadsworth.org/labcert/const.html. Accessed on 2007 Mar 22.
163. IGeneX Laboratory. Available at: http://www.igenex.com/about.htm.
164. Harris N. The IGeneX Western Blot: Better By Design. Available at: http://igenex.com/innovations3.htm.
165. Burrascano J, et al. The International Lyme and Associated Diseases Society. Evidence-based guidelines for the management of Lyme disease. Expert Rev Anti Infect Ther 2004;2(1 Suppl): S1-13. [66 references]. 2004. Available at: www.ilads.org.
166. Lawrence C, Lipton RB, Lowy FD, Cole PK. Seronegative chronic relapsing neuroborreliosis. Eur Neurol. 1995;35(2):113-7. Available at: http://www.ncbi.nlm.nih.gov. Accessed 2007 Mar 29.
167. Central Florida Research, Inc. Information page. [web site]. Available at: http://www.centralfloridaresearch.com/lab/. Accessed 2007 Mar 29.
168. Whitaker JA. New Test for Identifying the Morphing Menace. Q-RIBb© "Quantitative-Rapid Identification of Borrelia Burgdorferi." NutraNews. 2003 Oct. 2003. p. 8-10.
169. IGeneX. Multiplex PCR Assay for B. burgdorferi. [web page]. Available at: http://www.igenex.com/lymeset5.htm. Accessed 2007 Mar 22.
170. NIAID. NIAID Research: Diagnostic Procedures. 2007. [web site] Available at: http://www3.niaid.nih.gov/research/topics/lyme/research/diagnostics/. Accessed 2007 Mar 20.
171. IGenex, Inc. Lyme Dot-Blot Assay (LDA) [web page]. Available at: http://www.igenex.com/lymeset8.htm. Accessed 2007 Mar 29.

172. Harris N. IGeneX Innovations. Available at: http://igenex.com/innovations1.htm.
173. Klempner MS, Schmid CH, Hu L, Steere AC, et al. Intralaboratory Reliability of Serologic and Urine Testing for Lyme Disease. The American Journal of Medicine. 2001;110:217-219.
174. Wormser GP, Dattwyler RJ, Shapiro ED, et al. The Clinical Assessment, Treatment, and Prevention of Lyme Disease, Human Granulocytic Anaplasmosis, and Babesiosis: Clinical Practice Guidelines by the Infectious Diseases Society of America. Clinical Infectious Diseases 2006;43:1089-1134.
175. CDC. Lyme Disease (Borrelia burgdorferi) 1995 Case Definition. [web page]. Updated 2006 Jan 13. Accessed 2007 Mar 21. Available at: http://www.cdc.gov/epo/dphsi/casedef/lyme_disease_1995.htm
176. CDC. Lyme Disease (Borrelia burgdorferi) 1995 Case Definition. [web page]. Updated 2006 Jan 13. Accessed 2007 Mar 21. Available at: http://www.cdc.gov/epo/dphsi/casedef/lyme_disease_1995.htm
177. Engstrom SM, Shoop E, Johnson RC. Immunoblot interpretation criteria for serodiagnosis of early Lyme disease. J Clin Microbiol 1995;33:419-22.
178. Dressler F, Whelan JA, Reinhart BN, Steere AC. Western blotting in the serodiagnosis of Lyme disease. J Infect Dis 1993;167:392-400.
179. CMR. Clinical Microbiology Reviews. [web page]. Available at: http://cmr.asm.org/misc/edboard.shtml. Accessed 2007 Mar 22.
180. IDSA. Board of Directors. [web page]. Available at: http://www.idsociety.org. Accessed 2007 Mar 29.
181. www.canlyme.com [web site]. Accessed 2007 Mar 21.
182. Wilson JM. Lyme Disease Guidelines. 2007 Feb 15. [letter] Available at: http://www.canlyme.com. Accessed 2007 Mar 20.
183. www.canlyme.com [web site]. Accessed 2007 Mar 21.
184. Vanderhoof-Forschner K. Everything You Need to Know About Lyme Disease and Other Tick-Borne Disorders. 2nd Edition (paperback). John Wiley and Sons, Inc., Hoboken, New Jersey 2003.
185. Reynolds B. Transcript of Proceedings, Motion Hearing Case No. 97FA00136. State of Wisconsin, Circuit Court Branch II, Walworth County. 2003 Mar 13. Pages 26,44-46,59

186. Reynolds B. Transcript of Proceedings, Motion Hearing Case No. 97FA00136. State of Wisconsin, Circuit Court Branch II, Walworth County. 2003 Mar 13. Pages 37,48,50-51,58,60-61.
187. Steere AC, Malawista SE, Newman JH, Spieler PN, Bartenhagen NH. Antibiotic Therapy in Lyme Disease. Annals of Inter Med 1980:93(part 1):1-8.
188. Pachner AR, Steere AC. The triad of neurologic manifestations of Lyme disease: meningitis, cranial neuritis, and radiculoneuritis. Neurology, 1985 Jan;35(1):47-53.
189. Reik L, Burgdorfer W, Donaldson JO. Neurologic abnormalities in Lyme disease without erythema chronicum migrans. AM J Med. 1986 Jul;81(1):73-8. Available at: www.pubmed.gov. Accessed 2007 Jun 10.
190. Rawlings JA, Fournier PV, Teltow GJ. Isolation of Borrelia Spirochetes from Patients in Texas. J Clin Microbiol. 1987 Jul;25(7):1148-1150.
191. Craft JE, Fischer DK, Shimamoto GT, Steere AC. Antigens of Borrelia burgdorferi recognized during Lyme disease. Appearance of a new immunoglobulin M response and expansion of the immunoglobulin G response late in the illness. J Clin Invest. 1986 Oct;78(4):934-9.
192. Masson C. Neurologic aspects of Lyme disease. Presse Med. 1987 Jan 24;16(2):72-5. [abstract, article in French]. Available at: www.pubmed.gov. Accessed 2007 Jun 16.
193. Pachner AR. Borrelia burgdorferi in the nervous system: the new "great imitator." Annals of the NY Acad Sci. 1988;539(1):56-64. Available at: http://www.annalsnyas.org/cgi/content/abstract/539/1/56. Accessed 2007 Jun 19.
194. Dattwyler RJ, Volkman DJ, Luft BJ, Halperin JJ, Thoma J, Golightly MG. Seronegative Lyme disease. Dissociation of specific T- and B-lymphocyte responses to Borrelia burgdorferi. N Engl J Med. 1988 Dec 1;319(22):1441-6. Comment in: N Engl J Med. 1989 May 11;320(19):1279-80. Available at: www.pubmed.gov. Accessed 2007 Jul 25.
195. Preac-Mursic V, Weber K, Pfister W, Wilske B, Gross B, Baumann A, Prokop J. Survival of Borrelia burgdorferi in Antibiotically Treated Patients with Lyme borreliosis. Infection. 1989;17(6):355-359.
196. Pachner AR. Neurologic manifestations of Lyme disease, the new

"great imitator." Rev Infect Dis. 1989 Sep-Oct;11 Suppl 6:S1482-6. [abstract]

197. Steere AC. Lyme disease. N Engl J Med. 1990 Aug 31;321(9):586-96. Comment in: N Engl J Med. 1990 Feb 15;322(7):474-5.
198. Aguero-Rosenfeld ME, Nowakowski J, McKenna DF, Carbonaro CA, Wormser GP. Serodiagnosis in Early Lyme Disease. J Clin Microbiol. 1993 Dec;31(12):3090-3095.
199. Corpuz M, Hilton E, Lardis MP, Singer C, Zolan J. Problems in the use of serologic test for the diagnosis of Lyme disease. 1991 Sep;151(9):1837-40. Comment in: Arch Intern Med 1992 Jun:152(6):1331.
200. Nadelman RB, Pavia CS, Magnarelli LA, Wormser GP. Isolation of Borrelia burgdorferi from the blood of seven patients with Lyme disease. Am J Med. 1990 Jan;88(1):21-6.
201. Moody KD, Barthold SW, et al. 1990. Experimental chronic Lyme borreliosis in Lewis rats. Am J Trop Med Hyg. 42:165-174.
202. Melchers W, Meis J, Rosa P, Claas E, et al. Amplification of Borrelia burgdorferi DNA in Skin Biopsies from Patients with Lyme Disease. J Clin Microbiol, 1991 Nov. 29(11):2401-2406.
203. Dattwyler RJ, Volkman DJ, Luft BJ, Halperin JJ, Thomas J, Golightly MG. Seronegative Lyme disease. Dissociation of specific T- and B-lymphocyte responses to Borrelia burgdorferi. N Engl J Med. 1988 Dec1;319(22):1441-6. Comment in: N Engl J Med. 1989 May 11;320(19):1279-80.
204. Hippocratic Oath. Wikipedia. Available at: http://en.wikipedia.org/wiki/ Hippocratic_Oath.

To the world, you are but one person.
But to one person, you are the world.

– Author unknown

FOR THOSE WISHING TO CONTRIBUTE

Monetary donations are appreciated for these worthy Lyme causes:

Ryan Guerin Fund
c/o PJ Langhoff
PO Box 444, Hustisford, WI 53034, USA

The *Ryan Guerin Fund* is a fund in memory of deceased Lyme patient Ryan Guerin, whose story is told by his family within the pages of this book. 100% of the funds donated will be used to defray the costs of Lyme diagnostic testing for patients who cannot otherwise afford these services, beginning in North Carolina, Ryan's home state.

Please write or email pjay@lymeleague.com for more information on this worthwhile cause.

TURN THE CORNER™
The Fight Against Lyme Disease

Please visit:

www.turnthecorner.org

Dedicated to the support of research, education, awareness and innovative treatments for Lyme disease and other tick-borne diseases.

Printed in Dunstable, United Kingdom

91220018R00212